MECHANISMS OF NEUROINFLAMMATION

Edited by **Gonzalo Emiliano Aranda Abreu**

Mechanisms of Neuroinflammation
http://dx.doi.org/10.5772/66067
Edited by Gonzalo Emiliano Aranda Abreu

Contributors

Cristoforo Scavone, Elisa M. Mitiko Kawamoto, Paula F. Kinoshita, Ana Maria Marques Orellana, Jacqueline Alves Leite, Natalia Prudente de Mello, Sharon DeMorrow, Matthew McMillin, Dr. Ricardo B. Maccioni, Víctor Andrade, Leonardo Guzmán-Martínez, Katiana Vergara-Pulgar, Attila Sas, Attila Valikovics, Csaba Olah, Verónica Pérez De La Cruz, Gustavo Ignacio Vázquez Cervantes, Benjamin Pineda, Nora Karen Olascoaga Arellano, Aleli Salazar Ramirez, Daniela Ramirez Ortega, Camilo Ríos, Dinora González Esquivel, Edward Tobinick, Tracey Ignatowski, Robert Spengler, Nibaldo Inestrosa, Juan Zolezzi, Chuang Wang, Christina Alves Peixoto, Ana Karolina Nunes, Catarina Rapôso, Rachelle Dugue, Frank Barone, Manan Nath, Andrew Dugue, Huanhuan Wang, Xizhen Wang

Published by InTech
Janeza Trdine 9, 51000 Rijeka, Croatia

Publishing Process Manager Viktorija Zgela
Technical Editor SPi Global
Cover InTech Design team

First published September, 2017
Printed in Croatia
Legal deposit, Croatia: National and University Library in Zagreb

Additional hard copies can be obtained from orders@intechopen.com

Mechanisms of Neuroinflammation, Edited by Gonzalo Emiliano Aranda Abreu
p. cm.
Print ISBN 978-953-51-3451-0
Online ISBN 978-953-51-3452-7

For EU product safety concerns:
IN TECH d.o.o., Prolaz Marije Krucifikse Kozulić 3, 51000 Rijeka, Croatia,
info@intechopen.com or visit our website at intechopen.com.

Meet the editor

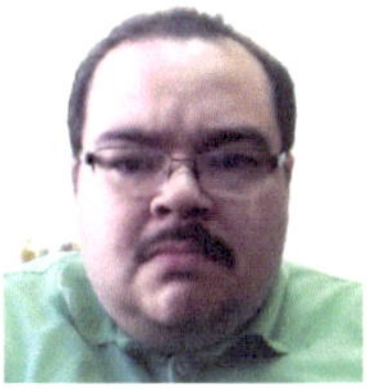

Professor Dr. Gonzalo Emiliano Aranda Abreu (Centro de Investigaciones Cerebrales, Universidad Veracruzana, Xalapa, Veracruz, Mexico) was born in 1968 in Ciudad del Carmen, Campeche, Mexico. He received his BSc (Experimental Biology) degree from the Universidad Autónoma Metropolitana, Iztapalapa, Mexico, in 1992; MSc (Molecular Biology and Genetics) degree from the Centro de Investigación y Estudios Avanzados, IPN, Mexico, in 1996; and PhD (Neurobiology) degree from Weizmann Institute of Science, Rehovot, Israel, in 2001. He has more than 20 years of experience in Alzheimer's disease research. He has written articles on tau mRNA transport in the neuronal axon and Alzheimer's disease, as well as book chapters where the main theme is brain rehabilitation. He is the president and member of the Southeastern Mexican Chapter of the Society for Neuroscience, USA. He is involved in the training of doctoral students. He teaches molecular and cellular neurobiology, and bioinformatics to PhD degree students.

Contents

Preface

"Mechanisms of Neuroinflammation" book offers a comprehensive analysis of how neurons become swollen due to brain injury. Each chapter describes in an elegant way how the neuroinflammatory process is carried out.

Neuroinflammation is a central process of the immune response to various acute and chronic diseases. The blood-brain barrier (BBB) is involved in the inflammation process, as it allows molecules such as tumor growth factor (TNF) and cytokines to enter the brain. TNF-α, IL-6, IL-1β, and other cytokines are able to make the BBB membrane more permeable and allow leukocytes to enter the brain. Cytokines have the ability to activate transcription of different genes in BBB cells including nuclear factor $\kappa\beta$ (NF-$\kappa\beta$) and cyclooxygenase-2 (COX-2), an enzyme involved in the formation of prostaglandins. Cyclooxygenase is involved in the synthesis of prostanoids, a large family of arachidonic acid metabolites comprising prostaglandins, prostacyclins, and thromboxanes. COX-2 is induced in response to growth factors, cytokines, and pro-inflammatory molecules and may lead to neurodegenerative diseases. Under normal conditions, these enzymes are involved in synaptic function, regulation of blood flow, apoptosis, angiogenesis, and gene expression. In pathological circumstances such as stroke, Alzheimer's disease, Parkinson's disease, they produce neuroinflammation involving vasodilation and vasoconstriction, platelet aggregation, leukocyte migration, and cytokine release, as well as oxidative stress.

I thank all the authors for contributing chapters that are part of this interesting book.

Dr. Gonzalo Emiliano Aranda Abreu
Center for Brain Research,
University of Veracruz,
Xalapa, Veracruz,
México

Section 1

Neuroinflammation and Psychiatric Disorders

Chapter 1

Reducing Neuroinflammation in Psychiatric Disorders: Novel Target of Phosphodiesterase 4 (PDE4) and Developing of the PDE4 Inhibitors

Chuang Wang, Zhen Wang, Mengmeng Li,
Chenli Li, Hanjie Yu, Dongsheng Zhou and
Zhongming Chen

Additional information is available at the end of the chapter

http://dx.doi.org/10.5772/intechopen.69154

Abstract

Multiple lines of evidence support the pathogenic role of neuroinflammation in psychiatric illness. Cyclic adenosine monophosphate (cAMP) is a critical regulator of microglia homeostasis; as the predominant negative modulator of cyclic AMP signaling within microglia, and phosphodiesterase 4 (PDE4) represents a promising target for modulating immune function. The approach for pharmacological manipulation of cAMP levels using specifc PDE4 inhibitors provokes an ant-iinflammatory response. Specifcally, PDE4 inhibitors have recently emerged as a potential therapeutic strategy for neuroinflammatory, neurodegenerative, and psychiatric diseases. Mechanistically, PDE4 inhibitors produce an anti-inflammatory and neuroprotection effect by increasing the accumulation of cAMP and activating protein kinase A (PKA), the signaling pathway of which is thought to play an important role in the development of psychiatric disorders. This chapter reviews present knowledge of the relationship between neuroinflammation and classical psychiatric disorders (major depressive disorder (MDD), bipolar disorder (BD), and schizophrenia) and demonstrates the signaling pathways that underlie the use of PDE4 inhibitors in neuroinflammation. In addition, among the four subtypes (A-D) of PDE4, it remains unclear which one exerts suppressive effects on neuroinflammation. Understanding how PDE4 and neuroinflammation interact can reveal pathogenic clues and help target new preventive and symptomatic therapies for psychiatric illness.

Keywords: cyclic adenosine monophosphate (cAMP), phosphodiesterase 4 (PDE4), psychiatric disorders, neuroinflammation

1. Introduction: the possibility that inflammation is the common mediator of psychiatric disorders

Classical psychiatric disorders, including major depressive disorder (MDD), bipolar disorder (BD), and schizophrenia, affect a significant percentage of the world population. More recently, inflammatory and immunological abnormalities have been documented in patients with classical psychiatric disorders, even though the exact mechanisms underlying this association are not known. A growing body of evidence suggests that activation of the immune response following systemic infection often results in neuroinflammation and consequently induces psychiatric symptoms in animal models and humans (as shown in **Figure 1**) [1–6]. Specifically, inflammation in the context of the nervous system termed "neuroinflammation" has been reported in patients with psychiatric disorders [7] and is typically associated with microglial activation.

Microglia, the resident phagocytes of the CNS, are ubiquitously distributed in the brain and are usually the first to be activated in response to tissue damage or brain infections [14]. At the same time, microglia are important players in the maintenance and plasticity of neuronal circuits, contributing to the protection and remodeling of synapses [15–16]. They provide ongoing immune surveillance and regulate developmental synaptic pruning [17–18]. Microglial activation can be divided into two distinct types: a classical M1 and an alternative M2 activation. Proinflammatory cytokines include interleukin-1β (IL-1β), interleukin-2 (IL-2), interleukin-6 (IL-6), tumor necrosis factor-α (TNF-α), interferon-gamma (IFN-γ), and they are secreted primarily by microglia [19–21]; [3]. In the M1 activation, microglial cells may become

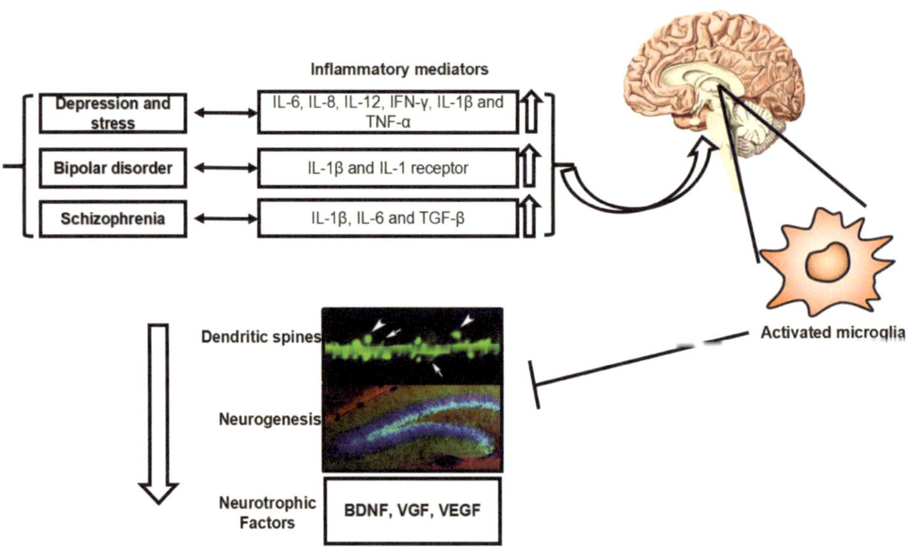

Figure 1. Summary of neuroinflammatory responses and microglial abnormalities observed in psychiatry disorders. A large body of evidence [8–13] supports the involvement of neuroinflammatory mechanisms, including microglial activation, downregulation of dendritic spines, neurogenesis, and neurotrophic factors in the pathophysiology of psychiatric disorders.

hyperramified or ameboid/phagocytic [22], and may synthesize proinflammatory molecules, superoxide radicals, glutamate [23–24], and nitric oxide (NO) and ultimately clear infections and repair tissues. Alternatively, M2 activation, which can be triggered by cytokines such as IL-4, IL-13, or IL-25 [25]; [22], has been associated with a release of antiinflammatory cytokines (e.g. IL-10, insulin-growth factor-1(IGF-1), transforming growth factor-β (TGF-β), and neurotrophic factors) [22], which facilitate healing and limit neuronal injury [7]. Cytokine response phenotypes are classified as either proinflammatory T-helper 1 (Th1) or antiinflammatory T-helper 2 (Th2) according to the immune functions they regulate. The key to neuroinflammation effects on psychiatric disorders appears to lie within the dysregulation of the control and release of pro- and antiinflammatory cytokines. In fact, Th1 and Th2, which are responsible for pathogen elimination and antibody regulation, respectively, were also found to be altered in untreated depressed patients [26]. Microglia activation is one of the mechanisms by which peripheral immune challenges can alter brain functioning [27, 28]; [1]. In fact, patients with psychiatric disorders have been shown to present an increase in serum levels of proinflammatory cytokines [29–32]; [8]. Interestingly, investigations involving animal models of depression and postmortem dorsal anterior cingulate matter from individuals suffering from MDD delineate altered expression of microglial activation markers, as well as chronicity-dependent fluctuations in microglial concentration in areas of the brain associated with mood regulation [33–36]; [10, 13]. Additionally, microglial activation was also greater in the ventral prefrontal white matter in individuals who committed suicide [37]. Altogether, these studies suggest that microglial activation may be considered as an important marker in MDD.

Bipolar disorder is a severe mood disorder characterized by recurrent episodes of mania followed by depression. The pathophysiology of BD is yet to be well understood, while recent studies have indicated that abnormal immunological functions may be a contributing factor [38–42]. Recently, positron emission tomography (PET) studies have shown microglial overactivation in the brain of patients with various psychiatric disorders [43–45]; [9] including bipolar disorder [42]. Consistent with the previous studies, it was revealed that in BD, the immune system is chronically activated by microglia, which in turn produces cytokines that render the brain to a vulnerable and unstable state, precipitating mood disturbances [45–47]. In fact, higher levels of IL-1β were associated with dysfunction and increased suicide risk in patients with BD [48].

Schizophrenia is a chronic and debilitating disorder that affects 0.5–1% of the world population [49]. Evidence suggests that the dopamine dysfunction hypothesis [50–51] has defined schizophrenia for many years, a growing number of research investigations and scientific curiosity have developed around the immune system and the role of neuroinflammation in precipitating psychotic symptoms in a subset of patients with psychosis [52–55]; [5, 6], providing a detailed review of the theories and mechanisms that support a role for inflammation in schizophrenia.

2. Cyclic nucleotide signaling and neuroinflammation

Several mechanisms can account for the high comorbidity of neuroinflammation and psychiatric disorders. These mechanisms include direct effects of cytokines on the neuronal environment or indirect effects via downregulation of cyclic nucleotide signaling [56–58].

Understanding cyclic nucleotide signaling mechanisms that underlie neuroinflammation and psychiatric disorder comorbidity may yield effective pharmaceutical targets that can treat both conditions simultaneously beyond traditional antipsychotic drugs. There is growing evidence that adenosine cyclic 3,5-monophosphate (cAMP) exerts many of its physiological effects by activating cAMP-dependent protein kinase (PKA), which in turn phosphorylates and regulates the functions of downstream protein targets including ion channels, enzymes, and transcription factors [59]. Specifically, cAMP is a ubiquitous regulator of the inflammatory response and is also a key second messenger that influences glial activity [60, 61]. Additionally, recent findings have also suggested that cAMP/cAMP response element-binding (CREB) signaling is closely involved in antiinflammatory responses [62] by suppressing the activation of glial cells (both microglia and astrocytes), decreasing the production of proinflammatory mediators, including tumor necrosis factor (TNF)-α, interleukin (IL)-1β, IL-6, IL-12, and nitric oxide, and increasing the expression of antiinflammatory factor IL-10 [63–65]. Therefore, previous work has shown that the application of cAMP analogs, adenylyl cyclase (AC) activators, or PDE inhibitors, to increase the levels of intracellular cAMP, antagonizes the changes in microglial cell morphology and their production of proinflammatory cytokines when they are exposed to inflammatory stimuli [66–67]. Intracellular cAMP signaling has been well established in the mediation of memory [68–71] and depression-like behaviors [72, 73]; [57]). cAMP activates protein kinase A (PKA), which phosphorylates and activates the subsequent downstream target CREB protein [74, 75] and is important for mediating synaptic plasticity [76, 77]; [74]. In addition, increases in cAMP levels during inflammation inhibit the production of proinflammatory cytokines and stimulate the formation of IL-10, an antiinflammatory factor [78, 79]. Conversely, inflammatory molecules, including lipopolysaccharide (LPS), interferon (IFN)-γ, and TNF-α, can dramatically reduce cyclic AMP levels in microglia, leading to changes in their phenotype and function [80]; [56]. Therefore, cAMP/CREB signaling may play a beneficial role in inflammatory responses and apoptosis of psychiatric disorders. Given that cAMP levels are regulated by a balance between the activities of two enzymes: AC and cyclic nucleotide phosphodiesterase (PDE), the pharmacological manipulation using specific PDE inhibitors, in particular, PDE4 inhibitors provoke profound antiinflammatory responses [81] and beneficial effects on psychiatric disorders [82]; [57]. Selective inhibitors of PDE4 are currently used in clinical practice for the treatment of cardiovascular disorders and erectile dysfunction, and other PDE inhibitors are under development for the treatment of CNS and inflammatory disorders. This chapter focuses on the development of PDE4 and PDE4 subtype inhibitors which have been reported as treatment for neuroinflammation.

3. PDE4 and specific PDE4 subtype inhibitors in neuroinflammation

3.1. PDE4 and the distribution of its subtypes in CNS

PDE4, one of the 11 PDE enzyme families, specifically catalyzes hydrolysis of cyclic AMP (cAMP); it has four subtypes (PDE4A–D) with at least 25 splice variants. Detailed analyses of the expression pattern of the human PDE4 isogenes have recently appeared [83, 84]. All four subtypes, PDE4A, PDE4B, PDE4C, and PDE4D, are found in most tissues although, notably, PDE4C is absent in blood (as shown in **Table 1**). PDE4 plays a critical role in the control of intracellular cAMP concentrations. PDE4 gene members are distributed throughout the brain and are expressed in various neurons. PDE4 specifically hydrolyzes cAMP to inactive AMP. High levels of cytosolic cAMP lead to the activation of PKA and further induce the phosphorylation of transcription factors, such as CREB and cAMP-dependent transcription factor-1 (ATF-1) to drive cAMP-driven genes, which involve in the regulation of proinflammatory and antiinflammatory pathways (as shown in **Figure 2**).However, the differential distribution of the four PDE4 subtypes (PDE4A–D) in the brain [85] may be attributed to the different regulation of cAMP-mediated signaling in CNS. PDE4A and PDE4D are highly expressed in the cortex, olfactory bulb, hippocampal formation, and brainstem, whereas PDE4B is mainly expressed in the amygdala, striatum, and hypothalamus [86–88]. By contrast, PDE4C exhibits a distribution different from those of PDE4A and PDE4D and appears to be limited to the thalamus and cerebellum [89, 90]. Because of the unique distribution of PDE4 isoform and its significance in various physiological functions in CNS, PDE4 presents promising pharmaceutical drug target treatment for psychiatric disorders.

3.2. Traditional PDE4 inhibitors

The search for selective inhibitors of PDE4 as novel antiinflammatory drugs has continued for more than 40 years. Recent findings have also suggested that cAMP/CREB/brain-derived neurotrophic factor (BDNF) signaling is closely involved in antiinflammatory responses [66], depression, and antidepressant actions [91]; [68]. PDE4 inhibition has been a target

Location	Level of expression			
	PDE4A	PDE4B	PDE4C	PDE4D
Brain	++	++	++	++
Liver	++	++	++	++
Lung	++	++	++	++
Trachea	++	++	++	++
Kidney	++	++	++	++
Placenta	++	++	++	++
Heart	++	++	++	++
Blood	++	++	–	++
Neutrophils	±	++	–	±
Eosinophils	++	++	–	++

++, expression.
±, very weak expression.
–, no expression.

Table 1. Expression patterns of mRNAs for the human phosphodiesterase 4 (PDE4) subtype genes.

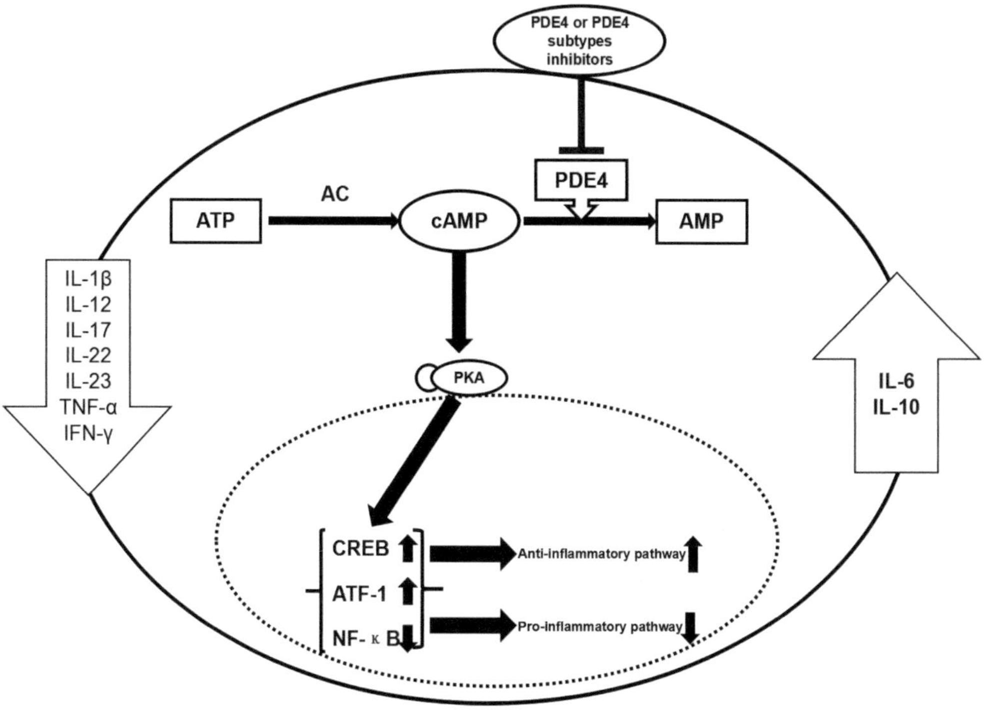

Figure 2. The antiinflammatory mechanisms of PDE4 and PDE4 subtype inhibitors. cAMP as a regulator of immunity. Adenylate cyclases (AC) produce cAMP from adenosin-tri-phosphate (ATP). High levels of cytosolic cAMP lead to the activation of protein kinase A (PKA) and further induce the phosphorylation of transcription factors, such as CREB and cAMP-dependent transcription factor-1 (ATF-1) to drive cAMP-driven genes. Phosphodiesterase 4 (PDE4) decreases intracellular cAMP levels and counterbalances the intracellular cAMP effect. However, PDE4 or subtype inhibitors block PDE4 or its subtypes. As PDE4 or subtypes degrade cAMP to AMP, cAMP levels rise during apremilast treatment. The elevation of intracellular cAMP leads to the activation of PKA. This results in the phosphorylation and activation of transcription factors like CREB and ATF-1. On the other hand, NF-κB is inactivated. This transcriptional regulation is responsible for the reduced production of proinflammatory mediators like IL-1β, IL-12, IL-17, IL-22, IL-23, TNF-α, and IFN-γ and the increased production of IL-6 and the antiinflammatory mediator IL-10.

of therapeutic drug research since the 1970s, with the prototypic PDE4 inhibitor, rolipram being tested in clinical trials in the 1980s [92]. Notably, PDE4 inhibitor rolipram that readily produces antidepressant-like actions [93, 94], which are associated with increased level of cAMP and its downstream targets of cAMP-dependent protein kinase A (PKA), CREB, and BDNF [95]; [68]. Therefore, the potential PDE4 inhibitors may be an efficient alternative strategy to play antidepressant action especially in depressive disorder induced by inflammation. Consistent with this hypothesis, the previous studies have demonstrated that rolipram reduces neuroinflammation and promotes axonal regeneration and functional recuperation following spinal cord injury [96–98]; [62]. More evidence have shown that PDE4 inhibitor rolipram reduces the production of proinflammatory cytokines and modulates the activity of cAMP-mediated signaling and thus regulates CREB phosphorylation and the downstream effectors [99]; [62, 68], showing that potential PDE4 inhibitors may be suitable to antagonize psychiatric disorders. Unfortunately, the development of PDE4 inhibitor rolipram for therapeutic purposes has been hindered by side effects, such as emesis [100, 101]. Based on the demonstration of significant efficacy in preclinical models, multiple PDE4 inhibitors have entered clinical development, and none have reached the market. Roflumilast and apremilast have been approved for peripheral inflammatory disorders, such as severe chronic obstructive pulmonary disease (COPD) and psoriatic arthritis (PA), respectively; however, their full immunomodulatory activity is limited to doses which are estimated to inhibit PDE4 by 50% due to the incidence of nausea and emesis at higher exposures. Unfortunately, the two PDE4 inhibitors (roflumilast and apremilast) approved for peripheral inflammatory disorders lack brain penetration and are dose limited by side effects making them unsuitable for modulating microglial function. Despite the challenges and complications that have been encountered during the development of PDE4 inhibitors, these drugs may provide a genuinely novel class of antineuroinflammatory agents, and there are several compounds in development that could fulfill that promise.

3.3. The novel potential PDE4 inhibitors

Notably, it has been recently reported that a pyrazolopyridine compound, etazolate, is a new-generation selective PDE4 inhibitor and is proven to be of particular significance in neuropsychiatric conditions [102, 103]; [94]. Previous studies reported that etazolate belongs to PDE4 inhibitor family and that treatment with etazolate restored cAMP levels [66, 94, 103]. In most of the clinical phase II or Phase IIb studies, etazolate has shown that it could be a potential candidate for the treatment of Alzheimer's disease [102]. Additionally, in several preclinical studies, etazolate has shown significant antidepressant- and anxiolytic-like effects in acute and chronic rodent models [104, 105]; [66, 103]. Specifically, it is reported that the expression of PDE4A, PDE4B, and PDE4D in the hippocampus was significantly increased by lipopolysaccharide (LPS) in mice. In addition, an etazolate significantly reversed the elevated IL-1β expression in hippocampus and prefrontal cortex induced by LPS [103], indicating significant antineuroinflammatory response. Although limited preclinical studies have been conducted on etazolate, the recent clinical trial results on its safety and tolerance are encouraging [106]. However, in March 2014, the development of the etazolate was stopped as the company transformed into a specialty in vitro diagnostics company.

Recently, more and more novel selective PDE4 inhibitors (as shown in **Table 2**) have been designed and explored in different rodent models, displaying a safer profile compared to traditional agents [107–111]; [66, 75], supporting further evaluation of these novel PDE4 inhibitors in a clinical setting.

3.4. PDE4 subtype inhibitors

Particular attention has been given to the PDE4 isoforms owing to the antiinflammatory effects observed after their inhibition in vitro and in vivo [81]. Of the four major phosphodiesterase 4 (PDE4) subtypes, PDE4A, PDE4B, or PDE4D, all of which are found to some extent in every inflammatory cell type studied, could be important regulators of inflammatory processes. Only PDE4C, which is present in the lung [112] but has only rarely and inconsistently been reported in any isolated inflammatory cell type, can be eliminated on the basis of its

Novel PDE4 inhibitors	Chemical structures	Active indications	Highest status
Etazolate	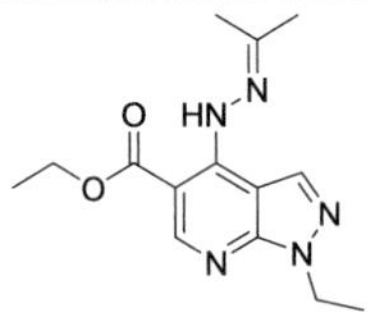	Depression, anxiety, traumatic brain injury	Phase 2 clinical to discontinued
EPPA-1	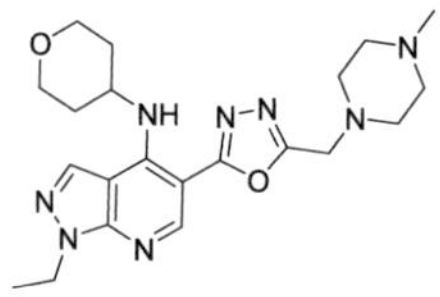	In vitro and in vivo anti inflammatory potencies	Discovery
GSK256066	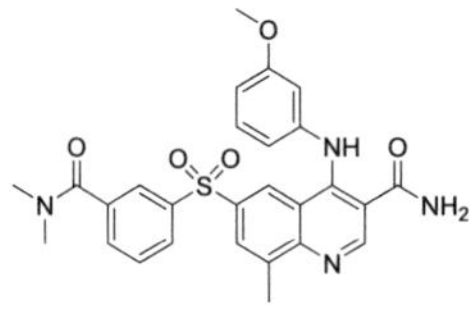	Antiinflammatory activities	Phase 2 clinical to discontinued
LASSBio-448	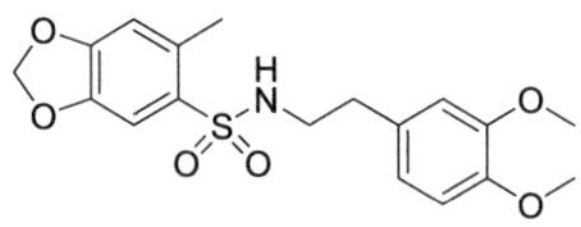	Antiinflammatory activities	Discovery
FFPM	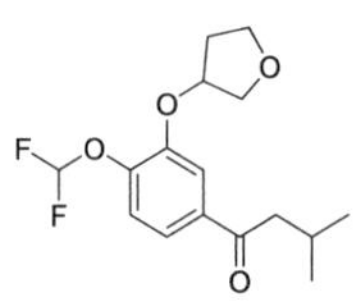	Reverses learning and memory deficits and appears to have potential antiinflammatory effects with little emetic potential	Discovery
Apremilast	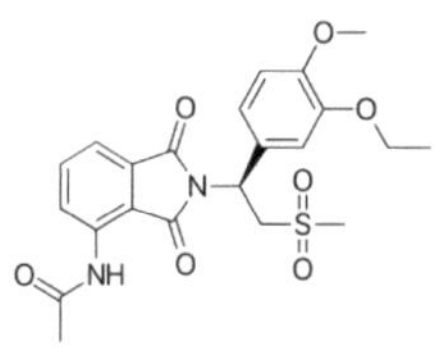	Ankylosing spondylitis; Atopic dermatitis; Behcet's disease; Hidradenitis suppurativa; Psoriasis; Psoriatic arthritis; Ulcerative colitis	Launched
HT-0712	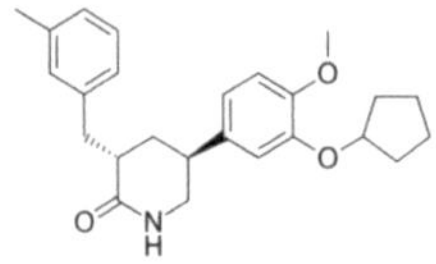	Cognitive disorder	Phase 2 clinical
Roflumilast	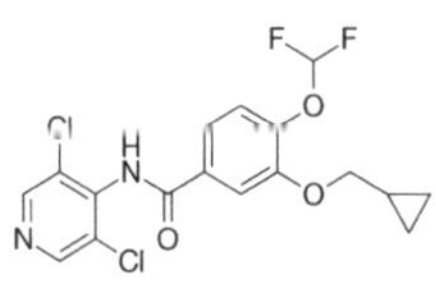	Alzheimer's disease; Asthma; Chronic obstructive pulmonary disease; Schizophrenia	Launched
Ibudilast	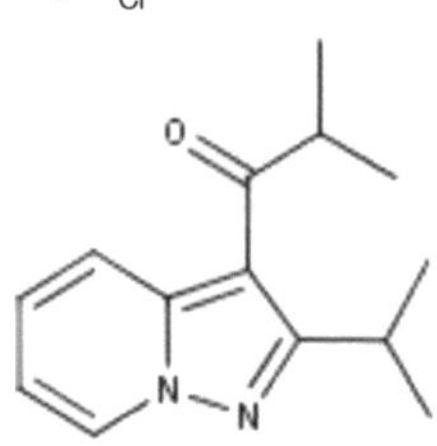	Alcoholism; Amphetamine dependence; Drug dependence; Neuropathic pain; Opiate dependence; Traumatic brain injury	Phase 2 clinical

Table 2. Development of novel PDE4 inhibitors.

distribution. This distribution characteristic provides many opportunities for selective therapeutic targeting [113, 114] and the potential to reduce the incidence of side effects attributed to PDE4 inhibition. The previous studies revealed that PDE4B might be the critical subtype that controls the inflammatory responses [115–117]. The work by Conti's group [115] identified PDE4B to be the primary PDE4 enzyme involved in proinflammatory responses to LPS in macrophages and leukocytes. Reports have suggested that mice deficient in PDE4A display anxiogenic-like behavior [118], while PDE4B is closely related with neuroinflammation [119]. Therefore, subtype selective inhibitors targeting PDE4B are of high interest given the critical role PDE4B plays in immune function versus the association of PDE4D with nausea and emesis. However, it is difficult to directly link PDE4 inhibitor-mediated efficacy to changes specifically in microglial cell function, and even more so whether these effects selectively involve PDE4B. The difficulty in establishing these links is because these investigations have almost exclusively used pharmacological inhibitors that are administered systemically and which show similar affinity toward all PDE4 family members, being designed largely to inhibit enzyme activity by binding to the catalytic site. Recently, the crystal structures of PDE4B have been exploited to develop subtype-selective PDE4 inhibitors [120]. The novel PDE4B inhibitor A33, which has an IC50 of 32 nM against PDE4B1, is 49-fold more selective for PDE4B versus PDE4D and does not appreciably inhibit any other PDEs [121]. Specifically, A33 inhibits all PDE4B isoforms and is 49-fold more selective toward PDE4B compared with PDE4D and does not appreciably inhibit other PDEs [120, 121]. Interestingly, TNF-α levels at 6-hour postsurgery of traumatic brain injury (TBI) were significantly reduced by A33, suggesting that an inflammatory pathway mediated by PDE4B is inhibited with A33 [122]; [115] (Jin and Conti; Jin et al.). However, further studies to determine the antineuroinflammatory mechanisms of A33 may yield insights into the processes involved in the improvements of psychiatric disorders with A33 treatment.

4. Conclusions

A large body of evidence supports the involvement of neuroinflammatory mechanisms in the pathophysiology of psychiatric disorders. Drugs that interfere with these mechanisms, such as PDE4 inhibitors, could be a novel and important new pathway for the treatment of these disorders. Furthermore, continued drug discovery efforts to identify safe and well-tolerated, brain-penetrant PDE4 inhibitors are a reflection of the confidence in the rationale for modulation of this target to produce meaningful therapeutic benefit in a wide range of neurological conditions and injury.

Acknowledgements

This research was supported by National Natural Science Foundation of China (No. 81671337; No.81201050; No.81541087); Natural Science Foundation of Zhejiang province (No. LQ12H09001); Natural Science Foundation of Ningbo (No. 2012A610251); Ningbo municipal innovation team of life science and health (2015C110026); new-shoot Talents

Program of Zhejiang province; and Student Research and Innovation Program of Ningbo University. This project is also sponsored by K.C. Wong Magna funded in Ningbo University and Li Dak Sum Yip Yio Chin Kenneth Li Marine Biopharmaceutical Development Fund, National 111 Project of China.

Author details

Chuang Wang[1,2,3,4*], Zhen Wang[6*], Mengmeng Li[1,2,3], Chenli Li[1,2,3], Hanjie Yu[1,2,3], Dongsheng Zhou[1,5] and Zhongming Chen[1,5]

*Address all correspondence to: wangchuang@nbu.edu.cn

1 Ningbo Key Laboratory of Behavioral Neuroscience, Ningbo University School of Medicine, Ningbo, Zhejiang, P.R. China

2 Zhejiang Provincial Key Laboratory of Pathophysiology, Ningbo University School of Medicine, Ningbo, Zhejiang, P.R. China

3 Department of Physiology and Pharmacology, Ningbo University School of Medicine, Ningbo, Zhejiang, P.R. China

4 Li Dak Sum Yip Yio Chin Kenneth Li Marine Biopharmaceutical Research Center, Ningbo University, Ningbo, Zhejiang, P.R. China

5 Ningbo Kangning Hospital, Ningbo, Zhejiang, P.R. China

6 CAS Key Laboratory for Receptor Research, Shanghai Institute of Materia Medica, Chinese Academy of Sciences, Shanghai, China

References

[1] Dantzer R, O'Connor JC, Freund GG, Johnson RW, Kelley KW. From inflammation to sickness and depression: When the immune system subjugates the brain. Nature Reviews Neuroscience. 2008;**9**(1):46-56. DOI: 10.1038/nrn2297

[2] Eisenberger NI, Berkman ET, Inagaki TK, Rameson LT, Mashal NM, Irwin MR.Inflammation-induced anhedonia: Endotoxin reduces ventral striatum responses to reward. Biological Psychiatry. 2010;68(8):748-754. DOI: 10.1016/j.biopsych.2010.06.010

[3] Haroon E, Raison CL, Miller AH. Psychoneuroimmunology meets neuropsychopharmacology: Translational implications of the impact of inflammation on behavior. Neuropsychopharmacology. 2012;**37**(1):137-162. DOI: 10.1038/npp.2011.205

[4] Cho HJ, Eisenberger NI, Olmstead R, Breen EC, Irwin MR. Preexisting mild sleep disturbance as a vulnerability factor for inflammation-induced depressed mood: A human experimental study. Translational Psychiatry. 2016;**6**:e750. DOI: 10.1038/tp.2016.23

[5] Notter T, Coughlin JM, Gschwind T, Weber-Stadlbauer U, Wang Y, Kassiou M, Vernon AC, Benke D, Pomper MG, Sawa A, Meyer U. Translational evaluation of translocator protein as a marker of neuroinflammation in schizophrenia. Molecular Psychiatry. 2017. DOI: 10.1038/mp.2016.248

[6] Miller BJ, Goldsmith DR. Towards an immunophenotype of schizophrenia: Progress, potential mechanisms, and future directions. Neuropsychopharmacology. 2017;**42**(1):299-317. DOI: 10.1038/npp.2016.211

[7] Najjar S, Pearlman DM, Devinsky O, Najjar A, Zagzag D. Neurovascular unit dysfunction with blood-brain barrier hyperpermeability contributes to major depressive disorder: A review of clinical and experimental evidence. Journal of Neuroinflammation. 2013;**10**:142. DOI: 10.1186/1742-2094-10-142

[8] Schiepers OJ, Wichers MC, Maes M. Cytokines and major depression. Progress in Neuro-Psychopharmacology & Biological Psychiatry. 2005;**29**(2):201-217. DOI: 10.1016/j.pnpbp.2004.11.003

[9] Suzuki K, Sugihara G, Ouchi Y, Nakamura K, Futatsubashi M, Takebayashi K, Yoshihara Y, Omata K, Matsumoto K, Tsuchiya KJ, Iwata Y, Tsujii M, Sugiyama T, Mori N. Microglial activation in young adults with autism spectrum disorder. JAMA Psychiatry. 2013;70(1):49-58. DOI: 10.1001/jamapsychiatry.2013.272

[10] Torres-Platas SG, Cruceanu C, Chen GG, Turecki G, Mechawar N. Evidence for increased microglial priming and macrophage recruitment in the dorsal anterior cingulate white matter of depressed suicides. Brain, Behavior, and Immunity. 2014;**42**:50-59. DOI: 10.1016/j.bbi.2014.05.007

[11] Cattaneo A, Cattane N, Begni V, Pariante CM, Riva MA. The human BDNF gene: peripheral gene expression and protein levels as biomarkers for psychiatric disorders. Translational Psychiatry. 2016;**6**(11):e958. DOI: 10.1038/tp.2016.214

[12] Apple DM, Fonseca RS, Kokovay E. The role of adult neurogenesis in psychiatric and cognitive disorders. Brain Research. 2017;**1655**:270-276. DOI: 10.1016/j.brainres.2016.01.023

[13] Churchward MA, Tchir DR, Todd KG. Microglial function during glucose deprivation: Inflammatory and neuropsychiatric implications. Molecular Neurobiology. 2017. DOI: 10.1007/s12035-017-0422-9

[14] Stertz L, Magalhaes PV, Kapczinski F. Is bipolar disorder an inflammatory condition? The relevance of microglial activation. Current Opinion in Psychiatry. 2013;**26**(1):19-26. DOI: 10.1097/YCO.0b013e32835aa4b4

[15] Ji K, Akgul G, Wollmuth LP, Tsirka SE. Microglia actively regulate the number of functional synapses. PLoS One. 2013;**8**(2):e56293. DOI: 10.1371/journal.pone.0056293

[16] Mosser CA, Baptista S, Arnoux I, Audinat E. Microglia in CNS development: Shaping the brain for the future. Progress in Neurobiology. 2017;**149-150**:1-20. DOI: 10.1016/j.pneurobio.2017.01.002

[17] Kettenmann H, Hanisch UK, Noda M, Verkhratsky A. Physiology of microglia. Physiological Reviews. 2011;**91**(2):461-553. DOI: 10.1152/physrev.00011.2010

[18] Tremblay MÈ1, Stevens B, Sierra A, Wake H, Bessis A, Nimmerjahn A. The role of microglia in the healthy brain. Journal of Neuroscience. 2011;**31**(45):16064-16069. DOI: 10.1523/JNEUROSCI.4158-11.2011

[19] Ehrhart J, Obregon D, Mori T, Hou H, Sun N, Bai Y, Klein T, Fernandez F, Tan J, Shytle RD. Stimulation of cannabinoid receptor 2 (CB2) suppresses microglial activation. Journal of Neuroinflammation. 2005;**2**:29. DOI: 10.1186/1742-2094-2-29

[20] Mattei D, Djodari-Irani A, Hadar R, Pelz A, de Cossio LF, Goetz T, Matyash M, Kettenmann H, Winter C, Wolf SA. Minocycline rescues decrease in neurogenesis, increase in microglia cytokines and deficits in sensorimotor gating in an animal model of schizophrenia. Brain, Behavior, and Immunity. 2014;**38**:175-84. DOI: 10.1016/j.bbi.2014.01.019

[21] Yu Z, Fukushima H, Ono C, Sakai M, Kasahara Y, Kikuchi Y, Gunawansa N, Takahashi Y, Matsuoka H, Kida S, Tomita H. Microglial production of TNF-alpha is a key element of sustained fear memory. Brain, Behavior, and Immunity. 2017;**59**:313-321. DOI: 10.1016/j.bbi.2016.08.011

[22] Boche D, Perry VH, Nicoll JA. Review: activation patterns of microglia and their identification in the human brain. Neuropathology and Applied Neurobiology. 2013;**39**(1):3-18. DOI: 10.1111/nan.12011

[23] Barger SW, Goodwin ME, Porter MM, Beggs ML. Glutamate release from activated microglia requires the oxidative burst and lipid peroxidation. Journal of Neurochemistry. 2007;**101**(5):1205-1213. DOI: 10.1111/j.1471-4159.2007.04487.x

[24] Takaki J, Fujimori K, Miura M, Suzuki T, Sekino Y, Sato K. L-glutamate released from activated microglia downregulates astrocytic L-glutamate transporter expression in neuroinflammation: The 'collusion' hypothesis for increased extracellular L-glutamate concentration in neuroinflammation. Journal of Neuroinflammation. 2012;**9**:275. DOI: 10.1186/1742-2094-9-275

[25] Maiorino C, Khorooshi R, Ruffini F, Lobner M, Bergami A, Garzetti L, Martino G, Owens T, Furlan R. Lentiviral-mediated administration of IL-25 in the CNS induces alternative activation of microglia. Gene Therapy. 2013;**20**(5):487-496. DOI: 10.1038/gt.2012.58

[26] Song C, Halbreich U, Han C, Leonard BE, Luo H. Imbalance between pro- and anti-inflammatory cytokines, and between Th1 and Th2 cytokines in depressed patients: the effect of electroacupuncture or fluoxetine treatment. Pharmacopsychiatry. 2009;**42**(5):182-188. DOI: 10.1055/s-0029-1202263

[27] Godbout JP, Moreau M, Lestage J, Chen J, Sparkman NL, O'Connor J, Castanon N, Kelley KW, Dantzer R, Johnson RW. Aging exacerbates depressive-like behavior in mice in response to activation of the peripheral innate immune system. Neuropsychopharmacology. 2008;**33**(10):2341-2351. DOI: 10.1038/sj.npp.1301649

[28] Patterson SL. Immune dysregulation and cognitive vulnerability in the aging brain: Interactions of microglia, IL-1β, BDNF and synaptic plasticity. Neuropharmacology. 2015;**96**(Pt A):11-18. DOI: 10.1016/j.neuropharm.2014.12.020

[29] Talaei A, Tavakkol Afshari J, Fayyazi Bordbar MR, Pouryousof H, Faridhosseini F, Saghebi A, Rezaei Ardani A, Talaei A, Tehrani M. A study on the association of interleukin-1 cluster with genetic risk in bipolar i disorder in Iranian patients: A case-control study. Iranian Journal of Allergy, Asthma and Immunology. 2016;**15**(6):466-475.

[30] Dunne PW, Roberts DL, Quinones MP, Velligan DI, Paredes M, Walss-Bass C. Immune markers of social cognitive bias in schizophrenia. Psychiatry Research. 2017;**251**:319-324. DOI: 10.1016/j.psychres.2017.02.030

[31] Wang AK, Miller BJ. Meta-analysis of cerebrospinal fluid cytokine and tryptophan catabolite alterations in psychiatric patients: Comparisons between schizophrenia, bipolar disorder, and depression. Schizophrenia Bulletin. 2017. DOI: 10.1093/schbul/sbx035

[32] Yoshimura R, Katsuki A, Atake K, Hori H, Igata R, Konishi Y. Influence of fluvoxamine on plasma interleukin-6 or clinical improvement in patients with major depressive disorder. Neuropsychiatric Disease and Treatment. 2017;**13**:437-441. DOI: 10.2147/NDT.S123121

[33] Hinwood M, Morandini J, Day TA, Walker FR. Evidence that microglia mediate the neurobiological effects of chronic psychological stress on the medial prefrontal cortex. Cerebral Cortex. 2012;**22**(6):1442-1454. DOI: 10.1093/cercor/bhr229

[34] Wohleb ES, Fenn AM, Pacenta AM, Powell ND, Sheridan JF, Godbout JP. Peripheral innate immune challenge exaggerated microglia activation, increased the number of inflammatory CNS macrophages, and prolonged social withdrawal in socially defeated mice. Psychoneuroendocrinology. 2012;**37**(9):1491-1505. DOI: 10.1016/j.psyneuen.2012.02.003

[35] Kreisel T, Frank MG, Licht T, Reshef R, Ben-Menachem-Zidon O, Baratta MV, Maier SF, Yirmiya R. Dynamic microglial alterations underlie stress-induced depressive-like behavior and suppressed neurogenesis. Molecular Psychiatry. 2014;**19**(6):699-709. DOI: 10.1038/mp.2013.155

[36] Lehmann ML, Cooper HA, Maric D, Herkenham M. Social defeat induces depressive-like states and microglial activation without involvement of peripheral macrophages. Journal of Neuroinflammation. 2016;**13**(1):224. DOI: 10.1186/s12974-016-0672-x

[37] Schnieder TP, Trencevska I, Rosoklija G, Stankov A, Mann JJ, Smiley J, Dwork AJ. Microglia of prefrontal white matter in suicide. Journal of Neuropathology & Experimental Neurology. 2014;**73**(9):880-890. DOI: 10.1097/NEN.0000000000000107

[38] Altamura AC, Buoli M, Pozzoli S. Role of immunological factors in the pathophysiology and diagnosis of bipolar disorder: Comparison with schizophrenia. Psychiatry and Clinical Neurosciences. 2014;68(1):21-36. DOI: 10.1111/pcn.12089

[39] Barbosa IG, Machado-Vieira R, Soares JC, Teixeira AL.The immunology of bipolar disorder. Neuroimmunomodulation. 2014;21(2-3):117-122.

[40] Miklowitz DJ, Portnoff LC, Armstrong CC, Keenan-Miller D, Breen EC, Muscatell KA, Eisenberger NI, Irwin MR. Inflammatory cytokines and nuclear factor-kappa B activation in adolescents with bipolar and major depressive disorders. Psychiatry Research. 2016;**241**:315-322. DOI: 10.1016/j.psychres.2016.04.120

[41] Nowakowski J, Chrobak AA, Dudek D. Psychiatric illnesses in inflammatory bowel diseases—psychiatric comorbidity and biological underpinnings. Psychiatria Polska. 2016;**50**(6):1157-1166. DOI: 10.12740/PP/62382

[42] Ohgidani M, Kato TA, Haraguchi Y, Matsushima T, Mizoguchi Y, Murakawa-Hirachi T, Sagata N, Monji A, Kanba S. Microglial CD206 gene has potential as a state marker of bipolar disorder. Frontiers in Immunology. 2017;**7**:676. DOI: 10.3389/fimmu.2016.00676

[43] van Berckel BN, Bossong MG, Boellaard R, Kloet R, Schuitemaker A, Caspers E, Luurtsema G, Windhorst AD, Cahn W, Lammertsma AA, Kahn RS. Microglia activation in recent-onset schizophrenia: a quantitative (R)-[11C]PK11195 positron emission tomography study. Biological Psychiatry. 2008;**64**(9):820-822. DOI: 10.1016/j.biopsych.2008.04.025

[44] Takano A, Arakawa R, Ito H, Tateno A, Takahashi H, Matsumoto R, Okubo Y, Suhara T. Peripheral benzodiazepine receptors in patients with chronic schizophrenia: A PET study with [11C]DAA1106. International Journal of Neuropsychopharmacology. 2010;**13**(7):943-950. DOI: 10.1017/S1461145710000313

[45] Dong XH, Zhen XC. Glial pathology in bipolar disorder: potential therapeutic implications. CNS Neuroscience & Therapeutics. 2015;**21**(5):393-397. DOI: 10.1111/cns.12390

[46] Réus GZ, Fries GR, Stertz L, Badawy M, Passos IC, Barichello T, Kapczinski F, Quevedo J. The role of inflammation and microglial activation in the pathophysiology of psychiatric disorders. Neuroscience. 2015;**300**:141-154. DOI: 10.1016/j.neuroscience.2015.05.018

[47] Klapal L, Igelhorst BA, Dietzel-Meyer ID. Changes in neuronal excitability by activated microglia: Differential Na(+) current upregulation in pyramid-shaped and bipolar neurons by TNF-α and IL-18. Frontiers in Neurology. 2016;**7**:44. DOI: 10.3389/fneur.2016.00044

[48] Monfrim X, Gazal M, De Leon PB, Quevedo L, Souza LD, Jansen K, Oses JP, Pinheiro RT, Silva RA, Lara DR, Ghisleni G, Spessato B, Kaster MP. Immune dysfunction in bipolar disorder and suicide risk: is there an association between peripheral corticotropin-releasing hormone and interleukin-1β? Bipolar Disorder. 2014;**16**(7):741-747. DOI: 10.1111/bdi.12214

[49] Tandon R, Keshavan MS, Nasrallah HA. Schizophrenia, "just the facts" what we know in 2008. 2. Epidemiology and etiology. Schizophrenia Research. 2008;**102**(1-3):1-18. DOI: 10.1016/j.schres.2008.04.011

[50] Brunelin J, Fecteau S, Suaud-Chagny MF. Abnormal striatal dopamine transmission in schizophrenia. Current Medicinal Chemistry. 2013;**20**(3):397-404.

[51] Laruelle M. Schizophrenia: From dopaminergic to glutamatergic interventions. Current Opinion in Pharmacology. 2014;**14**:97-102. DOI: 10.1016/j.coph.2014.01.001

[52] Potvin S, Stip E, Sepehry AA, Gendron A, Bah R, Kouassi E. Inflammatory cytokine alterations in schizophrenia: a systematic quantitative review. Biological Psychiatry. 2008;**63**(8):801-808. DOI: 10.1016/j.biopsych.2007.09.024

[53] Drexhage RC, Knijff EM, Padmos RC, Heul-Nieuwenhuijzen LV, Beumer W, Versnel MA, Drexhage HA. The mononuclear phagocyte system and its cytokine inflammatory networks in schizophrenia and bipolar disorder. Expert Review of Neurotherapeutics. 2010;**10**(1):59-76. DOI: 10.1586/ern.09.144

[54] Upthegrove R, Manzanares-Teson N, Barnes NM. Cytokine function in medication-naive first episode psychosis: A systematic review and meta-analysis. Schizophrenia Research. 2014;**155**(1-3):101-108. DOI: 10.1016/j.schres.2014.03.005

[55] Inta D, Lang UE, Borgwardt S, Meyer-Lindenberg A, Gass P. Microglia activation and schizophrenia: Lessons from the effects of minocycline on postnatal neurogenesis, neuronal survival and synaptic pruning. Schizophrenia Bulletin. Schizophr Bull. 2017; **43**(3):493-496. DOI:10.1093/schbul/sbw088

[56] Patrizio M. Tumor necrosis factor reduces cAMP production in rat microglia. Glia. 2004;**48**(3):241-249. DOI: 10.1002/glia.20074

[57] Garcia AM, Martinez A, Gil C. Enhancing cAMP levels as strategy for the treatment of neuropsychiatric disorders. Current Topics in Medicinal Chemistry. 2016;**16**(29):3527-3535.

[58] Ghosh M, Xu Y, Pearse DD. Cyclic AMP is a key regulator of M1 to M2a phenotypic conversion of microglia in the presence of Th2 cytokines. Journal of Neuroinflammation. 2016;**13**:9. DOI: 10.1186/s12974-015-0463-9

[59] Yang H, Yang L. Targeting cAMP/PKA pathway for glycemic control and type 2 diabetes therapy. Journal of Molecular Endocrinology. 2016;**57**(2):R93-R108. DOI: 10.1530/JME-15-0316

[60] Taskén K, Aandahl EM. Localized effects of cAMP mediated by distinct routes of protein kinase A. Physiological Reviews. 2004;**84**(1):137-167. DOI: 10.1152/physrev.00021.2003

[61] Liou JT, Liu FC, Hsin ST, Yang CY, Lui PW. Inhibition of the cyclic adenosine monophosphate pathway attenuates neuropathic pain and reduces phosphorylation of cyclic adenosine monophosphate response element-binding in the spinal cord after partial sciatic nerve ligation in rats. Anesthesia & Analgesia. 2007;**105**(6):1830-1837. DOI: 10.1213/01.ane.0000287652.42309.5c

[62] Wang C, Yang XM, Zhuo YY, Zhou H, Lin HB, Cheng YF, Xu JP, Zhang HT. The phosphodiesterase-4 inhibitor rolipram reverses Aβ-induced cognitive impairment and neuroinflammatory and apoptotic responses in rats. International Journal of Neuropsychopharmacology. 2012;**15**(6):749-766. DOI: 10.1017/S146114711000836

[63] Ottonello L, Morone MP, Dapino P, Dallegri F. Cyclic AMP-elevating agents downregulate the oxidative burst induced by granulocyte-macrophage colony-stimulating factor (GM-CSF) in adherent neutrophils. Clinical & Experimental Immunology. 1995;**101**(3):502-506.

[64] Pearse DD, Pereira FC, Marcillo AE, Bates ML, Berrocal YA, Filbin MT, Bunge MB. cAMP and Schwann cells promote axonal growth and functional recovery after spinal cord injury. Nature Medicine. 2004;**10**(6):610-616. Epub 2004 May 23. DOI: 10.1038/nm1056

[65] Min KJ, Yang MS, Jou I, Joe EH. Protein kinase A mediates microglial activation induced by plasminogen and gangliosides. Experimental & Molecular Medicine. 2004;**36**(5):461-467. DOI: 10.1038/emm.2004.58

[66] Guo J, Lin P, Zhao X, Zhang J, Wei X, Wang Q, Wang C. Etazolate abrogates the lipopolysaccharide (LPS)-induced downregulation of the cAMP/pCREB/BDNF signaling, neuroinflammatory response and depressive-like behavior in mice. Neuroscience. 2014;**263**:1-14. DOI: 10.1016/j.neuroscience.2014.01.008

[67] Serezani CH, Ballinger MN, Aronoff DM, Peters-Golden M. Cyclic AMP: Master regulator of innate immune cell function. The American Journal of Respiratory Cell and Molecular Biology. 2008;**39**(2):127-132. DOI: 10.1165/rcmb.2008-0091TR

[68] Li YF, Cheng YF, Huang Y, Conti M, Wilson SP, O'Donnell JM, Zhang HT. Phosphodiesterase-4D knock-out and RNA interference-mediated knock-down enhance memory and increase hippocampal neurogenesis via increased cAMP signaling. Journal of Neuroscience. 2011;**31**(1):172-183. DOI: 10.1523/JNEUROSCI.5236-10.2011

[69] Poppinga WJ, Muñoz-Llancao P, González-Billault C, Schmidt M. A-kinase anchoring proteins: cAMP compartmentalization in neurodegenerative and obstructive pulmonary diseases. British Journal of Pharmacology. 2014;**171**(24):5603-5623. DOI: 10.1111/bph.12882

[70] Lee D. Global and local missions of cAMP signaling in neural plasticity, learning, and memory. Frontiers in Pharmacology. 2015;**6**:161. DOI: 10.3389/fphar.2015.00161

[71] Peng S, Yang X, Liu GJ, Zhang XQ, Wang GL, Sun HY. From the camp pathway to search the ketamine-related learning and memory. European Review for Medical and Pharmacological Sciences. 2015;**19**(1):161-164.

[72] Zhou L, Ma SL, Yeung PK, Wong YH, Tsim KW, So KF, Lam LC, Chung SK. Anxiety and depression with neurogenesis defects in exchange protein directly activated by cAMP 2-deficient mice are ameliorated by a selective serotonin reuptake inhibitor, Prozac. Translational Psychiatry. 2016;**6**(9):e881. DOI: 10.1038/tp.2016.129

[73] Zhang C, Xu Y, Zhang HT, Gurney ME, O'Donnell JM. Comparison of the pharmacological profiles of selective PDE4B and PDE4D inhibitors in the central nervous system. Scientific Reports. 2017;**7**:40115. DOI: 10.1038/srep40115

[74] Li QQ, Shi GX, Yang JW, Li ZX, Zhang ZH, He T, Wang J, Liu LY, Liu CZ. Hippocampal cAMP/PKA/CREB is required for neuroprotective effect of acupuncture. Physiology & Behavior. 2015;**139**:482-490. DOI: 10.1016/j.physbeh.2014.12.001

[75] Guo H, Cheng Y, Wang C, Wu J, Zou Z, Niu B, Yu H, Wang H, Xu J. FFPM, a PDE4 inhibitor, reverses learning and memory deficits in APP/PS1 transgenic mice via cAMP/PKA/

CREB signaling and anti-inflammatory effects. Neuropharmacology. 2017;**116**: 260-269. DOI: 10.1016/j.neuropharm.2017.01.004

[76] Vitolo OV, Sant'Angelo A, Costanzo V, Battaglia F, Arancio O, Shelanski M. Amyloid beta -peptide inhibition of the PKA/CREB pathway and long-term potentiation: Reversibility by drugs that enhance cAMP signaling. Proceedings of the National Academy of Sciences of the United States of America. 2002;**99**(20):13217-13221. DOI: 10.1073/pnas.172504199

[77] Forero DA, Herteleer L, De Zutter S, Norrback KF, Nilsson LG, Adolfsson R, Callaerts P, Del-Favero J. A network of synaptic genes associated with schizophrenia and bipolar disorder. Schizophrenia Research. 2016;**172**(1-3):68-74. DOI: 10.1016/j.schres.2016.02.012

[78] Kast RE.Tumor necrosis factor has positive and negative self regulatory feed back cycles centered around cAMP. International Journal of Immunopharmacology. 2000;**22**(11):1001-1006.

[79] Miao Y, He T, Zhu Y, Li W, Wang B, Zhong Y. Activation of Hippocampal CREB by Rolipram partially recovers balance between TNF-α and IL-10 levels and improves cognitive deficits in diabetic rats. Cell Molecular Neurobiology. 2015;**35**(8):1157-1164. DOI: 10.1007/s10571-015-0209-3

[80] Patrizio M, Costa T, Levi G. Interferon-gamma and lipopolysaccharide reduce cAMP responses in cultured glial cells: Reversal by a type IV phosphodiesterase inhibitor. Glia. 1995;**14**(2):94-100. DOI: 10.1002/glia.440140204

[81] Banner KH, Trevethick MA. PDE4 inhibition: A novel approach for the treatment of inflammatory bowel disease. Trends in Pharmacological Sciences. 2004;**25**(8):430-436. DOI: 10.1016/j.tips.2004.06.008

[82] Duinen MV, Reneerkens OA, Lambrecht L, Sambeth A, Rutten BP, Os JV, Blokland A, Prickaerts J. Treatment of cognitive impairment in schizophrenia: Potential value of phosphodiesterase inhibitors in prefrontal dysfunction. Current Pharmaceutical Design. 2015;**21**(26):3813-3828.

[83] Engels P, Fichtel K, Lübbert H. Expression and regulation of human and rat phosphodiesterase type IV isogenes. FEBS Letters. 1994;**350**(2-3):291-295.

[84] Bolger GB, Rodgers L, Riggs M. Differential CNS expression of alternative mRNA isoforms of the mammalian genes encoding cAMP-specific phosphodiesterases. Gene. 1994;**149**(2):237-244.

[85] Pérez-Torres S, Miró X, Palacios JM, Cortés R, Puigdoménech P, Mengod G. Phosphodiesterase type 4 isozymes expression in human brain examined by in situ hybridization histochemistry and[3H]rolipram binding autoradiography. Comparison with monkey and rat brain. Journal of Chemical Neuroanatomy. 2000;20(3-4):349-374.

[86] Miró X, Pérez-Torres S, Artigas F, Puigdomènech P, Palacios JM, Mengod G. Regulation of cAMP phosphodiesterase mRNAs expression in rat brain by acute and chronic fluoxetine treatment. An in situ hybridization study. Neuropharmacology. 2002;**43**(7):1148-1157.

[87] Fatemi SH, King DP, Reutiman TJ, Folsom TD, Laurence JA, Lee S, Fan YT, Paciga SA, Conti M, Menniti FS. PDE4B polymorphisms and decreased PDE4B expression are associated with schizophrenia. Schizophrenia Research. 2008;**101**(1-3):36-49. DOI: 10.1016/j.schres.2008.01.029

[88] Reyes-Irisarri E, Pérez-Torres S, Miró X, Martínez E, Puigdomènech P, Palacios JM, Mengod G. Differential distribution of PDE4B splice variant mRNAs in rat brain and the effects of systemic administration of LPS in their expression. Synapse. 2008;**62**(1):74-79. DOI: 10.1002/syn.20459

[89] Zhang KY, Ibrahim PN, Gillette S, Bollag G. Phosphodiesterase-4 as a potential drug target. Expert Opinion on Therapeutic Targets. 2005;**9**(6):1283-1305. DOI: 10.1517/14728222.9.6.1283

[90] Zhang HT. Cyclic AMP-specific phosphodiesterase-4 as a target for the development of antidepressant drugs. Current Pharmaceutical Design. 2009;**15**(14):1688-1698.

[91] D'Sa C, Duman RS. Antidepressants and neuroplasticity. Bipolar Disorder. 2002;**4**(3): 183-194.

[92] Bertolino A, Crippa D, di Dio S, Fichte K, Musmeci G, Porro V, Rapisarda V, Sastre-y-Hernández M, Schratzer M. Rolipram versus imipramine in inpatients with major, "minor" or atypical depressive disorder: a double-blind double-dummy study aimed at testing a novel therapeutic approach. International Clinical Psychopharmacology. 1988;**3**(3):245-253.

[93] Fujita M, Hines CS, Zoghbi SS, Mallinger AG, Dickstein LP, Liow JS, Zhang Y, Pike VW, Drevets WC, Innis RB, Zarate CA Jr. Downregulation of brain phosphodiesterase type IV measured with 11C-(R)-rolipram positron emission tomography in major depressive disorder. Biological Psychiatry. 2012;**72**(7):548-554. DOI: 10.1016/j.biopsych.2012.04.030

[94] Jindal A, Mahesh R, Bhatt S. Type 4 phosphodiesterase enzyme inhibitor, rolipram rescues behavioral deficits in olfactory bulbectomy models of depression: Involvement of hypothalamic-pituitary-adrenal axis, cAMP signaling aspects and antioxidant defense system. Pharmacology Biochemistry & Behavior. 2015;**132**:20-32. DOI: 10.1016/j.pbb.2015.02.017

[95] Manji HK, Duman RS. Impairments of neuroplasticity and cellular resilience in severe mood disorders: implications for the development of novel therapeutics. Psychopharmacology Bulletin. 2001;**35**(2):5-49.

[96] Atkins CM, Oliva AA Jr, Alonso OF, Pearse DD, Bramlett HM, Dietrich WD. Modulation of the cAMP signaling pathway after traumatic brain injury. Experimental Neurology. 2007;**208**(1):145-158. DOI: 10.1016/j.expneurol.2007.08.011

[97] Hannila SS, Filbin MT. The role of cyclic AMP signaling in promoting axonal regeneration after spinal cord injury. Experimental Neurology. 2008;**209**(2):321-332. DOI: 10.1016/j.expneurol.2007.06.020

[98] Whitaker CM, Beaumont E, Wells MJ, Magnuson DS, Hetman M, Onifer SM. Rolipram attenuates acute oligodendrocyte death in the adult rat ventrolateral funiculus following contusive cervical spinal cord injury. Neuroscience Letters. 2008;**438**(2):200-204. DOI: 10.1016/j.neulet.2008.03.087

[99] Reneerkens OA, Rutten K, Steinbusch HW, Blokland A, Prickaerts J. Selective phosphodiesterase inhibitors: A promising target for cognition enhancement. Psychopharmacology (Berl). 2009;**202**(1-3):419-43. DOI: 10.1007/s00213-008-1273-x

[100] Robichaud A, Savoie C, Stamatiou PB, Tattersall FD, Chan CC. PDE4 inhibitors induce emesis in ferrets via a noradrenergic pathway. Neuropharmacology. 2001;**40**(2):262-269.

[101] Dyke HJ, Montana JG. Update on the therapeutic potential of PDE4 inhibitors. Expert Opinion on Investigational Drugs. 2002;**11**(1):1-13. DOI: 10.1517/13543784.11.1.1

[102] Drott J, Desire L, Drouin D, Pando M, Haun F. Etazolate improves performance in a foraging and homing task in aged rats. The European Journal of Pharmacology. 2010;**634**(1-3):95-100. DOI: 10.1016/j.ejphar.2010.02.036

[103] Jindal A, Mahesh R, Bhatt S, Pandey D. Molecular modifications by regulating cAMP signaling and oxidant-antioxidant defence mechanisms, produce antidepressant-like effect: A possible mechanism of etazolate aftermaths of impact accelerated traumatic brain injury in rat model. Neurochemistry International. 2016. pii: S0197-0186(16)30114-0. DOI: 10.1016/j.neuint.2016.12.004

[104] Jindal A, Mahesh R, Gautam B, Bhatt S, Pandey D. Antidepressant-like effect of etazolate, a cyclic nucleotide phosphodiesterase 4 inhibitor—an approach using rodent behavioral antidepressant tests battery. The European Journal of Pharmacology. 2012;**689**(1-3):125-131. DOI: 10.1016/j.ejphar.2012.05.051

[105] Jindal A, Mahesh R, Bhatt S. Etazolate rescues behavioral deficits in chronic unpredictable mild stress model: modulation of hypothalamic-pituitary-adrenal axis activity and brain-derived neurotrophic factor level. Neurochemistry International. 2013;**63**(5):465-475. DOI: 10.1016/j.neuint.2013.08.005

[106] Vellas B, Sol O, Snyder PJ, Ousset PJ, Haddad R, Maurin M, Lemarié JC, Désiré L, Pando MP; EHT0202/002 study group. EHT0202 in Alzheimer's disease: A 3-month, randomized, placebo-controlled, double-blind study. Current Alzheimer Research. 2011;**8**(2):203-212.

[107] Davis TG, Peterson JJ, Kou JP, Capper-Spudich EA, Ball D, Nials AT, Wiseman J, Solanke YE, Lucas FS, Williamson RA, Ferrari L, Wren P, Knowles RG, Barnette MS, Podolin PL. The identification of a novel phosphodiesterase 4 inhibitor, 1-ethyl-5-{5-[(4-methyl-1-piperazinyl)methyl]-1,3,4-oxadiazol-2-yl}-N-(tetrahydro-2H-pyran-4-yl)-1H-pyrazolo[3,4-b]pyridin-4-amine (EPPA-1), with improved therapeutic index using pica feeding in rats as a measure of emetogenicity. Journal of Pharmacology and Experimental Therapeutics. 2009;**330**(3):922-931. DOI: 10.1124/jpet.109.152454

[108] Tralau-Stewart CJ, Williamson RA, Nials AT, Gascoigne M, Dawson J, Hart GJ, Angell AD, Solanke YE, Lucas FS, Wiseman J, Ward P, Ranshaw LE, Knowles RG. GSK256066, an exceptionally high-affinity and selective inhibitor of phosphodiesterase 4 suitable for administration by inhalation: In vitro, kinetic, and in vivo characterization. Journal of Pharmacology and Experimental Therapeutics. 2011;**337**(1):145-154. DOI: 10.1124/jpet.110.173690

[109] Zhang MZ, Zhou ZZ, Yuan X, Cheng YF, Bi BT, Gong MF, Chen YP, Xu JP. Chlorbipram: a novel PDE4 inhibitor with improved safety as a potential antidepressant and cognitive enhancer. The European Journal of Pharmacology. 2013;**721**(1-3):56-63. DOI: 10.1016/j.ejphar.2013.09.055

[110] Rutter AR, Poffe A, Cavallini P, Davis TG, Schneck J, Negri M, Vicentini E, Montanari D, Arban R, Gray FA, Davies CH, Wren PB.GSK356278, a potent, selective, brain-penetrant phosphodiesterase 4 inhibitor that demonstrates anxiolytic and cognition-enhancing effects without inducing side effects in preclinical species. Journal of Pharmacology and Experimental Therapeutics. 2014;**350**(1):153-163. DOI: 10.1124/jpet.114.214155

[111] Nunes IK, de Souza ET, Cardozo SV, Carvalho VF, Romeiro NC, Silva PM, Martins MA, Barreiro EJ, Lima LM. Synthesis, pharmacological profile and docking studies of new sulfonamides designed as phosphodiesterase-4 inhibitors. PLoS One. 2016;**11**(10):e0162895. DOI: 10.1371/journal.pone.0162895

[112] Obernolte R, Ratzliff J, Baecker PA, Daniels DV, Zuppan P, Jarnagin K, Shelton ER. Multiple splice variants of phosphodiesterase PDE4C cloned from human lung and testis. Biochimica et Biophysica Acta. 1997;**1353**(3):287-297.

[113] Siuciak JA, Chapin DS, McCarthy SA, Martin AN. Antipsychotic profile of rolipram: Efficacy in rats and reduced sensitivity in mice deficient in the phosphodiesterase-4B (PDE4B) enzyme. Psychopharmacology (Berl). 2007;**192**(3):415-424. DOI: 10.1007/s00213-007-0727-x

[114] Contreras S, Milara J, Morcillo E, Cortijo J. Selective inhibition of phosphodiesterases 4A, B, C and D isoforms in chronic respiratory diseases: Current and future evidences. Current Pharmaceutical Design. 2017. DOI: 10.2174/1381612823666170214105651.

[115] Jin SL, Conti M. Induction of the cyclic nucleotide phosphodiesterase PDE4B is essential for LPS-activated TNF-alpha responses. Proceedings of the National Academy of Sciences of the United States of America. 2002;**99**(11):7628-7633. DOI: 10.1073/pnas.122041599

[116] Ma H, Shi J, Wang C, Guo L, Gong Y, Li J, Gong Y, Yun F, Zhao H, Li E. Blockade of PDE4B limits lung vascular permeability and lung inflammation in LPS-induced acute lung injury. Biochemical and Biophysical Research Communications. 2014;**450**(4):1560-1567. DOI: 10.1016/j.bbrc.2014.07.024

[117] Huang H, Hong Q, Tan HL, Xiao CR, Gao Y. Ferulic acid prevents LPS-induced up-regulation of PDE4B and stimulates the cAMP/CREB signaling pathway in PC12 cells. Acta Pharmacologica Sinica. 2016;**37**(12):1543-1554. DOI: 10.1038/aps.2016.88

[118] Hansen RT 3rd, Conti M, Zhang HT. Mice deficient in phosphodiesterase-4A display anxiogenic-like behavior. Psychopharmacology (Berl). 2014;**231**(15):2941-2954. DOI: 10.1007/s00213-014-3480-y

[119] Pearse DD, Hughes ZA. PDE4B as a microglia target to reduce neuroinflammation. Glia. 2016;**64**(10):1698-1709. DOI: 10.1002/glia.22986

[120] Naganuma K, Omura A, Maekawara N, Saitoh M, Ohkawa N, Kubota T, Nagumo H, Kodama T, Takemura M, Ohtsuka Y, Nakamura J, Tsujita R, Kawasaki K, Yokoi H, Kawanishi M. Discovery of selective PDE4B inhibitors. Bioorganic & Medicinal Chemistry Letters. 2009;**19**(12):3174-3176. DOI: 10.1016/j.bmcl.2009.04.121

[121] Fox D 3rd, Burgin AB, Gurney ME. Structural basis for the design of selective phosphodiesterase 4B inhibitors. Cell Signal. 2014;**26**(3):657-663. DOI: 10.1016/j.cellsig.2013.12.003

[122] Jin SL, Lan L, Zoudilova M, Conti M. Specific role of phosphodiesterase 4B in lipopolysaccharide-induced signaling in mouse macrophages. The Journal of Immunology. 2005;**175**(3):1523-1531

Chapter 2

Neuroinflammation and Neurotransmission Mechanisms Involved in Neuropsychiatric Disorders

Jacqueline A. Leite, Ana Maria M. Orellana,
Paula F. Kinoshita, Natália P. de Mello,
Cristoforo Scavone and Elisa M. Kawamoto

Additional information is available at the end of the chapter

http://dx.doi.org/10.5772/intechopen.69343

Abstract

Some classical psychiatric disorders, such as schizophrenia, autism, major depression, bipolar and obsessive-compulsive disorders, have been related to neuroinflammatory process, immunological abnormalities, and neurotransmission impairment beyond genetic mutations. Neuroinflammation is mostly regulated by glial cells, which respond to physiological and pathological stimuli by anti- and pro-inflammatory cytokine and chemokine signaling; moreover, recent studies have indicated that glial cells also respond to the neurotransmitters. Neurotransmitters regulate many biological processes, such as cell proliferation and synaptogenesis, which contribute to the formation of functional circuits. Alterations in the neurotransmission can lead to many pathological changes that occur in brain disorders. For example, studies have shown that neuroinflammation can alter the metabolism of glutamate as well as the function of its transporters, resulting in cognitive, behavioral, and psychiatric impairments. Cytokines as IL-1β and IL-6 appear to have an important influence in the dopaminergic and serotoninergic neurons. These data together suggest that glial cells via cytokines and abnormal regulation of neurotransmitters can influence psychiatric disorders. The present knowledge about this issue does not allow answering whether neuroinflammation is the cause or the consequence of neurotransmission imbalance and emphasizes the importance to improve in vivo imaging methods and models to elucidate this enigma.

Keywords: neuroinflammation, neurotransmitters, psychiatric disorders

1. Introduction

The processing and the transmission of information by the neurons depend on intracellular and intercellular signaling, which occur, respectively, due to the conduction of an action potential and the neurotransmission across a synapse [1]. The action potential alters the membrane voltage and causes the opening of ion channels and, consequently, the entering of Ca^{2+} inside the neuron. This Ca^{2+}influx leads to neurotransmitters release from the synaptic vesicle into the synaptic space where they can bind to their receptors and activate signaling cascades, be recaptured by presynaptic transporters and astrocytes, or be degraded by specific enzymes that are present in the synaptic space [2]. Neurotransmitters are molecules responsible for the transmission of information from one neuron (presynaptic) to another (postsynaptic) on chemical synapses. There are different kinds of neurotransmitters, which are classified according to their structure and function, and each one has its own mechanism of synthesis and action [2]. In this way, after being released in the synaptic space, they bind to their respective receptors and activate signaling cascades that will result in the clinical effects that are already well known. The neurotransmitters with greater clinical relevance are mainly the acetylcholine, norepinephrine (NE), glutamate (Glu), gamma-amino butyric acid (GABA), dopamine and serotonin (5-HT). Neuroinflammation refers to an inflammatory response that leads to accumulation of glial cells in the central nervous system (CNS) [3], and it is mainly constituted by CNS cells (neuron and glia) together with cytokines, pattern-recognition receptors (PRRs), and peripheral immune cells [4]. The sustained neuroinflammation, for example, is capable of altering membrane expression of neurotransmitter receptors, glutamate and GABA and, consequently, impairing spatial learning, cognitive and motor functions by altering neurotransmission [5]. Therefore, neuroinflammation seems to be involved in different neurodegenerative diseases [4] and psychiatric disorders including autism, schizophrenia, and major depression [6–8]. Also, as will be better explained ahead, altered neurotransmission appears to be related to several neurological diseases such as autism spectrum disorders (ASD), obsessive-compulsive disorder (OCD), bipolar disorder (BD), depression, and schizophrenia, which exhibit alterations of one or more neurotransmitters and either their absence or their excess may result in a pathological situation.

2. Microglia and neurotransmission alterations

Neurotransmission alterations are the etiological hypothesis for many neuropsychiatric diseases, and, in general, the hypotheses are based on the observations of agents that acting on the synaptic concentrations of neurotransmitters can improve the symptoms of the disease [9]. Actually, hypothesis previously postulated has been updated due to the finding of several studies. The monoamine hypothesis, for example, was the first one established to explain the symptoms of depression [9]. According to it, the reduction in the monoamine neurotransmitters, as serotonin and norepinephrine, is the main cause of the depressive symptoms. However, based on more recent data, the etiology of depression can also be related to impairments in the amino neurotransmission, such as glutamate and GABA [9]. Another example is the dopaminergic hypothesis about schizophrenia, which attributes the main cause of this disease to excessive stimulation of dopamine D2 receptors in the associative striatum and decreased stimulation of dopamine D1 receptors in prefrontal cortex [10]. Indeed, more recent studies have shown that the glutamate and its N-methyl-D-aspartate (NMDA) receptor, as well the GABAergic, opioid, cholinergic, and serotonergic systems, seem also to be related with etiology of schizophrenia [10]. Alterations in the glutamatergic signaling were also already linked to ASD, a group of neurodevelopmental disorders characterized by neurobehavioral and neurological dysfunctions [11]. Besides genetic propensity, inflammation is another factor that is involved with neurotransmission alterations, as well as neurodegenerative and neuropsychiatric diseases [12, 13]. The acute inflammatory response has the goal to help the organism in the combat of pathogens and repair the damages caused by them. However, when this process remains persistent in time and becomes chronic, it generates a condition of cumulative damage, resulting in neuronal degeneration and in the development of a neurodegenerative disease [4]. According to studies, the use of anti-inflammatory drugs was related to lower incidence of Alzheimer's disease [3]. On the other hand, chronic inflammatory processes such as cancer, infections, and autoimmune syndromes increase the risk of developing neuropsychiatric deviations [14].

For many years, it was assumed that cerebrum was an organ immunologically privileged owed to the existence of the blood-brain barrier (BBB) (reviewed in [15]). However, a number of evidence suggests that peripheral inflammation could generate a brain inflammation by activating microglia and releasing some pro-inflammatory cytokines, as interleukin (IL)-6, IL-1β, and tumor necrosis factor α (TNFα) [16]. The communication between immune system and brain occurs via cytokines and pathogen-associated molecular patterns (PAMPs) that activate afferent nerves, such as the vagus nerve, or it could access the brain through regions that lack intact BBB, known as circumventricular organs (CVOs), thereby promoting activation of microglia that secretes cytokines and chemokines, leading to the recruitment of cells, such as monocytes and lymphocytes to the brain [17, 18].

In the brain, resident macrophages are known as microglia and comprise approximately 15% of the cells of the CNS, being important in the regulation of inflammatory response, neuronal development, and maintenance of tissue homeostasis [19, 20]. These cells have receptors for serotonin, norepinephrine, GABA, acetylcholine, AMPA, and NMDA glutamate receptor, as well for group I, II, and III metabotropic glutamate receptors, variations in the concentrations of these mediators could interfere with microglial function and morphology, as well as in the recognition of neuronal activity by the microglia [21, 22]. Glutamate, an important excitatory neurotransmitter of the CNS, acts mostly in the hippocampus, cortex, and caudate nucleus through its metabotropic and ionotropic receptors, NMDA, AMPA, and Kainate and plays an important role in the processes of learning and memory formation, as well as in motor behavior and brain development [23]. The hyperglutamatergic hypothesis of autism is based on studies that showed high levels of glutamate in the serum, lower levels of the enzymes glutamate acid decarboxylase 65 and 67 (GAD65 and GAD67) [24, 25], and the presence of increased gliosis in these patients [11]. Moreover, studies in autism genome found genetic abnormalities in the gene GluR6, which is involved in brain development through the regulation of a member of the ionotropic receptor kainite family [26]. GABA is an important neurotransmitter in inhibitory synaptic transmissions, which is synthesized from glutamate via the action of enzyme glutamic acid decarboxylase (GAD) [27]. Inflammation induced by lipopolysaccharide (LPS) and polyI:C during the gestational period reduces GABA-producing enzyme, GAD important for development of schizophrenia in animal models [28, 29]. In addition, TNF-α leads to endocytosis of GABA receptors in rat hippocampus while IL-1 and IL-6 reduced GABAergic currents [30–32]. Beyond the decrease in the synaptic availability of monoamines, inflammatory cytokines upregulate the activity of the indoleamine 2,3-dioxygenase (IDO) [14], which alters the neurotransmission by increasing catabolism of tryptophan, the precursor of serotonin, into kynurenine, which can be converted into the metabolite quinolinic acid by activated microglia [33]. Some neurodegenerative and neuropsychiatric disorders [34], as well mood and cognitive impairments [35], present high quantities of kynurenine and its neurotoxic metabolites in the brain or cerebrospinal fluid (CSF). More recently, it has also been shown to influence the neurogenesis in the human hippocampal [36]. Moreover, these cytokines are capable of decreasing the availability of tetrahydrobiopterin (BH4), which is a co-factor to the production of all monoamines [37].

Despite the etiology of all of these neurodegenerative and neuropsychiatric disorders remaining unclear, growing and strong evidence supports the important roles of the neuroinflammation and the neurotransmission alterations in theses clinical situations. All these findings and new discoveries allow the improvement of the drug therapy and, consequently, the life of these patients, as well as contribute to the progress in the search for healing.

3. Inflammation: a key factor for mood disorders

Lately, the relationship between inflammation and mood disorders became more evident [38]. In fact, it seems that the immune dysregulation plays an important role in mood disorders during life and is also one of the main factors for the development of the disease. It has been shown that inflammation during prenatal or childhood can trigger the development of mood disorder [39]. A study showed that high levels of IL-6 during childhood can be related to a higher risk of depression during adulthood [40]. The higher levels of IL-6 and Il-1β can be also an indicative of more susceptibility to commit suicide [41, 42]. Major depressive disorder (MDD) and bipolar disorder (BD) have in common the presence of activated microglia, and hypothalamus-pituitary-adrenal (HPA) axis alterations are highly frequent as well as can modulate synapses and monoaminergic and glutamatergic systems [43].

4. Bipolar disorder (BD)

Bipolar disorder (BD) is a multisystem disorder characterized by depressive phases that alternate with mania or hypomania. However, the presence of some mixed episodes with those two phases is also a possibility. This disorder affects mood, cognition, behavior, and social functioning [44]. BD can be classified in BD-I and BD-II. BD-I is a severe type of BD and the individual usually presents a manic episode for a week or more with an intense mood disturbance that needs hospitalization or psychotic features. BD-II is classified if the individual had a depressive and a hypomanic episode for at least 4 days with a change in functioning without a manic episode. The prevalence of BD is approximately 1% (BD I and BD II) [45]. This low rate can be explained by the fact that it is hard to diagnose hypomania. BD is also a disabling disease with a high mortality mainly because of comorbid medical conditions [46].

Inflammation is present in BD and is a good parameter to evaluate the prognosis of the impact on social and occupational life of patients and many other comorbidities are associated with higher rates of BD, such as autoimmune disorders, multiple sclerosis (MS), migraine, cardiovascular disorders, obesity, and diabetes which can reduce the life expectancy from 9 to 20 years [47]. There is no consensus whether autoimmune diseases and psychiatric diseases have a common origin pathway; however, it is well known that patients with autoimmune diseases have more often psychiatric symptoms [48]. BD is associated with autoimmune diseases such as Guillain-Barré syndrome (GBS), autoimmune hepatitis, rheumatoid arthritis, multiple sclerosis, systemic lupus erythematosus, psoriasis, and autoimmune thyroiditis [49].

A chronic low-grade inflammation can disrupt the endothelial barrier permeability and lead to the exposure of bacteria and other compounds to the blood, which could be the first step to the development of autoantibodies that are also described in BD [50]. The presence of anti-NMDA receptor autoantibody has been found in blood and cerebrospinal fluids of patients, which has as main target GluN1 subunit. This autoantibody can impair the receptor dynamics and as a result, synapses can be disrupted, being capable to lead to mood disorders and to cognitive problems that are commonly related to these disorders [51]. During BD phases, pro-inflammatory cytokines in serum can be elevated and levels can be different in each phase and serum cytokines can cross the blood-brain barrier, subsequently causing neuroinflammation [52, 53]. Although it is not yet known if there is causality between CNS and peripheral levels of pro-inflammatory cytokines, the increased levels of these cytokines may be a consequence of rupture of CNS, loss of immune system integrity, and some unsolved inflammatory responses during the development [44].

In animal models, the deleterious effect of TNF-α occurs via excess of glutamate that can cause LTP impairment [54] and the soluble TNF-α receptor type 1 (sTNFR1) is more expressed in serum during euthymia, mania, and depressive episodes in comparison with healthy patients and becomes an important marker for BD [55]. Furthermore, inflammation can also modulate the neurotransmitter levels. For example, IL-2, TNF-α, and IL-6 can decrease 5-HT levels. IL-2 increases the cleavage of tryptophan by modulating indoleamine 2,3-dioxygenase activity, which leads to a decrease in 5-HT levels, while TNF-α and IL-6 increases the metabolization of 5-HT to 5-hydroxyindoleacetic acid (5-HIAA) that also leads to low 5-HT levels. The low availability of 5-HT is also a main characteristic of BD and also MDD [43, 56].

Activated microglia also seems to present a very important feature in BD [57]. Serum TNF-α and IL-1β can overactivate microglial cells that increase apoptosis, oxidative stress and result in a neuronal dysfunction [58]. In *postmortem* brain of BD patients, the levels of IL-1β, MyD88 (key factor in TRL4 signaling), NF-κB subunits (p65 and p50), and activation glial markers were elevated in the prefrontal cortex which is an important region for cognitive control and affective regulation [59]. Some structural brain changes such as the lateral ventricular enlargement and functional changes in subgenual prefrontal cortex activity and mesolimbic connectivity were also found [60]. BD chronic inflammatory state also activates chronically hypothalamic-pituitary-adrenal (HPA) axis. BD peripheral cortisol levels are increased in patients during the mania/depression episodes and euthymia. Cortisol levels are an indicator of the severity of BD [61]. This increase in cortisol (hypercortisolemia) has also implications in weight gain, insulin resistance, and hypothyroidism [62]. In physiological conditions, the acute glucocorticoid receptor (GR) activation leads to anti-inflammatory effect and in pathological conditions; the chronic activation has the opposite effect by preventing the negative feedback of the immune response which is caused by the modulation of GR. GR expression and sensitivity are decreased in hypothalamus and pituitary which maintain a pro-inflammatory environment that trigger impaired neuroplasticity. All these changes lead to alterations in mood and cognition [63]. Childhood is a critical phase for the development of BD. In this period, the CNS and immune system are not entirely developed and this could be highly affected by psychological stress. Traumatic experiences in childhood increase the chances to develop BD and correlate with earlier onset and severity. It is also related to an inflammatory dysregulation that continues through adulthood which shows that an early trauma can have permanent consequences that could lead to a psychiatric disorder [64]. This intense psychological stress could lead to impairments in GR signaling and in HPA hyperactivity which are associated with the lack of inflammation control [65]. Other factors in trauma also cause immune imbalance such as sleep disturbance, metabolic syndrome, gut microbiota leakage, and drug abuse [49, 66]. The susceptibility to the development of psychiatric disorder is also a result of genetic background together with priming events in early life [67, 68]. BD has a high rate of inheritance that could explain the differences between individuals against the same inflammatory stimulus. So far, the major histocompatibility complex (MHC) was identified in BD as highly polymorphic protein especially in the region of the HLA locus [69].

A correlation between TLR4 and TLR2 with BD has also been shown. Some genotypes of TLR4 and one specific genotype for TLR2 are an indicative of BD's early onset and are associated with a poor inflammatory response. The impairment of important inflammatory response protein shows that inflammatory impairment is an important factor for BD and may somehow lead the individual to be more susceptible to other risk factors like infections and childhood traumas [70, 71]. Studies in BD patients showed that they have more alterations in genes related to IL-6, IL-8, and IFN pathway [72]. The gut microbiota can play an important role in BD because some prebiotics can increase the expression of BDNF and NMDA and also regulate immune system by decreasing hypersensitivity and better immune response [73]. BD patients usually do not practice physical exercises, which are a good tool to improve metabolic parameters that are important characteristics in BD and to have an antidepressant effect [74].

There is still a lot of debate concerning the role of immune dysfunction in the neuropsychiatric disease. However, this immune dysfunction can be an important target in therapeutics and the control of immune system could have a relevant synergic effect during treatment. Many different studies showed the anti-inflammatory concomitant antidepressants, mood stabilizers, and antipsychotics treatment could help the patients. On the other hand, other studies showed that some antipsycotics have pro-inflammatory properties which could help during the acute state [75]. Even though there is no consensus of the benefits of adjunctive therapy with anti-inflammatory drugs. A study with TNF-α inhibitors in BD patients without any antidepressant therapy showed only effect in patients with high levels of CRP and TNF-α which shows how important is a more effective and individual treatment for BD in following the levels of different cytokines [76].

5. Major depressive disorder (MDD)

Major depressive disorder (MDD) is known as the most relevant disability cause worldwide and is one of the most frequent DSM-IV disorder and the prevalence is of approximately 17% [77]. MDD occurs more in women than in men and its etiology is multifactorial although MDD could be 35% heritable [78]. MDD is characterized by patients having major depressive episodes for at least 2 weeks. The episodes can be recurrent or isolated depending on the intensity and number of symptoms. This could lead to a huge impact on occupational and social life. The long-lasting depressive episodes are followed by anxiety, feelings of guilt, and suicidal thoughts [79]. MDD has a similar profile to BD such as the increase of the risk to develop the disorder is higher if the individual had a trauma during childhood and this could also lead to an increase in the severity and in the lack of response to the treatment [80].

Studies suggest that control of stress-coping is impaired which can be a result of poor communication between a range of brain areas that are related to stress and emotions. It was also found that the volume of basal ganglia, hippocampus, and thalamus are smaller than healthy individuals [81]. In MDD patients, there is a hyper-reactivity of amygdala not only during emotional process but also at resting state. Some important areas of control of amygdala in prefrontal cortex are not able to regulate hyperactivity in amygdala during a negative stimulus in MDD. This hyperactivity is related to a hyperexcitability and enhanced firing rate in stress-response regions [82]. Thus, neurotransmitters regulation in the synaptic cleft plays an important role in MDD.

Monoamine hypothesis is an important mechanism involved in depression where there is a reduced activity of the catecholaminergic and/or serotoninergic systems [83]. The dopamine (DA) hypothesis considers the malfunctioning of the system of reward in mesolimbic system by the decrease of dopaminergic transmission that is the result of a decrease in the DA in the synaptic cleft that decreases the dopamine transporter expression and increases the D2 availability in neurons membrane [84]. Noradrenaline (NA) hypothesis shows that noradrenergic neurons control important brain areas such as the medial orbitofrontal cortex that responds to positive stimuli and lateral prefrontal cortex, anterior cingulate, and anterior insula respond to negative stimulus. 5-HT is important for the regulation of emotional behavior. It was previously showed that the decrease of 5-HT in synapse could impact negatively in mood of subjects which have MDD family history [85]. Therapeutic monoamine theory is supported because the drugs available can lead to DA, 5HT, and/or NA increase in synaptic cleft by blocking these monoamines reuptake. These monoamine transporters blockage help several patients; however, in more than 50% patients, they do not show any anti-depressive effect and also need 3–6 weeks to observe the changes in mood [86]. Although the monoamine theory is well established, it is understandable that this change in neurotransmitters can also lead to changes in other neurotransmitters, for instance, GABA, acetylcholine, histamine, and glutamate [87]. It has been also shown that the levels of glutamate in CSF and blood are increased in MDD patients compared to healthy controls. These higher glutamate levels can be reduced by the use of antidepressants. In postmortem studies, the elevated levels of glutamate in the brain and important alterations in the expression and function of NMDA receptor which is a relevant target for the treatment of MDD. Recently, ketamine, a NMDA inhibitor, could be a promisor treatment for the MDD. Thus, an impairment in glutamate pathway both in the neurotransmitter levels and in its receptor´s expression and function is present in MDD [88].

MDD patients presented elevation in serum levels of IL-1β, IL-6, and TNF-α and an increased microglial activation in some regions of cortex and insula [75, 89]. Although the microglial activation is present, there is also important loss of glia in prefrontal cortex (PFC) and also that chronic stress may lead to MDD by impairing PFC's astrocytes [90]. Almost all the important features observed in BD are also found in MDD, for example, the leaky gut is also seen in MDD which has higher concentrations of IgM and IgA and the presence of high levels of C-reactive protein [91]. MDD is related to neurodegenerative diseases especially because of the presence of neuroinflammation, a common factor between all neurodegenerative diseases. There is a higher probability of Alzheimer's disease (AD) patients developing MDD and vice-versa. Since increased pro-inflammatory cytokines in CSF can lead to depression in AD patients, elevated levels of IL-10 are associated with lower depression scores, showing the relevance of inflammation in the severity of MDD. The Aβ40/Aβ42 ratio in serum was increased in MDD patients in comparison with healthy controls which show that the Aβ cleavage control is also impaired. MDD and AD are associated with impaired signaling pathways involving the decrease of BDNF expression, an important growth factor in CNS, and changes in the volume of regions in the brain related to limbic system. However, the exact mechanism involving MDD and AD is still unknown [92–94].

Parkinson's disease (PD) patients present impairment in monoaminergic systems (dopamine, serotonin, and noradrenaline) which can lead to MDD. However, the glutamatergic system is also impaired in PD which could also lead to MDD and cognitive deficits that is also frequently related to MDD [95]. There is also strong evidence suggesting MDD being associated with Huntington's disease (HD), maybe because of high rates of suicide in HD patients compared to the population in general, and that the HD patients can develop MDD during the disease course [96]. Amyotrophic lateral sclerosis as all other neurodegenerative diseases has also an association with MDD. The ALS progression occurs faster if the patients have a high depressive score [97].

Aging can also be an important factor for MDD, because older adults are more vulnerable to MDD. During aging process, there is a reduction in some neurotransmitters such as dopamine and noradrenaline, decrease of BDNF expression, and also increased levels of cortisol due to the imbalance of HPA axis [98]. There is also the involvement of glial activation and expression of pro-inflammatory cytokines that affect the synaptic activity and also are found in MDD patients [99].

6. Obsessive-compulsive disorder

Obsessive-compulsive disorder (OCD) is an anxiety disorder with a prevalence of 2.3% and does not present any correlation between gender [100]. This disorder is characterized by recurrent intrusive thoughts or images that become obsessions and cause a huge distress that lead the individuals to present repetitive behaviors or mental ritual. In OCD, there is an overlap between cortico-striato-thalamic circuits [76]. The repetitive behavior is maybe due to a communication disruption between cortex and dorsal striatum. Studies suggested that the reward system and processing emotional stimuli are impaired in OCD. Thus, the emotional states are dysregulated and the proportion of response is also lost [101]. The precise cause of OCD onset is still not revealed and this disorder can appear during childhood or adulthood. OCD share some features with MDD and BD such as autoimmunity, genetic factors and the comorbid diseases; however some different comorbidities are specific for OCD, such as Tourette's syndrome and eating disorders [102]. The role of microglia in OCD has not been completely elucidated. However, an OCD mouse model called Hoxb8 KO seems to present microglial impairment, but new studies in patients should appear to contribute with this idea. This possible mechanism could be a result of dysregulation of glutamatergic system [103]. OCD has been also related to streptococcal infections in early life [104]. Pro-inflammatory cytokines IL-6, IL-2, IL-4, and TNF-α are increased in plasma of OCD subjects suggesting an important role of inflammation also in OCD [105].

7. Schizophrenia

Schizophrenia comprises a group of closely related chronic psychotic disorders that are characterized by a particular type of disordered thinking, behavior, and in affectionate relationships. The most common abnormalities are a special disorder in the perception of one's self in relation to the external world and hallucinations that differ from delirium and other confusional states, sometimes observed in dementia and depression [106]. Before the onset of schizophrenic disease that usually happens in the end of the childhood or early adulthood or when in remission, the individuals can be considered normal except by their vague and concerned appearance with their own thoughts. There is also a difficulty to fully understand figurative statements or to discern irrelevant to relevant data, to respect the logical limit of time and space and opposite things can be considered as identical as conceptual relationships are distorted. Schizophrenic patients are usually unable to clearly communicate an idea. All these symptoms can be categorized as cognitive symptoms because it directly reflects in executive functions including inability to sustain attention and working memory impairment [57]. Such confused thoughts reflect in the patient's behavior that can manifest as social withdrawal, idleness, aimlessness, aloof, and self-absorption. These are referred to as negative symptoms. Finally, schizophrenic patients can also present auditory and visual hallucinations, bizarre actions, aggression, agitation, delusion, paranoia, and major thought disorders that are symptoms categorized as positive. Cognitive and negative symptoms seem to precede positive symptoms, however, although their distinct clinical manifestations, it is possible that they usually can co-exist. The prevalence of this syndrome worldwide is about 0.5–1.0% and seems to be related to industrialization, urbanization, and increasing population density [107, 108].

In vivo imaging studies suggest common macroscopic brain abnormalities associated with schizophrenia, also present in drug-naïve patients with first episode psychosis, that include ventricular enlargement, decreased cortical and hippocampal volume, and reduced neuronal size. Furthermore, functional neuroimaging in patients with schizophrenia detected aberrant activity of neuronal circuits in prefrontal cortex, hippocampus, and also some subcortical structures [109]. In accordance with these findings, there was observed a decrease in NMDA receptor expression in postmortem analysis of prefrontal cortex of schizophrenic patients [110], and, in addition, preclinical and clinical data support the theory of stage-specific glutamatergic abnormalities in this illness because analysis of in vivo proton magnetic resonance spectroscopy (1H-MRS) to measure glutamine concentrations in the brain of schizophrenic patients compared to control subjects suggests that early-stage schizophrenia appeared to be associated with abundant glutamatergic activity whereas late-stage schizophrenia showed decreased glutamatergic activity [111].

Furthermore, growing evidence suggests a myelination dysfunction and altered oligodendrocyte number, as well as myelin, N-acetylaspartate (NAA), and fatty-acid biosynthesis dysfunction in prefrontal cortex of postmortem schizophrenia patients, possibly as a mechanism underlying the observed reductions in white mater volume. NAA can also be considered a function neuronal marker because it acts as an osmolyte and donate its acetate group in myelin synthesis [112]. Other metabolites were also analyzed, in vivo, by fractional anisotrophy (FA), as myo-inositol, that is associated with aging and neuroinflammation. This metabolite is highly expressed in astrocytes and is also a precursor for the cell signaling phosphatidylinositol and for synthesis phospholipids in cellular membrane. During chronic inflammation and/or slow virus infections of the brain, during glial activation and macrophage infiltration, an increase in myo-inositol is observed. Indeed, myo-inositol increase may contribute to hypomyelination disorders associated with inflammation on white matter microstructure in general [113].

The immune system can contribute to the pathogenic process by generating reactive nitrogen and oxygen species, releasing cytokines via microglia and lymphocytes that promote neuroinflammation. Specifically, the heme oxygenase (HO) system that acts as a sensor for oxidative stress as well as a key modulator of redox homeostasis is composed by two major isoforms, the heme oxygenase 1 (HO-1) that is inducible and the heme oxygenase 2 (HO-2) that is constitutive. Recently, there are some lines of evidence suggesting the involvement of HO-1 in the pathogenesis of schizophrenia [114]. Furthermore, sustained increase of HO-1 in the brain during the pre- or perinatal period could lead to activation of HO-1 in astrocytes prior to the maturation of offspring mesolimbic and nigrostriatal system, what induces changes in DA network structure and function predisposing to neurodevelopmental phenotypes of schizophrenia observed in early adulthood [114]. In the adult, one of the most important and well-established disturbances recognized in schizophrenia is in the dopaminergic neurotransmission, therefore the actual antipsychotics classified as typical and atypical that are effective in schizophrenic positive symptoms are antidopaminergic drugs, that are not effective on cognitive, negative, and other deficits found in schizophrenic patients [115]. The dopaminergic dysfunction can be a consequence of glutamatergic hypofunction in schizophrenia, being glutamatergic system closely related to the immune system [115].

Some in vitro studies proposed that after antipsychotics therapy, some cytokine levels become normalized, such as IFN-γ, that is blunted in the illness, as well as IL-2, ICAM-1, and the ICAM-1 ligand leukocyte function antigen-1, TNF-α, and TNF-α receptors (for more details [119]). Furthermore, medicated schizophrenics patients presented an increase in IL-18 serum levels that play a pivotal role in immunological response type-1 and a decrease in IL-6, one important cytokine of type-2 immune response, suggesting a role for antipsychotics in cytokine levels balance [119]. In schizophrenic patient's blood sample, it is possible to observe the predominance of type-2 immune response due to activated monocytes releasing IL-6, high levels of Th2 type lymphocytes, immunoglobulin E and IL-10 serum levels. In CSF of juvenile schizophrenic patients it was observed an increase in IL-4 levels, one of the most important cytokines in type-2 response indicating that this predominance is not only an exclusive peripheral immune response phenomenon [115].

Science is still far from an effective answer and treatment to offer to schizophrenic patients and, therefore, is still hurried to consider the pro-inflammatory cytokines as a possible target to psychosis treatment. There are many preclinical trials being performed in the world focusing on schizophrenia and major depression treatment with monoclonal antibodies to anti- and pro-inflammatory cytokine (infliximab, tocilizumab) [116], but the Janus face of inflammation mechanisms still needs to be carefully and detailed understood especially in the psychotic brain.

8. Autism spectrum disorders (ASDs)

Disorders on the autism spectrum are classified as neurodevelopmental disorders including childhood disintegrative syndrome, autism itself, pervasive developmental disorder not-otherwise specified (PDD-NOS) and Asperger syndrome, Rett's syndrome [11]. Autism itself is a debilitating neurodevelopmental disorder that starts at early childhood with genetic and environmental causes and immune influence. The ASD symptoms comprise impaired language and communication, impaired social relationship, repetitive behaviors, and a narrow range of interests and many autistics also have intellectual disability [117]. Intellectual disability (ID) comprises significant limitations in both intellectual functioning and adaptive behavior starting in childhood. The stable incidence of ASD in children has been estimated in 0.5–1.0% B [117, 11].

In the brain, neuropathologic alterations observed in ASD correlates to cytoarchitecture abnormalities that affect many structures as cortex, limbic system, and cerebellum, leading to hypoplasia of the inferior vermis of the cerebellum with loss of Purkinje cells, asymmetrical enlargement of the amygdala, and increased gliosis (GFAP), whereas biochemical abnormalities include altered energy metabolism, dysregulated amino acid metabolism with increased aspartate and glutamate serum levels in the amygdala and hippocampus [117]. It is well known that in ASD pathology, abnormalities in genes that regulate the expression of glutamatergic receptors are involved, as mutations in chromosome 6q21, where GluR6 gene is located [26]. The GluR6 genes codify the family of kainite receptors that are ionotropic glutamatergic receptors very important during development [117].

The degree of ASD severity appears to be related to the intensity and period that excitotoxic or immune insult occurs. Woman exposed to ethanol during pregnancy, as well as ketamine, phencyclidine, benzodiazepines, barbiturates, anticonvulsants, or anesthetics can have GluR activity altered. During development, CNS neurons are more susceptible to synaptic environment, and disturbances that increase NMDA receptors activity can easily trigger neurodegeneration due to excitotoxicity [11]. During development of the neural systems, an excess of extraneural glutamate can alter the migratory neuronal pattern, differentiation, and synaptic development, leading to different abnormal brain architecture degrees. A postnatal injury seems to produce lesser ASD syndromes compared to prenatal, as human brain continues to develop during the first 2 years of childhood. In older children, injury due to elevated levels of heavy metals, glutamate, and inflammatory cytokines secondary to microglial activation can affect postnatal brain development [11]. Based on observations made from adult brain exposed to elevated inflammatory cytokines, the capacity of immune system to reestablish a homeostatic state is the major determinant factor as abnormalities of immune system function is always reported in ASD, being overactivation the most commonly seen [11].

According to the literature, immunological abnormalities reported in ASD include a shift in T-helper cells,Th1/Th2, balance, abnormal reactivity of lymphocytes, increased levels of cytokines as IL-1β and TNF-α, and finally elevated levels of anti-brain antibodies, specifically antibodies against neurotransmitter receptors. In the autistic brain, a considerable loss of Purkinje cells is observed in the cerebellum, the most damaged area, followed by glial activation widespread all over the brain. There is also an increase in macrophage IL-6 and chemoattractant protein-1, which play an important role in the response of innate immune system including monocytes and T-cell activation [11].

Therewithal, there are considerable data proposing that prolonged and excessive microglial activation can impair either neurodevelopment or neurogenesis due to the increase in cytokine release by microglia and excitotoxicity as already observed in CSF, brain tissue, and blood of autistic child with high levels of cytokines and glutamate [118]. The co-localization of NMDA receptors with TNFR was also reported, implicating that GluR can interact with inflammatory cytokine membrane receptors allowing a cross talk that can lead to excitotoxicity especially through TNFR1. Furthermore, TNF can increase the glial release of glutamate by upregulating glutaminase [119].

As in schizophrenia, elevated cytokines during pregnancy have a very important role in ASD as proposed by human studies that found increased levels of INF-γ, IL-4, IL-5, and MCP-1 in mid-gestational mother sera and IL-4 and TNF in amniotic fluid [120]. Elevated levels of inflammatory chemokines such as granulocyte macrophage colony-stimulating factor (GM-CSF) and cytokines as TNF, INF-γ, IL-1β, IL-4, and IL-6 during mid-gestation have been more related to ASD subphenotype that presents intellectual disability (ID) than to ASD alone or developmental delay (DD) without autism [121].

Moreover, the production of maternal autoantibodies reactive to seven developmentally regulated proteins in the fetal brain has only been measured in blood of women whose children were later diagnosed with ASD. The seven proteins are Y-box binding protein 1 (YBX1), stress-induced phosphoprotein-1 (STIP1), lactate dehydrogenase A and B (LDH-A and LDH-B), cypin, and collapsing response mediator proteins 1 and 2 (CRMP1 and CRMP2) [120]. However, in order to determine the predictive value of the maternal autoantibodies for autism risk and diagnose, additional studies need to be done, because at this moment it seems to influence, if not define, ASD.

During postnatal period, individuals with ASD could present an increase in endogenous circulating anti-brain auto-immunoglobulins correlating with aberrant behaviors, impaired development and with immune dysregulation (increased IL-6, IL-8, and MCP-1) leading to an increase in the pro-inflammatory Th1/Th2 ratio. Besides the observed increased baseline activity of (natural killer) NK cells, there is a decrease in response to activation suggesting dysfunctional activity and a shift in T-cell population that is decreased [120]. However, the role of IL-17 is still obscure in ASD despite some temptations of explanation in rodent maternal immune activation (MIA) models [122]. The relationship between autoimmune diseases and ASD has long been described. Autism has itself been considered an autoimmune disorder [123, 124] due to the findings that family history of autoimmune disorders is a risk factor for autism and autoantibodies can also be found in multiple sclerosis, systemic lupus erythematosus (SLE), and schizophrenia. These autoantibodies can also cross-react with N-methyl-D-aspartate receptors [124].

9. Schizophrenia and autism spectrum disorders (ASDs), a common source: neurodevelopmental hypothesis of maternal immune activation

There are many evidences linking the etiology and pathophysiology of schizophrenia, with immunological changes especially during prenatal lifetime. During pregnancy, MIA that can be triggered by many common viruses seems to be enough to cause offspring brain function lifelong changes and behavior, in both animal models and humans [125, 126]. In 1964, after rubella pandemic, the incidence of two neurodevelopmental disorders, autism and schizophrenia, increased abruptly from less than 1% to about 13 and 20%, respectively [127]. Subsequent to this first observation, other studies revealed an association with outbreaks of influenza, chicken pox, polio and mumps, and schizophrenia or autism [120, 128, 129] as well as bacterial infections and parasite such as *Toxoplasma gondii* [125, 127]. Furthermore, any environmental insult or genetic predisposition that elevates immune responses above a threshold, like allergies, acute stress, asthma, and exposure to environmental pollutants, have been related to enhanced risk of schizophrenia and autism [125, 126].

According to this theory, during pregnancy, a maternal infection due to viral or bacterial invasion leads to pathogen recognition by peripheral immune cell through the action of the family of toll-like receptors (TLRs), classified as pattern-recognition receptors that is responsible, in peripheral immune system, for the generation and fast release of inflammatory cytokines, among others. The cytokines can cross the placenta barrier arriving in the fetal blood circulation according to the cytokine structure, gestational stage, and the physiological conditions of both mother and fetus [107]. The placenta from vertebrates is a very complex organ that plays the important role of fetus protection from pathogenic invasion and maintenance of a normal development hormonal environment. In physiological conditions, cytokines are constitutively expressed in placenta and seem to play important roles in the healthy environmental maintenance [130]. The expression of toll-like receptors (TLR) type 2 and 4 on normal human chorionic villi of placenta suggests that placenta can constitute an immunological barrier prepared to sustain and respond a pathogenic attack being also considered a pregnancy-specific component of the innate immune system. However, during maternal infection, a dangerous increase in environmental pro-inflammatory cytokines can strike an increase in placental cytokines that can become threat to the normal development of fetal brain [130]. During the CNS development, different classes of cytokines have different important roles. In the normal development of dopaminergic phenotype, IL-1β is the cytokine that can induce the mesencephalic progenitor cells conversion, whereas in embryonic hippocampal neural stem cells (NSCs) this cytokine can exert anti-proliferation, anti-neurogenesis, and pro-gliogenesis effects. Furthermore, IL-6 can modulate serotoninergic neurons viability, decreasing its survival in fetal brain, in an in vitro model of serotoninergic neurons from the rostral raphe embryonic cell culture. During development, TNF-α, in turn, can not only act as a neurotrophic factor in dopaminergic ventral mesencephalic neurons but also it can be neurotoxic at the beginning of brain development [126].

Due to the dificulty of clinical research in identify the molecular pathways downstream of maternal infection, animal models of research became a valuable tool once through this model it become clear the critical roles of cytokines in this process together with oxidative stress, zinc deficiency and hypoferremia, mediating in prenatal lifetime the neurodevelopmental effects of infection [106, 126]. In animal models, pregnant rodents and non-human primate (NHP) can be exposed to immunological manipulation, and brain structures of offspring can easily be compared to control offspring [131]. The behavior of the offspring can manifest a broad range of schizophrenia and autism-related abnormalities and also decreased ability of the brain to filter out extraneous information, deficits in cognitive flexibility, working memory, and increased anxiety behavior [125, 127, 131]. There are two different protocols that are very well established in MIA models, one that consists in pregnant female exposure to LPS, a bacterial endotoxin (lipopolysaccharide) and other that is based in exposure to polyriboinosinic-polyribocytidilic acid (polyI:C), a synthetic analog of viral double-stranded RNA. Both of them are recognized by toll-like receptors (TLRs), a class of receptors that recognize pathogen, being LPS recognized by TLR4 and polyI:C by TLR3. The female exposure to LPS or polyI:C during pregnancy notably enhances pro-inflammatory cytokine levels in many gestational structures as amniotic fluid and placenta and latter in fetal brain, leading to fetal microglia activation and an increase in transcription factor nuclear factor-κB (NF-κB) activity in both fetal and neonatal brains [106, 132] at the same time as white matter injury is observed by evident hypomyelination together with precursor cells of oligodendrocytes death and increased rate of apoptotic neurons during fetal and neonatal brain development. The activation of microglia together with this entire pro-inflammatory scenario is sufficient to induce a delayed increase of AMPA receptor expression and activity in excitatory synapses [132].

http://dx.doi.org/10.5772/intechopen.69343

When pregnant rodents are exposed to a model of viral infection with poly(I:C) injection, offspring tend to manifest autism spectrum disease behavioral symptoms, as abnormal communication, social interaction, and an increase in repetitive behaviors [126, 131]. When offspring reach adulthood they also exhibit other neuropathologies associated to schizophrenia, as reduced hippocampal volume and cortical thickness as well as and increased ventricular size, deficits in synaptic protein levels, in dendritic spine density, in long-term plasticity and cortical malformation [122, 129], and associated to ASD, aberrant Purkinje cells [125, 127, 129]. Altered serotoninergic and dopaminergic signaling was also observed additionally to specific changes in inhibitory neurotransmission and a decrease in several components of the γ-aminobutyric acid (GABA) system, related to both schizophrenia and ASD [125, 126, 129, 131]. Transposed to humans, it seems that most of maternal infections do not lead to ASD or schizophrenia in offspring, but it can act as a disease primer making individual more susceptible to the effects of this maternal infection in the presence of more than one risk factor along adult life, such as familiar historic of schizophrenia or autoimmune diseases [125–127].

Notwithstanding, to bridge the gap between humans and rodents, several groups have established *rhesus* macaque in MIA models to validate remarkably strong finding in rodents. As rodents and humans, these models display behavior symptoms of schizophrenia and ASD that increase in intensity along with age, as repetitive behavior, abnormal communication, and impaired social interactions [129, 131]. Gray and white matter volume is also altered in MIA non-human primate (NHP) models as well as changes in dendritic branching in neonatal offspring [129].

There are some theories made from animal observation suggesting that IL-6 can cross the rodent placental barrier in early and middle gestation but not in the late. It was observed that a maternal viral-like immune activation during the first half of mouse gestation could elevate IL-6 protein levels not followed by an increase in endogenous interleukin production in fetal brain [133] suggesting that IL-6, opposite to IL-1β and TNFα, can easily cross the placental barrier also in humans. As a matter of fact, to develop and establish a functional immune system, a series of very well-coordinated events during fetal development, that only in late gestational and postnatal stages will achieve the highest functional maturation period, seems to be necessary. In summary, the fetal cytokine reaction observed due to maternal infection is absolutely dependent on the precise gestational stage [107]. However, the mechanism by which this cytokines alter brain development is still unknown. There is an assumption that these cytokines can regulate the expression of immune molecules expressed in neurons, as histocompatibility complex I (MHCI) where it negatively regulates synapse formation, and the synaptic plasticity required for activity-dependent synaptogenesis and dendritic branching [126, 134], that are both altered in neurodevelopmental disorders and are thought to be important in etiology of schizophrenia and ASD [135].

Actually, MIA changes dramatically neuronal levels of MHCI, in brain of neonatal offspring [126], but it is still unknown whether these changes are long-lasting and related to the behavior changes related to disease in later stages of development. Alterations in the MHCI levels may be acute and directly reflecting the nature, intensity and duration of infection, that can

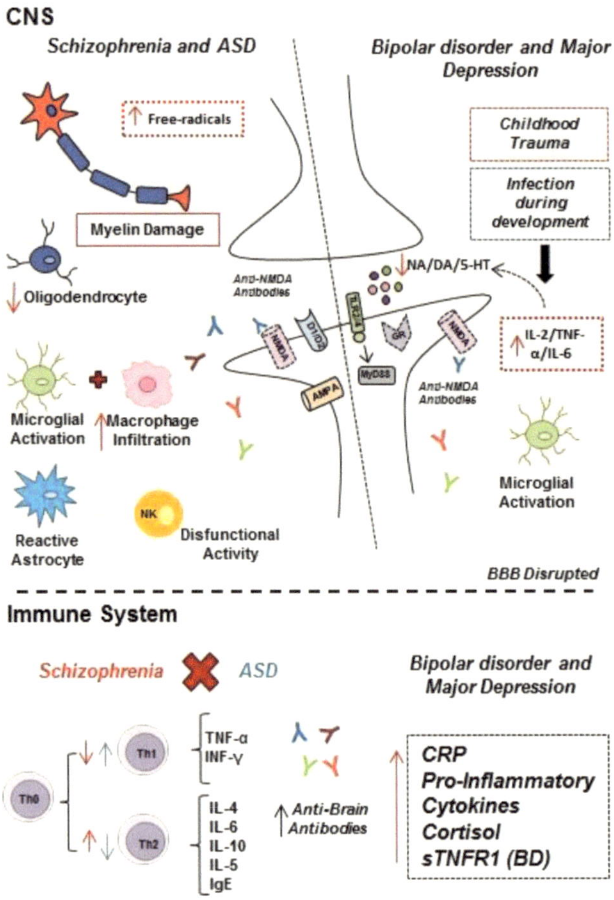

Figure 1. Main changes observed in neuropsychiatric diseases. On left, major immune changes related to schizophrenia and autism spectrum diseases (ASD) observed in central nervous system (CNS). A direct interchange is observed from cellular and molecular components of peripheral system and CNS due to blood brain barrier (BBB) disruption leading to an increase in macrophage infiltration, in microglia activation, and in astrocyte reactivity. There is also an increased inflammatory signaling responsible for higher levels of free radicals that together with decreased oligodendrocyte numbers favors the myelin damage process [112]. An increase in natural killer (NK) cells can be observed; however, its activity is dysfunctional [120]. Altered neurotransmission due to an increased expression of dopaminergic receptors (D1/D2) [111] and a decrease in N-methyl-d-aspartate (NMDA) receptors expression can be found in part as a consequence of the presence of anti-brain antibodies that among other cerebral targets can recognize NMDA receptors [11]. AMPA activity is also disrupted [132]. In peripheral system, a decrease in the shift Th1/Th2 is observed in schizophrenia, whereas an increase in Th1/Th2 relation is observed in autism spectrum disorders (ASDs) [11, 115, 120]. Anti-brain antibodies are also detected in peripheral system. On the right, the main changes in inflammatory response in mood disorders: bipolar disorder (BD) and major depression disorder (MDD) [38]. Most of the changes are consequence of traumas during childhood and/or infections during the development [39]. These diseases have important inflammatory markers such as microglia activation [57, 58], HPA (hypothalamic-pituitary-adrenal) axis impaired [43, 61, 65] and increase in pro-inflammatory cytokines which are related to each other [72, 75, 89]. The increase of C-reactive protein (CRP) and pro-inflammatory cytokines could lead to an increase in cortisol levels and also in the BBB disruption that could also lead to microglia activation. Since TNF-α levels are elevated, there is also a modulation of sTNFR1 in BD [55]. The chronic high levels of cortisol decrease the GR expression, which contributes to the inflammatory imbalance. High levels of cytokines also modulate the amount of neurotransmitters in the synaptic cleft. The levels of noradrenaline (NA), dopamine (DA), and serotonin (5-HT) are downregulated that conducts to the mood changes [85]. TLR4 and TLR2 pathways are also changed in BD [70, 71], for instance, the MyD88 is increased [59]. The presence of auto-antibodies is also an important feature in BD and MDD, especially anti-NMDA antibody that impairs glutamatergic pathway and could lead to cognitive impairment [51].

http://dx.doi.org/10.5772/intechopen.69343

become chronic, due to epigenetic changes that might synergize with other risk factors at different stages of life. Furthermore, as a convergent signaling pathway to cytokines, synaptic scaffolding proteins, and trophic factors, the literature now is trying to understand the role of mammalian target of rapamycin (mTOR) signaling pathway in individuals with schizophrenia, ASD and MIA offspring, as well as schizophrenia-associated DISC-1 mutation in animal models. Changes in physiological mTOR signaling can implicate in neuronal morphology changes, as well as synaptic plasticity and synaptic protein and glutamate receptor synthesis [113].

Several phenotypes related to schizophrenia and ASD, in MIA offspring, can also be prevented with probiotics, environmental enrichment, or maternal supplementation with zinc, several phenotypes related to schizophrenia and ASD, in MIA offspring, can also be prevented with probiotics, environmental enrichment, or maternal supplementation with zinc, specific antibodies to cytokines [122] and later during adolescence MIA rats treated with COX2 inhibitor were protected to develop several schizophrenic behavior aberrations, as well as the treatment with minocycline (a microglia modulator) during a stress condition in adolescence could prevent adult offspring to develop schizophrenic behavior [125, 127]. In particular, autism shares many significant similarities with schizophrenia, including genetic variants and neuroinflammation in early development and chronic inflammatory process affecting especially pregnant woman [111, 120] leading to aberrant neuronal connectivity, synaptic plasticity, and altered neurotransmission in both. Indeed, defects in inhibitory (GABAergic) and excitatory (glutamatergic, dopaminergic) neurotransmission leading to an imbalance of inhibition/excitation can be found in ASD and schizophrenia [111]. A summary of the most relevant similarities between ASD and schizophrenia concerning neuroinflammation in CNS as well as bipolar disorders and major depression are illustrated in **Figure 1**. However, in the immune system some differences can be observed between ASD and schizophrenia.

10. Conclusion

Therefore, a better comprehension about the pathophysiology of inflammation and immune system especially during fetal and neonatal brain development in psychiatric disorders remains an exciting field in science. The hypothesis of finding some answers that lead to a potentially preventable or treatable neurodevelopmental disorders is welcome in a field where current therapeutics are far from an ideal outcome.

Acknowledgements

J.A.L., P.F.K., and N.P.M. are supported by graduate fellowship from Fundação de Amparo à Pesquisa do Estado de São Paulo-FAPESP (2014/10171-0; 2014/01435-3; 2015/25491-2, respectively), and A.M.M.O. is supported by post-doc fellowship from Coordenação de Aperfeiçoamento de Pessoal de Nível Superior (CAPES). C.S.: grant from FAPESP (2016/07427-8) and CNPq. E.M.K.: grant from FAPESP (2011/21308-8).

Author details

Jacqueline A. Leite, Ana Maria M. Orellana, Paula F. Kinoshita, Natália P. de Mello, Cristoforo Scavone and Elisa M. Kawamoto*

*Address all correspondence to: kawamotoe@gmail.com

Pharmacology Department, Institute of Biomedical Sciences, University of São Paulo, Brazil

References

[1] Lodish H, Berk A, Zipursky SL, et al. Molecular Cell Biology. 5th edition. New York: W. H. Freeman; 2003. Section 7.8, Neurotransmitters and Receptor and Transport Proteins in Signal Transmission at Synapses. p.287

[2] Golan DE, et al. Principles of Pharmacology: The Pathophysiologic Basis of Drug Therapy. 3rd ed. Philadelphia: Lippincott Williams & Wilkins; 2011. p. 954

[3] Morales I, et al. Neuroinflammation in the pathogenesis of Alzheimer's disease. A rational framework for the search of novel therapeutic approaches. Frontiers in Cellular Neuroscience. 2014;**8**(112):1-9

[4] Shastri A, Bonifati DM, Kishore U. Innate immunity and neuroinflammation. Mediators of Inflammation. 2013;**342931**:1-19

[5] Wang DS, et al. Memory deficits induced by inflammation are regulated by alpha5-subunit-containing GABAA receptors. Cell Reports. 2012;**2**:488-496

[6] Cohly HH, Panja A. Immunological findings in autism. International Review of Neurobiology. 2005;**71**:317-341

[7] Fineberg AM, Ellman LM. Inflammatory cytokines and neurological and neurocognitive alterations in the course of schizophrenia. Biological Psychiatry. 2013;**73**:951-966

[8] Maes M, et al. The effects of psychological stress on humans: Increased production of pro-inflammatory cytokines and TH1-Like response in stress induced anxiety. Cytokine. 1998;**10**:313-318

[9] Pasquini M, Berardelli I, Biondi M. Ethiopathogenesis of depressive disorders. Clinical Practice & Epidemiology in Mental Health. 2014;**10**:166-171

[10] Laruelle M. Schizophrenia: From dopaminergic to glutamatergic interventions. Current Opinion in Pharmacology. 2014;**14**:97-102

[11] Blaylock RL, Strunecka A. Immune-glutamatergic dysfunction as a central mechanism of the autism spectrum disorders. Current Medicinal Chemistry. 2009;**16**(2):157-170

[12] Müller N, et al. The role of inflammation in schizophrenia. Frontiers in Neuroscience. 2015;**9**(372):1-9

[13] Leonard BE. Impact of inflammation on neurotransmitter changes in major depression: An insight into the action of antidepressants. Progress in Neuro-Psychopharmacology and Biological Psychiatry. 2014;**48**:261-267

[14] Sperner-Unterweger B, Kohl C, Fuchs D. Immune changes and neurotransmitters: Possible interactions in depression? Progress in Neuro-Psychopharmacology and Biological Psychiatry. 2014;**48**:268-276

[15] Xao BG, Watkins LR. Immune regulation within the central nervous system. Journal of the Neurological Sciences. 1998;**157**(1):1-12

[16] Quan N, Whiteside M, Herkenham M. Time course and localization patterns of interleukin-1beta messenger RNA expression in brain and pituitary after peripheral administration of lipopolysaccharide. Neuroscience. 1998;**83**:281-293

[17] Dantzer R, et al. Neural and humoral pathways of communication from the immune system to the brain: Parallel or convergent? Autonomic Neuroscience: Basic and Clinical. 2000;**85**(1-3):60-65

[18] Miller AH, Maletic V, Raison CL. Inflammation and its discontents: The role of cytokines in the pathophysiology of major depression. Biological Psychiatry. 2009;**65**(9):732-741

[19] Tremblay ME. The role of microglia in the healthy brain. Journal of Neuroscience. 2011;**31**:16064-16069

[20] Wake H. Microglia: Actively surveying and shaping neuronal circuit structure and function. Trends in Neurosciences. 2013;**36**:209-217

[21] Gundersen V, Storm-Mathisen J, Bergersen LH. Neuroglial transmission. Physiological Reviews. 2015;**95**(3):695-726

[22] Pocock JM, Kettenmann H. Neurotransmitter receptors on microglia. Trends in Neurosciences. 2007;**30**:527-535

[23] Kinoshita PF, et al. The influence of Na+, K+-ATPase on glutamate signaling in neurodegenerative diseases and senescence. Frontiers in Physiology. 2016;**7**(195):1-19

[24] Laurence JA, Fatemi SH. Glial fibrillary acidic protein is elevated in superior frontal, parietal and cerebellar cortices of autistic subjects. Cerebellum. 2005;**4**:206-210

[25] Vargas DL, et al. Neuroglial activation and neuroinflammation in the brain of patients with autism. Annals of Neurology. 2005;**57**(1):67-81

[26] Purcell AE, et al. Postmortem brain abnormalities of the glutamate neurotransmitter system in autism. Neurology. 2001;**57**(9):1618-1628

[27] Soghomonian JJ, Martin DL. Two isoforms of glutamate decarboxylase: Why? Trends in Pharmacological Sciences. 1998;**19**:500-505

[28] Harvey L, Boksa P. A stereological comparison of GAD67 and reelin expression in the hippocampal stratum oriens of offspring from two mouse models of maternal inflammation during pregnancy. Neuropharmacology. 2011;**62**:1767-1776

[29] Richetto J, et al. Prenatal immune activation induces maturation-dependent alterations in the prefrontal GABAergic transcriptome. Schizophrenia Bulletin. 2014;**40**:351-361

[30] Pribiag H, Stellwagen D. TNF-α downregulates inhibitory neurotransmission through protein phosphatase 1-dependent trafficking of GABA(A) receptors. Journal of Neuroscience. 2013;**33**:15879-15893

[31] Wang S, et al. Interleukin-1beta inhibits gamma-aminobutyric acid type A (GABAA) receptor current in cultured hippocampal neurons. Journal of Pharmacology and Experimental Therapeutics. 2000;**292**:497-504

[32] Garcia-Oscos F, et al. The stress-induced cytokine interleukin-6 decreases the inhibition/excitation ratio in the rat temporal cortex via transsignaling. Biological Psychiatry. 2012;**71**:574-582

[33] Miller AH, Raison CL. The role of inflammation in depression: From evolutionary imperative to modern treatment target. Nature Reviews Immunology. 2016;**16**:22-34

[34] Capuron L, Castanon N. Role of inflammation in the development of neuropsychiatric symptom domains: Evidence and mechanisms. Current Topics in Behavioral Neurosciences. 2016;**31**:31-44

[35] Stone TW, et al. Involvement of kynurenines in Huntington's disease and stroke-induced brain damage. Journal of Neural Transmission. 2012;**119**(2):261-274

[36] Savitz J, et al. Neuroprotective kynurenine metabolite indices are abnormally reduced and positively associated with hippocampal and amygdalar volume in bipolar disorder. Psychoneuroendocrinology. 2015;**52**:200-211

[37] Neurauter G. Chronic immune stimulation correlates with reduced phenylalanine turnover. Current Drug Metabolism. 2008;**9**:622-627

[38] Najjar S, et al. Neuroinflammation and psychiatric illness. Journal of Neuroinflammation. 2013;**10**(1):43

[39] McNamara RK, Lotrich FE. Elevated immune-inflammatory signaling in mood disorders: A new therapeutic target? Expert Review of Neurotherapeutics. 2012;**12**(9):1143-1161

[40] Khandaker GM, et al. Association of serum interleukin 6 and C-reactive protein in childhood with depression and psychosis in young adult life: A population-based longitudinal study. JAMA Psychiatry. 2014;**71**(10):1121-1128

[41] Lindqvist D, et al. Interleukin-6 is elevated in the cerebrospinal fluid of suicide attempters and related to symptom severity. Biological Psychiatry. 2009;**66**(3):287-292

[42] Monfrim X, et al. Immune dysfunction in bipolar disorder and suicide risk: Is there an association between peripheral corticotropin-releasing hormone and interleukin 1β? Bipolar Disorders. 2014;**16**(7):741-747

[43] Dunn AJ, Swiergiel AH, de Beaurepaire R. Cytokines as mediators of depression: What can we learn from animal studies? Neuroscience and Biobehavioral Reviews. 2005;**29**(4):891-909

[44] Leboyer M, et al. Is it time for immunopsychiatry in psychotic disorders? Psychopharmacology. 2016;**9**:1651-1660

[45] Merikangas KR, et al. Prevalence and correlates of bipolar spectrum disorder in the world mental health survey initiative. Archives of General Psychiatry. 2011;**68**(3):241-251

[46] Roshanaei-Moghaddam B, Katon W. Premature mortality from general medical illnesses among persons with bipolar disorder: A review. Psychiatric Services. 2009;**60**(2):147-156

[47] Leboyer M, et al. Can bipolar disorder be viewed as a multi-system inflammatory disease? Journal of Affective Disorders. 2012;**14**(1):1-10

[48] Kayser MS, Dalmau J. The emerging link between autoimmune disorders and neuropsychiatric disease. Journal of Neuropsychiatry and Clinical Neurosciences. 2011;**23**(1):90-97

[49] SayuriYamagata A, et al. Medical comorbidity in bipolar disorder: The link with metabolic-inflammatory systems. Journal of Affective Disorders. 2017;**211**:99-106

[50] Diamond B, et al. Brain-reactive antibodies and disease. Annual Review of Immunology. 2013;**31**:345-385

[51] León-Caballero J, et al. Bipolar disorder and antibodies against the N-methyl-d-aspartate receptor: A gate to the involvement of autoimmunity in the pathophysiology of bipolar illness. Neuroscience and Biobehavioral Reviews. 2015;**55**:403-412

[52] Muneer A. Bipolar disorder: Role of inflammation and the development of disease biomarkers. Psychiatry Investigation. 2016;**13**(1):18-33

[53] Patel JP, Frey BN. Disruption in the blood-brain barrier: The missing link between brain and body inflammation in bipolar disorder? Neural Plasticity. 2015;**2015**(708306):1-12. DOI: 10.1155/2015/708306

[54] Brietzke E, Kapczinski F. TNF-α as a molecular target in bipolar disorder. Progress in Neuro-Psychopharmacology and Biological Psychiatry. 2008;**32**(6):1355-1361

[55] Rosenblat JD, Gregory JM, McIntyre RS. Pharmacologic implications of inflammatory cmorbidity in bipolar disorder. Current Opinion in Pharmacology. 2016;**29**:63-69

[56] Zhang JJ, et al. Peripheral interleukin-6 administration increases extracellular concentrations of serotonin and the evoked release of serotonin in the rat striatum. Neurochemistry International. 2001;**38**(4):303-308

[57] Panaccione I, Spalletta G, Sani G. Neuroinflammation and excitatory symptoms in bipolar disorder. System. 2015;**36**:40

[58] Watkins CC, Sawa A, Pomper MG. Glia and immune cell signaling in bipolar disorder: Insights from neuropharmacology and molecular imaging to clinical application. Translational Psychiatry. 2014;**4**(1):e350

[59] Rao JS, et al. Increased excitotoxicity and neuroinflammatory markers in postmortem frontal cortex from bipolar disorder patients. Molecular Psychiatry. 2010;**15**(4):384-392

[60] Drevets WC, Price JL, Furey ML. Brain structural and functional abnormalities in mood disorders: Implications for neurocircuitry models of depression. Brain Structure and Function. 2008;**213**(1-2):93-118

[61] Murri MB, et al. The HPA axis in bipolar disorder: Systematic review and meta-analysis. Psychoneuroendocrinology. 2016;**63**:327-342

[62] Tsigos C, Chrousos GP. Hypothalamic–pituitary–adrenal axis, neuroendocrine factors and stress. Journal of Psychosomatic Research. 2002;**53**(4):865-871

[63] Anacker C, et al. The glucocorticoid receptor: Pivot of depression and of antidepressant treatment? Psychoneuroendocrinology. 2011;**36**(3):415-425

[64] Baumeister D, et al. Childhood trauma and adulthood inflammation: A meta-analysis of peripheral C-reactive protein, interleukin-6 and tumour necrosis factor-α. Molecular Psychiatry. 2016;**21**(5):642-649

[65] Linthorst AC, et al. Glucocorticoid receptor impairment alters CNS responses to a psychological stressor: An in vivo microdialysis study in transgenic mice. European Journal of Neuroscience. 2000;**12**(1):283-291

[66] Danese A, Lewis SJ. Psychoneuroimmunology of early-life stress: The hidden wounds of childhood trauma? Neuropsychopharmacology. 2017;**42**(1):99-114. DOI: http://dx.doi.org/10.1038/npp.2016.198

[67] Caspi A, et al. Genetic sensitivity to the environment: The case of the serotonin transporter gene and its implications for studying complex diseases and traits. Focus. 2010;**8**(3):398-416

[68] Giovanoli S, et al. Stress in puberty unmasks latent neuropathological consequences of prenatal immune activation in mice. Science. 2013;**339**(6123):1095-1099

[69] Purcell SM, et al. Common polygenic variation contributes to risk of schizophrenia and bipolar disorder. Nature. 2009;**460**(7256):748-752

[70] Oliveira J, et al. Polymorphism of toll-like receptor 4 gene in bipolar disorder. Journal of Affective Disorders. 2014;**152**:395-402

[71] Oliveira J, et al. Combined effect of TLR2 gene polymorphism and early life stress on the age at onset of bipolar disorders. PloS One. 2015;**10**(3):e0119702

[72] Drago A, et al. Enrichment pathway analysis. The inflammatory genetic background in bipolar disorder. Journal of Affective Disorders. 2015;**179**:88-94

[73] Savignac HM, et al. Prebiotic feeding elevates central brain derived neurotrophic factor, N-methyl-d-aspartate receptor subunits and d-serine. Neurochemistry International. 2013;**63**(8):756-764

[74] Janney CA, et al. Are adults with bipolar disorder active? Objectively measured physical activity and sedentary behavior using accelerometry. Journal of Affective Disorders. 2014;**152**:498-504

[75] Rosenblat JD, et al. Inflammation as a neurobiological substrate of cognitive impairment in bipolar disorder: Evidence, pathophysiology and treatment implications. Journal of Affective Disorders. 2015;**188**:149-159

[76] Soczynska JK, et al. The effect of tumor necrosis factor antagonists on mood and mental health-associated quality of life: Novel hypothesis-driven treatments for bipolar depression? Neurotoxicology. 2009;**30**(4):497-521

[77] Kessler RC, et al. The epidemiology of major depressive disorder: Results from the National Comorbidity Survey Replication (NCS-R). Journal of the American Medical Association. 2003;**289**(23):3095-3105

[78] Otte C, et al. Major depressive disorder. Nature Reviews Disease Primers. 2016;**2**:16065

[79] Association AP. Diagnostic and statistical manual of mental disorders (DSM-5®), Section II: Depressive disorders. 2013;155-188

[80] Miller S, et al. Cognition-childhood maltreatment interactions in the prediction of antidepressant outcomes in major depressive disorder patients: Results from the iSPOT-D trial. Depression and Anxiety. 2015;**32**(8):594-604

[81] Kempton MJ, et al. Structural neuroimaging studies in major depressive disorder: Meta-analysis and comparison with bipolar disorder. Archives of General Psychiatry. 2011;**68**(7):675-690

[82] Limon A, et al. Targets of polyamine dysregulation in major depression and suicide: Activity-dependent feedback, excitability, and neurotransmission. Neuroscience and Biobehavioral Reviews. 2016;**66**:80-91

[83] Nikolaus S, et al. Key players in major and bipolar depression: A retrospective analysis of in vivo imaging studies. Behavioural Brain Research. 2012;**232**(2):358-390

[84] Willner P. Dopamine and depression: A review of recent evidence. I. Empirical studies. Brain Research Reviews. 1983;**6**(3):211-224

[85] Moret C, Briley M. The importance of norepinephrine in depression. Neuropsychiatric Disease and Treatment. 2011;**7**(Suppl 1):9-13

[86] Al-Harbi KS. Treatment-resistant depression: Therapeutic trends, challenges, and future directions. Patient Preference and Adherence. 2012;**6**:369-388

[87] Murrough JW, Abdallah CG, Mathew SJ. Targeting glutamate signalling in depression: Progress and prospects. Nature Reviews Drug Discovery. 2017. advance online publication.

[88] Lener MS, et al. Glutamate and gamma-aminobutyric acid systems in the pathophysiology of major depression and antidepressant response to ketamine. Biological Psychiatry. 2017;**81**(10):886-897. DOI: 10.1016/j.biopsych.2016.05.005

[89] Setiawan E, et al. Role of translocator protein density, a marker of neuroinflammation, in the brain during major depressive episodes. JAMA Psychiatry. 2015;**72**(3):268-275

[90] Rial D, et al. Depression as a glial-based synaptic dysfunction. Frontiers in Cellular Neuroscience. 2016;**9**:521

[91] Bankier B, et al. Association between major depressive disorder and C-reactive protein levels in stable coronary heart disease patients. Journal of Psychosomatic Research. 2009;**66**(3):189-194

[92] Réus GZ, et al. Neurochemical correlation between major depressive disorder and neurodegenerative diseases. Life Sciences. 2016;**158**:121-129

[93] O'shea DM, et al. Examining the association between late life depressive symptoms, cognitive function, and brain volumes in the context of cognitive reserve. International Journal of Geriatric Psychiatry. 2015;**30**(6):614-622

[94] Rodrigues R, Petersen RB, Perry G. Parallels between major depressive disorder and Alzheimer's disease: Role of oxidative stress and genetic vulnerability. Cellular and Molecular Neurobiology. 2014;**34**(7):925-949

[95] Martínez-Martín P, Damián J. Parkinson disease: Depression and anxiety in Parkinson disease. Nature Reviews Neurology. 2010;**6**(5):243-245

[96] Pla P, et al. Mood disorders in Huntington's disease: From behavior to cellular and molecular mechanisms. Frontiers in Behavioral Neuroscience. 2014;**8**:135

[97] Rabkin JG, et al. Depression and wish to die in a multicenter cohort of ALS patients. Amyotrophic Lateral Sclerosis and Frontotemporal Degeneration. 2015;**16**(3-4):265-273

[98] Stilling RM, et al. De-regulation of gene expression and alternative splicing affects distinct cellular pathways in the aging hippocampus. Frontiers in Cellular Neuroscience. 2014;**8**:373. DOI: 10.3389/fncel.2014.00373

[99] Pickering M, Cumiskey D, O'Connor JJ. Actions of TNF-α on glutamatergic synaptic transmission in the central nervous system. Experimental Physiology. 2005;**90**(5):663-670

[100] Ruscio AM, et al. The epidemiology of obsessive-compulsive disorder in the National Comorbidity Survey Replication. Molecular Psychiatry. 2010;**15**(1):53-63

[101] Pérez-Vigil A, et al. The link between autoimmune diseases and obsessive-compulsive and tic disorders: A systematic review. Neuroscience and Biobehavioral Reviews. 2016;**71**:542-562

[102] Davis LK, et al. Partitioning the heritability of Tourette syndrome and obsessive compulsive disorder reveals differences in genetic architecture. PLoS Genetics. 2013;**9**(10): e003864

[103] Frick L, Pittenger C. Microglial dysregulation in OCD, Tourette syndrome, and PANDAS. Journal of Immunology Research. 2016;**2016**:8606057. DOI:http://dx.doi.org/10.1155/2016/8606057.

[104] Mell LK, Davis RL, Owens D. Association between streptococcal infection and obsessive-compulsive disorder, Tourette's syndrome, and tic disorder. Pediatrics. 2005;**116**(1):56-60

[105] Rao NP, et al. Plasma cytokine abnormalities in drug-naïve, comorbidity-free obsessive–compulsive disorder. Psychiatry Research. 2015;**229**(3):949-952

[106] Meyer U. Developmental neuroinflammation and schizophrenia. Progress in Neuro-Psychopharmacology and Biological Psychiatry. 2013;**42**:20-34

[107] Meyer U, Feldon J, Yee BK. A review of the fetal brain cytokine imbalance hypothesis of schizophrenia. Schizophrenia Bulletin. 2009;**35**(5):959-972

[108] Tandon R, Keshavan MS, Nasrallah HA. Schizophrenia, "just the facts" what we know in 2008. 2. Epidemiology and etiology. Schizophrenia Research. 2008;**102**(1-3):1-18

[109] Zetterberg H. Psychosis and biological markers. Lancet Psychiatry. 2017;**4**(1):3-5

[110] Catts VS, et al. A quantitative review of the postmortem evidence for decreased cortical N-methyl-d-aspartate receptor expression levels in schizophrenia: How can we link molecular abnormalities to mismatch negativity deficits? Biological Psychology. 2016;**116**:57-67

[111] Liu X, et al. Genetics implicate common mechanisms in autism and schizophrenia: Synaptic activity and immunity. Journal of Medical Genetics. 2017. DOI: 10.1136/jmedgenet-2016-104487

[112] Chiappelli J, et al. Alterations in frontal white matter neurochemistry and microstructure in schizophrenia: Implications for neuroinflammation. Translational Psychiatry. 2015;**5**(4):e548

[113] Santini E, Klann E. Reciprocal signaling between translational control pathways and synaptic proteins in autism spectrum disorders. Science Signaling. 2014;**7**(349):re10

[114] Calabrese V, et al. Hormesis cellular stress response and neuroinflammation in schizophrenia early onset versus late onset state. Journal of Neuroscience Research. 2017;**95**(5):1182-1193

[115] Muller N, Myint AM, Schwartz MJ. Inflammation in schizophrenia. Advances in Protein Chemistry and Structural Biology. 2012;**88**:49-68

[116] Raison CL, et al. A randomized controlled trial of the tumor necrosis factor-alpha antagonist infliximab in treatment resistant depression: Role of baseline inflammatory biomarkers. JAMA Psychiatry. 2013;**70**(1):31-41

[117] Mefford HC, Batshaw ML, Hoffman EP. Genomics, intellectual disability, and autism. New England Journal of Medicine. 2012;**366**(8):733-743

[118] Singh VK, et al. Abnormal measles-mumps-rubella antibodies and CNS autoimmunity in children with autism. Journal of Biomedical Science. 2002;**9**(4):359-364

[119] Yang L, et al. Target depletion of distinct tumor necrosis factor receptor subtypes reveals hippocampal neuron death and survival through different signal transduction pathways. Journal of Neuroscience. 2002;**22**(8):3025-3032

[120] Meltzer A, Van de Water J. The role of the immune system in autism spectrum disorder. Neuropsychopharmacology. 2017;**42**(1):284-298

[121] Jones KL, et al. Autism with intellectual disability is associated with increased levels of maternal cytokines and chemokines during gestation. Molecular Psychiatry. 2017;**22**(2):273-279

[122] Choi GB, et al. The maternal interleukin-17a pathway in mice promotes autism-like phenotypes in offspring. Science. 2016;**351**(6276):933-939

[123] Singh VK. Phenotypic expression of autoimmune autistic disorder (AAD): A major subset of autism. Annals of Clinical Psychiatry. 2009;**21**(3):148-161

[124] Coutinho E, Vincent A. Autoimmunity in neuropsychiatric disorders. Handbook of Clinical Neurology. 2016;**133**:269-282

[125] Knuesel I, et al. Maternal immune activation and abnormal brain development across CNS disorders. Nature Reviews Neurology. 2014;**10**(11):643-660

[126] Estes ML, McAllister AK. Immune mediators in the brain and peripheral tissues in autism spectrum disorder. Nature Reviews Neuroscience. 2015;**16**(8):469-486

[127] Patterson PH. Immune involvement in schizophrenia and autism: Etiology, pathology and animal models. Behavioural Brain Research. 2009;**204**(2):313-321

[128] Atladottir H, et al. Maternal infection requiring hospitalization during pregnancy and autism spectrum disorders. Journal of Autism and Developmental Disorders. 2010;**40**(12):1423-1430

[129] Reisinger S, et al. The poly(I:C)-induced maternal immune activation model in preclinical neuropsychiatric drug discovery. Pharmacology and Therapeutics. 2015;**149**:213-226

[130] Jonakait GM. The effects of maternal inflammation on neuronal development: Possible mechanisms. International Journal of Developmental Neuroscience. 2007;**25**(7):415-425

[131] Meyer U. Prenatal poly(i:C) exposure and other developmental immune activation models in rodent systems. Biological Psychiatry. 2014;**75**(4):307-315

[132] Roumier A, et al. Prenatal activation of microglia induces delayed impairment of glutamatergic synaptic function. PLoS One. 2008;**3**(7):e2595

[133] Meyer U, et al. The time of prenatal immune challenge determines the specificity of inflammation-mediated brain and behavioral pathology. Journal of Neuroscience. 2006;**26**(18):4752-4762

[134] Glynn MW, et al. MHC class I negatively regulates synapse density during the establishment of cortical connections. Nature Neuroscience. 2011;**14**(4):442-451

[135] Sekar A, et al. Schizophrenia risk from complex variation of complement component 4. Nature. 2016;**530**(7589):177-183

Section 2

Neuroinflammation in Alzheimer's Disease

Comprehensive Overview of Alzheimer's Disease Neurodegeneration, from Amyloid-β to Neuroinflammatory Modulation

Juan M. Zolezzi and Nibaldo C. Inestrosa

Additional information is available at the end of the chapter

http://dx.doi.org/10.5772/intechopen.69463

Abstract

Alzheimer's disease (AD) constitutes a major health threat to elder people. Despite the great advances achieved regarding our knowledge of the disease, we are far to successfully treat this pathology. Molecular alterations, immune/inflammatory response, and cell death are some of the processes involved during the pathology. Moreover, AD affects the whole brain. In this regard, we must not only consider the health status of neurons, of course, but also pay attention to the status of the glial cells and additional surrounding structures, such as the blood-brain barrier (BBB). Several groups have demonstrated how the molecular alterations occurring during AD alter neurons, glial, and endothelial cells. This situation has become so relevant that different groups are currently working to unveil the blank spaces in our understanding about the co-involvement of these elements in AD. Based in our experience, we believe that this kind of approach will lead to the design and development of more comprehensive therapeutical interventions. The present chapter summarizes the relevant aspects of state of the art regarding AD, from its molecular genesis to the recent advances in neuroinflammatory modulation, including nuclear receptors (NR), such as peroxisome proliferator-activated receptors (PPARs), and the Wnt pathway involved in the AD neurodegeneration.

Keywords: Alzheimer's disease, neurodegeneration, amyloid-β, neuroinflammation, Toll-like receptors, glial activation, TREM2

1. Introduction

Scientific progress has given enormous benefits to human population. In this regard, the continuous advances in biomedicine have constituted one of the more relevant achievements of the last centuries. Increased rate of newborn survival, control of devastating infectious pathologies, chirurgical management of systemic pathologies, and increased life expectancy of the world population are some of the milestones reached because of science development.

Although positive, the increased longevity of world population has led to two critical events, which have huge implications in human health. On one side, our biological system must work for a longer period of time. Considering that no machine can work indefinitely without failure, the alteration/impairment of our cellular and molecular mechanisms should be considered as part of the price to live longer and as an open door for the development of several diseases. On the other side, we must consider that a longer life span also implies an increased exposition time to different kinds of xenobiotics. Environmental pollutant levels have increased along with the population growth, and although huge efforts have been committed to reduce the usage of the more toxic chemicals worldwide, just a rapid revision of the lists published by the International Agency for Research on Cancer (http://www.iarc.fr) allows us to understand and to dimension the threats usually faced during our life span. Accordingly, the increased incidence and prevalence of several chronic-degenerative pathologies, including cancer and neurodegenerative disorders, should not be a surprise. Indeed, age and the exposition to environmental pollutants are considered as the main risk factors for the establishment and progression of these pathologies. Thus, to properly face this specific type of alterations, a complex equation should be solved, including deep knowledge of the cellular and molecular mechanisms behind each disorder and the environmental elements able to induce, perpetuate, and/or accelerate the pathophysiological processes.

In the present chapter, we will focus our efforts to summarize the most relevant aspects regarding Alzheimer's disease (AD) and the key elements of its pathophysiological process. Moreover, we will include relevant information and discussion about some aspects of neuroinflammatory modulation.

2. Alzheimer's disease

Described more than a century ago, Alzheimer's disease (AD) constitutes nowadays an extremely complex public health threat. With up to 10% of people over 65 years old affected by this pathology and up to 50% of people over 85, AD is the most common form of dementia worldwide. Moreover, the cost associated to AD has been estimated in USD 818 billion. Additionally, the social implications should be considered when the total impact of the disease is addressed. Indeed, according to Alzheimer's Research International, in most cases, the relatives of an AD patient are those who take care of the patient health, causing a huge impact in the familial economy as well as social stress [1].

To date, two presentation forms have been reported for AD: the familial or early-onset AD (EOAD) and the late-onset AD (LOAD). As suggested by its name, the main characteristic of EOAD is its presentation before the 65 years old, with cases reported from the 30s to 60s and with a high genetic background at least in three genes (amyloid precursor protein, *APP*; presenilin 1, *PSEN1*; and presenilin 2, *PSEN2*). Although no consensus has been agreed, several

http://dx.doi.org/10.5772/intechopen.69463

researchers have defined that EOAD might reach the 5% of total AD cases worldwide. On the other hand, the LOAD occurs after the 65 years old, and age and life style are considered as the main factors leading to AD insurgence. Importantly, in both presentation forms, the apolipoprotein E (*ApoE*) ε4 gene allele has been identified as a relevant risk factor (**Figure 1**) [2].

Clinically, AD progresses from the compromise of the short-term memory to long-term memory loss and cognitive impairment. The selective neuronal death within memory and learning brain areas is at the basis of these clinical alterations. Indeed, frontal cortex, limbic area, and hippocampus atrophies along with extracellular accumulation of amyloid-β (Aβ) plaques and intra-neuronal neurofibrillary tangles (NFTs), constituted by hyperphosphorylated *tau* protein, are pathological hallmarks of the disease [3]. Additionally, increased oxidative stress status, mitochondrial dysfunction, impaired energy metabolism, and altered autophagy process have also been demonstrated during the disease. Importantly, the spread of these alterations across the different brain areas ultimately leads to neuronal network failure, affecting the synapses critically, and to the loss of function of these areas [3, 4].

On the other hand, it is important to realize that AD affects the whole brain. In this regard, we must consider the health status of neurons, of course, but also pay attention to the status of

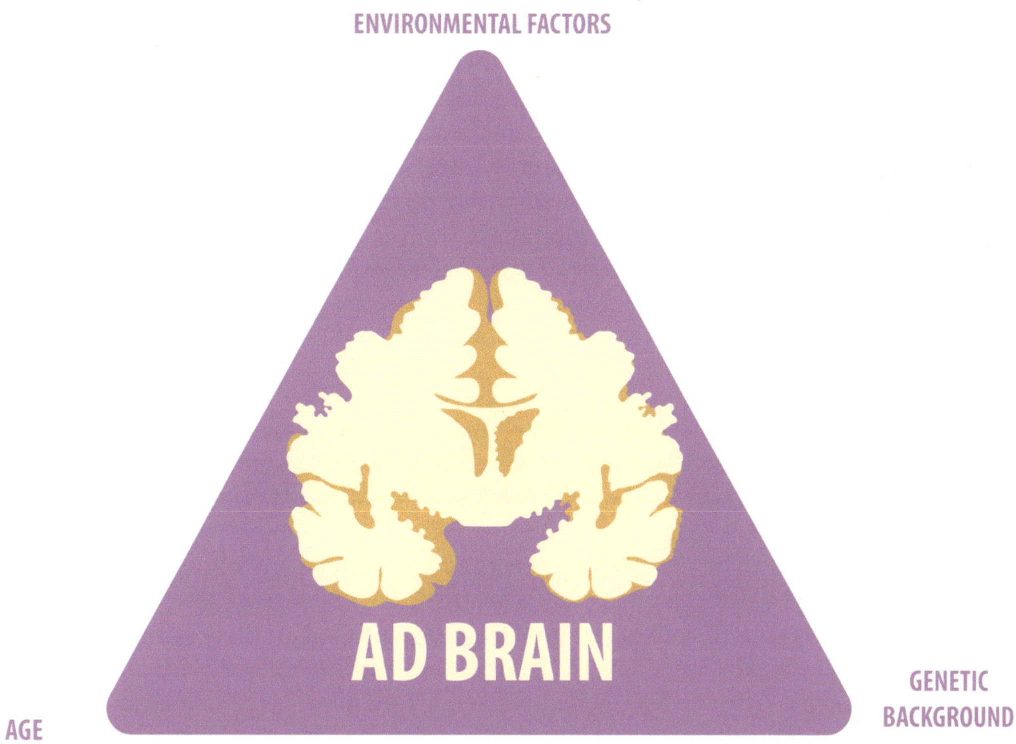

Figure 1. Etiological factors of AD. A simplified view. Alzheimer's disease is a highly complex disease. Although several risk factors have been identified, the etiology of this disorder remains elusive. Environmental factors, such as exposure to common pollutants; aging, which not only accounts for a decrease in the natural defenses of the organism but also increases the exposure time to the environmental contaminants; and the genetic susceptibility, such as the ApoE ε4 allele or presenilin mutations, create the perfect conditions to facilitate the establishment and progression of AD.

the glial cells and additional surrounding structures, such as the blood-brain barrier (BBB) [5]. Several research groups have demonstrated that the molecular alterations occurring during AD not only alter neurons but also microglia, astrocytes, pericytes, and endothelial cells, as well; and more importantly, each of these cells will respond to the molecular insults triggering a subsequent series of molecular events able to affect itself as well as the neighboring cells and tissues [5–7]. Whether these subsequent events are just the consequence or part of the cause/progression of AD is still matter of research.

2.1. Alzheimer's disease amyloid hypothesis

Since its description in 1906 by Dr. Alois Alzheimer, several hypotheses have been proposed to explain the pathobiology of the disease. Based on initial neurochemical studies of AD brains, an altered metabolism of acetylcholine (ACh) in the basal forebrain of AD patients was reported. This finding leads to the formulation of the "cholinergic hypothesis" of AD in which the ACh deficiency at the cortical level is considered responsible, at least in part, of the cognitive and behavioral impairment observed during disease progression. Moreover, ACh deficiency has been linked to NFT formation, and an increased activity of the ACh-esterase (AChE) has been found surrounding the Aβ plaques [8]. On the other hand, "*tau* hypothesis" was proposed in attention to the presence of NFTs across the brain and because this alteration seems to correlate better with the cognitive impairment observed as disease progress. In the same way, *tau* hyperphosphorylation and aggregation can also explain several of the molecular and physiological events related to the pathology, including synaptic failure, mitochondrial dysfunction, Aβ aggregation, and neuronal death, among others. Other relevant features of AD, the senile plaques, have also lead to its own hypothesis. Indeed, already in 1985, it was suggested that AD was an amyloidosis phenomenon, similar to other pathological processes, in which the Aβ accumulation starts a series of event leading to neuronal death and cognitive impairment. The observations of such events have led to the "amyloid hypothesis" of AD and, to date, constitute the main axis behind AD-oriented basic and applied research [4, 9].

As mentioned previously, the amyloid hypothesis states that AD will result from the increased accumulation of Aβ within the brain. Accordingly, several authors have suggested that the accumulation will result from an altered equilibrium between the production and elimination rate of Aβ from the brain [10–12]. Aβ constitutes a small posttranscriptional processing product of the ubiquitous amyloid precursor protein (APP), a transmembrane protein, coded in chromosome 21, which has been linked to nerve differentiation and cell adhesion and signaling. Physiologically, APP can undergo two clearly defined processing pathways. The non-amyloidogenic processing is carried out by the alpha (α) and gamma (γ) secretases, which lead to the release of the soluble APPα (sAPPα) and the p3 fragment. On the other hand, when this process is carried out by the beta (β) and γ secretases, the amyloidogenic pathway is established and leads to the release of the sAPPβ and the neurotoxic Aβ peptide (**Figure 2**) [9, 12].

Ranging from 37 to 49 amino acids, Aβ constitutes the critical molecular event at the basis of the AD establishment and progression [9]. Although Aβ can interact with other molecular elements and organelles, a relevant feature of this peptide is its ability to self-aggregate, being able to constitute monomers, oligomers, fibrils, or bigger aggregates, such as plaques [3, 8].

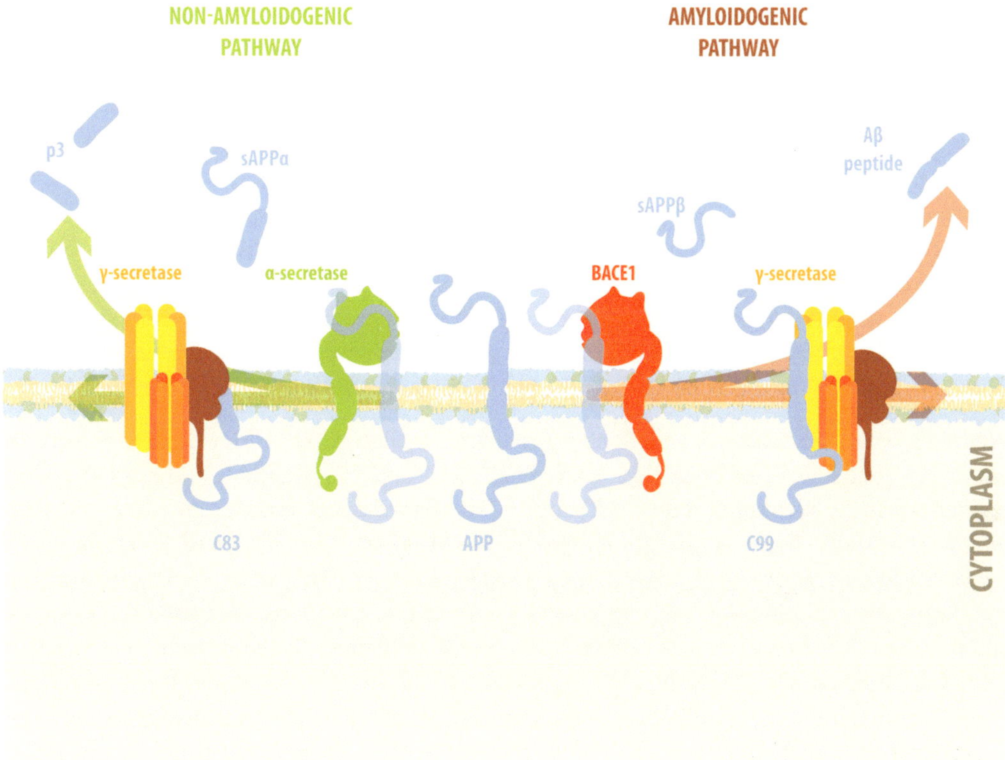

Figure 2. Apolipoprotein processing pathways. APP can be processed according two known paths. The non-amyloidogenic pathway will require α- and γ-secretase activity and will lead to the release of the sAPPα and the p3 peptide, both small peptides with a poorly understood function. On the other hand, when β- and γ-secretases work sequentially, the formation of the sAPPβ and the Aβ peptide, the main neurotoxic agent described in AD, will be favored. Importantly, external factors can increase the expression levels/activity of β-secretase, suggesting the potential upregulation of the amyloidogenic processing of the APP. sAPPα/β, soluble APP fragment α/β; p3, 3-KDa peptide; BACE, β-site APP cleaving enzyme.

Importantly, each of these forms has its own implications in terms of reactivity and toxicity. During several years, the plaques were considered the most harmful element of the AD pathophysiology. Indeed, the dystrophic neurites, reactive astrocytes and microglia, and increased activity of AChE commonly found around the plaques were considered as clear indicators that these formations were responsible for the progression of the pathology [8]. However, currently, it has been accepted that the oligomeric Aβ is the most neurotoxic form, which needs to be controlled to avoid AD progression. Evidently, any circumstance able to favors the amyloidogenic processing of the APP, would increase the risk of developing AD due to increased levels of Aβ [9, 11]. Down syndrome (chromosome 21 trisomy leads to an additional copy of the APP gene), upregulation of γ-secretase activity (presenilins 1 and 2), upregulation of the β-site APP cleaving enzyme (BACE, β-secretase) activity, downregulation of non-amyloidogenic APP processing enzyme (A disintegrin and metalloprotease, ADAM, 9–10 and 17) activity, and increased APP enzymatic processing hotspots within the plasma membrane (lipid raft) are some of the conditions able to increase the Aβ production rate within the brain, causing its subsequent accumulation [11–16].

On the other hand, the Aβ removal occurs mainly through the blood stream and, in a lesser extent, through the cerebrospinal fluid (CSF). Apolipoprotein E (ApoE) constitutes the Aβ chaperone, necessary to mobilize the peptide from the interstitial fluid (ISF) to the blood-brain barrier (BBB) transport system and/or to the choroid plexus to its final elimination from the brain [9, 10]. Although several members of the ATP-binding cassette family of transporters, such as ABCB1, ABCC2, and ABCG4, can be linked to the Aβ removal, the low-density lipoprotein receptor-related protein/ApoE receptor (LRP/APOER) is the main responsible of the Aβ clearance through the BBB. Contrarily, the receptor for advanced glycation end products (RAGE), a transmembrane receptor of the immunoglobulin superfamily located at the luminal side of the cerebral microvasculature, allows the influx of Aβ from the blood stream to the brain parenchyma [5, 6, 9, 17].

When the balance between production and clearance is altered, the Aβ levels start to increase within the brain interstitial fluid (ISF) where finally it will start to aggregate and exert its neurotoxic effects in the surrounding cells. Although Aβ-derived damage is considered as an extracellular process, it has been also suggested that the intracellular accumulation of Aβ might play a relevant role at the early stages of the disease. In this regard, APP has been found in different cell compartments including the Golgi apparatus, endoplasmic reticulum, endosomes, lysosomes, and mitochondria. Moreover, cell uptake has been also evidenced through the $\alpha 7$ nicotinic acetylcholine receptor, suggesting that in the presence of increased extracellular levels of Aβ, the peptide can enter the cell and starts to accumulate within the intracellular space, probably causing the first cellular alterations, including *tau* hyperphosphorylation and neurite atrophy [9].

Although no hypothesis can be discarded, amyloid hypothesis is considered as the most relevant one because the molecular cascade and cellular effects observed during AD can be tracked backward to the Aβ peptide. Moreover, in vitro, in vivo, and human studies have evidenced that Aβ-directed interventions can prevent or slow the progression of the disease. In the same way, more recently, studies focused to improve the clearance of Aβ from the brain have shown promising results as potential AD drugs [4, 10, 18].

As pointed previously, AD pathophysiology is a very complex disease, with a multifactorial etiology which, to date, is still matter of intense research. Moreover, even when we have been able to establish that the clinical signs correlate with the impairment of the neuronal network and neuronal loss, the broad range of molecular alterations still seem like little islands in the sea. In this regard, Aβ has been proposed as a central element in the pathology and as the starting point for all the molecular and cellular alterations found at the different stages of the disease. However, several questions, like how disease spreads across the brain, are still open. During the recent years, the neuroinflammatory response has been identified as a relevant feature of the AD brain, and it has been suggested that disease progression might be due, at least in part, to a chronic neuroinflammatory state of the brain [19–21]. Again, Aβ can be located at the center of this process leading to additional alterations which can further promote an exacerbated inflammatory response within the brain.

3. Aβ: the core of the immune/neuroinflammatory response in Alzheimer's disease

Inflammation is a fundamental physiological process to solve tissue damage. In general, pathogens and/or toxic elements disturb the cellular environment, triggering a whole range of responses including complement cascade activation and cytokine release from the injured cell and from the immune cells located at the site of the insult. The final goal of such response is to eliminate the initial cause of distress and cell debris and to repair of the damaged tissue. In this regard, pro-inflammatory and anti-inflammatory cytokines, such as tumor necrosis factor 1 (TNF-1α), interleukins (IL-1, IL-8, IL-10), interferon (INF-γ), and transforming growth factor 1 (TGF-1), along with complement proteins, develop a coordinated response to constitute a solid first line of defense against many unspecific damaging agents [19, 21]. Although this mechanism is common to the whole organism, the central nervous system (CNS) and the brain possess some particularities, which need to be addressed.

The CNS is a highly specialized structure, and neurons are recognized to require specific microenvironmental conditions to carry out its functions and to ensure that neuronal network is properly functioning. Although the CNS is partially isolated, preventing both external and internal elements to alter the brain homeostasis, eventually, some external insults, such as pathogens or environmental pollutants, and/or endogenous conditions, such as autoimmune diseases, sterile pathological processes, and aging, among others, will reach the brain parenchyma and induce neuronal damage that will require an efficient immune response to control and to prevent the spreading of the damage. It is important to consider that the brain parenchyma constitutes an anti-inflammatory environment with high expression of relevant anti-inflammatory mediators, such as transforming growth factor b (TGFb) and interleukin (IL)-10 [22, 23]. Although common systemic immune cells and molecules, such as cluster of differentiation 11b- and 11c (CD11b, CD11c)-positive cells, can be found in the CNS during the immune/inflammatory response, these factors mainly localize close to BBB-damaged areas, suggesting that its migration might be due to an increased BBB permeability [24]. Interestingly, an important feature of the anti-inflammatory molecules localized in the brain is to prevent peripheral immune cell proliferation. This condition establishes microglia and astrocytes as the specialized cells responsible to carry out the immune surveillance and to act as the first line of response against harmful events within the brain. Even when these characteristics might prompt us to consider the brain, and the CNS, as an immune-incompetent organ, it has been proposed that the mentioned conditions are necessary to prevent strong and uncontrolled immune/inflammatory responses, which can cause further neuronal damage [24]. However, under pathologic conditions, such as AD, in which a harmful molecule, such as Aβ, accumulates and aggregates within the neurons and ISF, a chronic inflammatory condition can still be triggered leading to the involvement of the different cells and structures within the brain, including neurons and brain microvasculature, among others (**Figure 3**). Interestingly, during

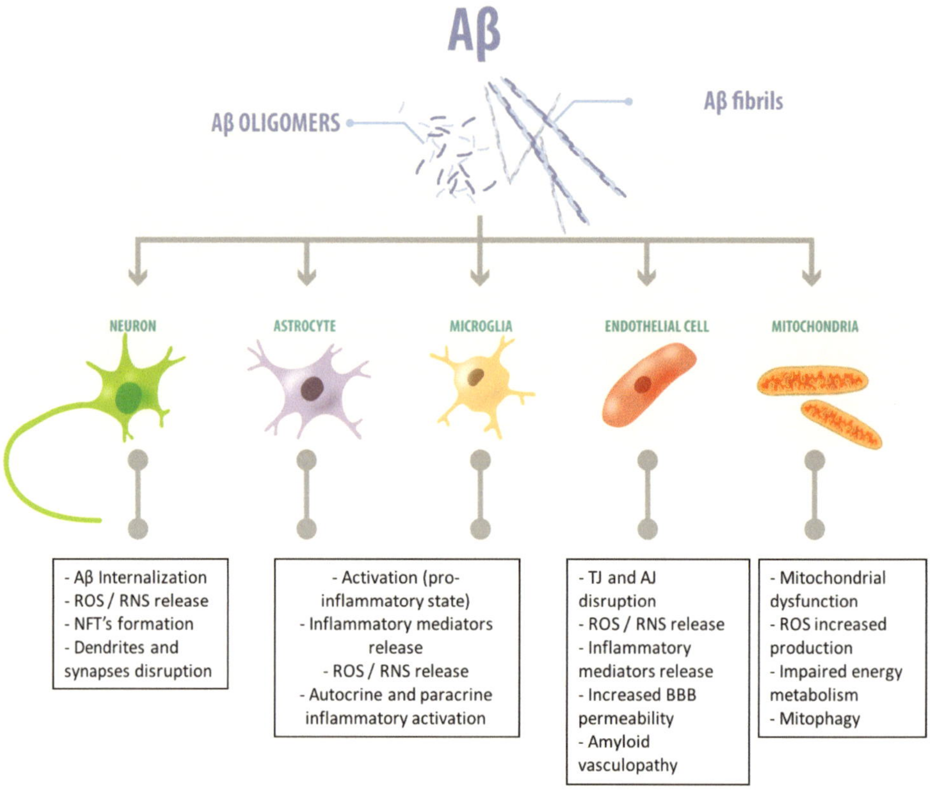

Figure 3. Amyloid-β-mediated effects on cells and organelles. Whether as oligomers or fibrils, Aβ is able to induce several effects on cells and on subcellular compartments. Aβ-derived damage and/or response will trigger a cascade of events, which ultimately will affect a wide range of CNS elements. Neuroinflammation is a common outcome of Aβ exposure. Upon Aβ challenge, neurons will release pro-inflammatory mediators. Moreover, neurons can internalize the Aβ affecting the neuronal trafficking and leading to cytoskeleton alterations, such as NFT formation. On the other hand, astrocytes and microglia will be activated inducing the production and release of pro-inflammatory mediators, which in turn can further activate surrounding glial cells and neurons. In the same way, Aβ will also deposit around cerebral microvasculature, leading not only to the release of additional inflammatory molecules but also to the disruption of the BBB sealing, allowing the extravasation of blood components to the brain parenchyma, altering the CNS microenvironment. Similarly, it has been demonstrated that Aβ can enter the mitochondria where it will cause mitochondrial dysfunction with an increased production of ROS, which will increase the oxidative stress within the surrounding cells, further inducing an inflammatory response. These events will occur simultaneously and together will sustain a persistent inflammatory response which will perpetuate and enhance the initial Aβ damage.

recent years, the Aβ-driven neuroinflammation has become significantly relevant and currently is considered as a critical target to control AD [5, 25]. Moreover, it has been demonstrated that permanent exposure to Aβ due to an increased production or deficient clearance from the brain will lead to a chronic inflammatory state, which results in a harmful environment for the neurons, causing additional damage and ultimately further neuronal death. Importantly, the inflammatory mechanisms triggered by Aβ are driven mostly through the Toll-like receptor (TLR) family [20].

3.1. Toll-like receptors (TLRs) and Aβ

The TLR family constitutes a relevant group of the pattern recognition receptors (PRRs), a subtype of the damage-associated molecular patterns (DAMPs), which are endogenous indicatives of cell damage. As PRRs, TLRs are necessary not only to unleash the initial immune response but also to connect this first unspecific defense with the secondary adaptive immunity [20]. In this regard, TLRs have been demonstrated to be present in several cell components and in immunocompetent cells of the brain, including astrocytes, microglia, neurons, and oligodendrocytes, suggesting that each of these cells can sense and react to harmful molecular patterns [26, 27]. Moreover, it has been demonstrated that microglia and neurons express all TLR subtypes, whereas astrocytes express a more limited repertoire, including TLR2, TLR3, TLR4, TLR9, and TLR11 [28, 29]. Several members of the TLR family have been described, depending on the species, and these can be divided into two main groups: those expressed on the plasma membrane, such as TLRs 1, 2, 4, 5, and 6, and those expressed on endosomes, such as TLR 3, 7, 8, and 9. In general terms, TLRs signal through the myeloid differentiation factor 88 (MyD88) pathway. Accordingly, MyD88 recruitment leads to the activation of interleukin 1 receptor-associated kinase (IRAK) family of proteins, which in turn results in the activation of tumor necrosis factor receptor-associated factor 6 (TRAF6), causing the recruitment of transforming growth factor-b-activated kinase-1 (TAK1). TAK1 along with TAK1-binding proteins (TABs) activates the IKK complex, resulting in the phosphorylation of IkB factor, which induces the release of nuclear factor-kB (NF-kB) and enables its translocation to the nucleus and subsequent expression of inflammatory-related genes. However, some TLRs, such as TLRs 3 and 4, can signal via an additional pathway mediated by TIR-containing adaptor inducing interferon-β (IFN-β) (TRIF). Although this pathway results in the release of NF-kB, it also causes, via the IKKe/TANK-binding kinase 1 (TBK1), the phosphorylation of interferon regulatory factors 3 and 7 (IRF3–IRF7), inducing IFN-β expression. At the end of these TLR-related molecular cascades, we observe the production and release of several molecular mediators, such as cytokines, chemokines, complement proteins, and enzymes, including IL-1, IL-6, IL-10, IL-11, IL-12, tumor necrosis factor (TNF), TGF, IFN, CCL2, CCL5, CXCL8, and CXCL10, among others [26–29]. Among the several effects exerted by these molecules, these can further activate the TLRs, reactivating the inflammatory cascade.

Relevantly, Aβ has been demonstrated to interact with several members of the TLR subfamily of receptors, including TLR2 and TLR4, inducing an immune response with the subsequent release of pro-inflammatory molecules, including several members of the interleukin family, such as IL-1β, IL-6, IL-12, TNFα, cyclooxygenase 2 (COX2), and inducible nitric oxide synthase (iNOS) [30]. As previously mentioned, microglia, astrocytes, neurons, and oligodendrocytes express several members of TLRs, making them able to respond both to the Aβ insult and to the inflammatory mediators released in response to Aβ [20]. In this regard, it has been demonstrated that IL-6 levels are significantly elevated in AD and that its increased expression can be achieved by both direct production after primary Aβ exposure of the microglia, astrocytes, and/or neurons and as a secondary response to pro-inflammatory mediators such as IL-1β [31].

3.2. Neurons

As mentioned, Aβ induces the secretion of pro-inflammatory molecules and/or exerts mechanical damage to the neurons, altering its delicate metabolism and leading to neuronal dead. Moreover, it will induce the release of additional inflammatory mediators, such as reactive oxygen and nitrogen species (ROS and RNS), which are able to interact with several biomolecules, including membrane lipids, nucleic acids, and proteins. As a result, synapses, dendritic projections, myelin sheath, and cell structure will be altered, compromising neuronal functionality [32–34]. Additionally, it is well known that increased BBB permeability is one of the primary alterations in AD, leading to the loss of brain isolation allowing systemic components to enter the brain parenchyma, altering the neuronal microenvironment [5]. As this condition is sustained in time, such variation will further damage neurons triggering and spreading the inflammatory response [9].

On the other hand, several authors have proposed that Aβ can also drive the hyperphosphorylation of *tau* protein, altering neuronal cytoskeleton and impairing the neuronal network. Indeed, it has been demonstrated that Aβ can be incorporated to the neurons, altering the synapses also through a *tau*-mediated mechanism. In this regard, it has been demonstrated that *tau* modifications lead to frontotemporal dementia without Aβ deposition, but Aβ alterations induce the full range of AD pathology, including NFTs. Importantly, this *tau*-mediated cytoskeleton alterations might induce neuronal apoptosis causing the release of DAMPs which will be sensed by the TLRs located in the surrounding cells, including glial cells and neurons, and triggering an inflammatory response [3, 4, 6, 8].

3.3. Astrocytes

Astrocytes are fundamental to sustain brain homeostasis. These cells carry out several critical functions for neuronal function including, but not limited to, offering metabolic support to neurons and synapses and regulation of the neurotransmitter concentration. Astrocytes also play a relevant role in the inflammatory response [35]. Indeed, reactive astrocytes are a common feature of neuroinflammation and are usually considered as an indicator of the inflammatory state of the brain. In this regard, it has been demonstrated that the activation of TLR and NF-κB within astrocytes induces the production of pro-inflammatory molecules including IL-1; IL-6; TNF; chemokines, such as CCL2 and CC3CL1; and proteins of the major histocompatibility complex (MHC). Additionally, astrocytes have been syndicated as the responsible for the excitotoxicity damage because of glutamate release during harmful stimuli [21, 36]. Importantly, in response to the inflammatory signals, astrocytes can proliferate, migrate, and produce further inflammatory mediators, some of which are able to act in a paracrine manner activating the surrounding cells, including microglia, neurons, resting astrocytes, and endothelial cells [37].

On the other hand, a particularity of astrocytes is that these cells produce the ApoE, the main Aβ chaperone which allows the removal of the peptide from the brain. Altered astrocytes or genetic conditions, such as ApoE ε4 allele expression, will cause an impaired ApoE activity leading to a reduced rate of Aβ clearance, facilitating its accumulation and triggering the inflammatory response observed upon Aβ exposure [10]. In the same way, it must be noticed that astrocytes are in close contact with the BBB through the astrocytic end-feet, being able to sense the intracerebral microenvironment but also to be the first to response to increased BBB permeability [5–7].

3.4. Microglia

Microglia reach the brain before the BBB closure and are defined as the main effectors of the immune response acting as the macrophages of the brain. Microglia remain in a "resting" state until diverse stimuli trigger the activation of these cells inducing the inflammatory response. It has been demonstrated that the resting state is maintained because of the interaction between the microglial chemokine (C-X-C motif) receptor 1 (CXCR1) and CD200L, with the neuronal CX3CL1 and CD200, respectively [38, 39]. As expected, activation of the microglia will be induced when these inhibitory interactions are loss or inflammatory signals are sensed by the resting microglia. In this regard, activated microglia is being able to phagocyte the surrounding tissue, proliferate, and migrate where needed. Moreover, activated microglia will release additional pro-inflammatory molecules, such as TNF-α or IL-1β, as well as ROS and RNS [37].

Among the several receptors that allow the microglia to sense the surrounding environment, the Toll-like receptors (TLR 1-9) and its co-receptor CD14 are the most important for microglial activation. Regarding Aβ, certainly, TLR2 and TLR4 are fundamental and drive main of the microglial reactions to Aβ, including phagocytosis [20]. Relevantly, during the last few years, an important genetic component has emerged regarding microglial response. Complement receptor 1 (CR1), cluster of differentiation 33 (CD33), and triggering receptor expressed on myeloid cells 2 (TREM2) have been related to microglial-mediated Aβ phagocytosis. Although it has been evidenced that these three genes help to sustain the phagocytic phenotype of the microglial cells, TREM2 has emerged as a potential biomarker due to its increased levels found in the CSF in AD [40–42]. Moreover, it has been reported that TREM2 mutations, such as arginine 47 to histidine (R47H), are critical for Aβ plaque formation because of an impaired function and expression of the receptor within the microglia. Indeed, such mutations seem to facilitate TREM2 ADAM/γ-secretase processing, as evidenced by the increased levels of the soluble TREM2 fragment within the plasma and CSF in AD [43]. The significance of such findings is just emerging, and intense research are focused to elucidate the roles of TREM2 and its soluble fragment in the pathophysiology of neurodegenerative disorders.

3.5. Blood-brain barrier

Although the concept of the BBB was proposed in the 1900s, only recently it has attracted high attention due to its relevance in the neurodegenerative disorders. Importantly, along with the blood-CSF barrier and the arachnoid epithelium, the BBB is a fundamental part of the brain isolation system. Indeed, several researchers have demonstrated, using hydrophilic compounds, that polar solutes were unable to cross the BBB because of occluding tight junctions (TJ) established between adjacent endothelial brain cells [5]. Moreover, brain endothelial cells evidenced the expression of a highly complex proteome, necessary to efficiently conduct the traffic of different molecules form the brain to the blood stream and vice versa. These characteristics clearly demonstrate that the BBB is an active player in maintaining the cerebral microenvironment. Furthermore, it is widely known that Aβ transport across the BBB is the main way to remove the Aβ from the brain. Due to its electrochemical characteristics, Aβ requires specialized transport to cross the BBB [6, 7]. The LRP1 and LRP2 and some members of the ABC family of transporters are related to brain Aβ clearance. Evidently, any pathological condition able to alter the brain microvasculature and, particularly, the endothelial cells will have a tremendous impact in the brain homeostasis and can affect the Aβ levels within the brain. In this regard, it has been demonstrated that Aβ accumulates around the blood vessels, leading to neurovascular dysfunction and cerebral amyloid angiopathy. Indeed, several changes take place in the cerebral blood vessels of AD patients, including loss of vascular density, decreased luminal diameter of vessels and capillaries, and thickness of vessel walls. More importantly, several of these alterations occur at the early stages of the disease. In attention to this observation, several authors have suggested that the BBB alteration might not be only a consequence of the neurodegenerative process but could be the basis of the pathological changes observed during the course of the disease [5–7, 9].

3.6. Mitochondria

Although an organelle, mitochondria should be addressed because one of the critical features of the Aβ-mediated damage precisely relates with mitochondrial dysfunction [3, 5]. Moreover, mitochondria constitute the power supply within cells, and each of the functions that have been reported in this section requires important amounts of energy to be carried out. In this regard, mitochondrial activity will depend on cellular status, and pathological conditions able to modify internal cell environment will absolutely have an impact on mitochondrial fate. Increased oxidative status or proapoptotic stimuli will trigger different cellular mechanisms conducted to control cell death and the destruction of cell organelles, such as the mitochondria. In this regard, it has been demonstrated that beyond inflammatory cascade, Aβ is able to induce several proapoptotic signaling including endoplasmic reticulum stress, with the intracellular release of Ca^{2+} which will overload the mitochondria, and ROS-mediated apoptosis through the apoptosis signal-regulated kinase (ASK1) and favors the apoptosis through the B-cell lymphoma 2 (BCL2)-beclin1 (BECN1) complex, among others [44, 45]. Moreover, it has been found that Aβ can also enter the mitochondria, leading directly to mitochondrial dysfunction and to altered energy metabolism within cells. Along with the reduction of available ATP, altered mitochondria will also increase the production of ROS contributing to increase the brain oxidative status and resulting in the production of additional pro-inflammatory mediators, such as IL-6 [44–47]. In this regard, once released to the extracellular compartment, ROS can further trigger the inflammatory pathways in the neighboring cells inducing the activation of the NF-kB-dependent pro-inflammatory cascade [20].

4. New insights of neuroinflammatory modulation in Alzheimer's disease

As evidenced previously, the inflammatory response has demonstrated to be highly relevant in several neurodegenerative disorders, including AD, Parkinson's disease, Huntington's disease, multiple sclerosis, and amyotrophic lateral sclerosis. In these disorders, inflammation verifies since the early stages of the neurodegenerative process, and it is believed that it can also accelerate the spread of the disease across different brain areas. Moreover, several experimental therapeutic approaches have evidenced that controlling neuroinflammation might improve the disease outcome. Accordingly, during the last decades, huge efforts have been committed to understand neuroinflammation and how to control such process. Although several molecular pathways can be tracked down to explain the neuroinflammatory cascade, some of these pathways, such as nuclear receptors (NR) and the Wnt signaling, seem to develop a critical role in this kind of processes because it usually plays a pivotal role in the cellular physiology.

4.1. Nuclear receptors

Nuclear receptors (NR) constitute a highly conserved superfamily of proteins [48]. These receptors act sensing the intra- and extracellular microenvironments and exert several functions including embryogenesis, reproduction, metabolism, inflammation, immunity, and lipid signaling. An important feature of its structure is that several domains can be recognized which upon activation, mainly through ligand binding, will induce conformational changes allowing the exposure of functional domains to the consensus nucleotide sequence present in the target genes, inducing their expression [49].

Peroxisome proliferator-activated receptors (PPARs) are classified as type II NR, which are characterized by the formation of heterodimers with the retinoid X receptor (RXR). PPARs possess a four-region structure including an amino terminal region, AF-1, which functions as a constitutive ligand-independent transactivation domain: the DNA-binding domain (DBD), constituted by two zinc fingers which recognize and bind the specific DNA nucleotide sequences termed peroxisome proliferator response element (PPRE), which consists of two AGGTCA sequences separated by a single nucleotide. Importantly, this domain contains the necessary elements to allow dimerization with the RXR. Next, the Hinge region is found and is believed to allow to connect the DBD to the ligand-binding domain (LBD). The LBD is a well-conserved domain among species, which is characterized by the presence of the ligand-binding pocket, a 12–13 anti-parallel α-helix structure. Within this region, there is also a ligand-dependent transactivation (AF-2) domain, which is intimately involved with both the generation of the ligand-binding pocket and interaction with transcription coactivators. Three PPAR isoforms have been described. Generally, PPARα is expressed in the liver, kidney, and skeletal muscle; PPARβ/δ is widely expressed, including the CNS; and PPARγ is highly expressed in fat tissue [49]. Importantly, several researchers have demonstrated the expression of the three PPAR isoforms within the brain, including the hippocampus, the critical brain area related to memory (**Figure 4**) [50].

Activation of the PPAR/RXR heterodimer will lead not only to the DNA binding but also to the exposure of the AF-2 domain, which will interact with the LXXLL motifs present in several PPAR coactivators, including the receptor family p160/steroid coactivator (SRC), p300/CREB-binding protein (CBP) complex, the switching/sucrose non-fermenting (SWI/SNF) chromatin remodeling complex, the PPAR interacting complex (PRIC) 285, and PRIC320/chromodomain helicase DNA-binding protein 9 (CHD9) [51]. Each of these coactivators, which have

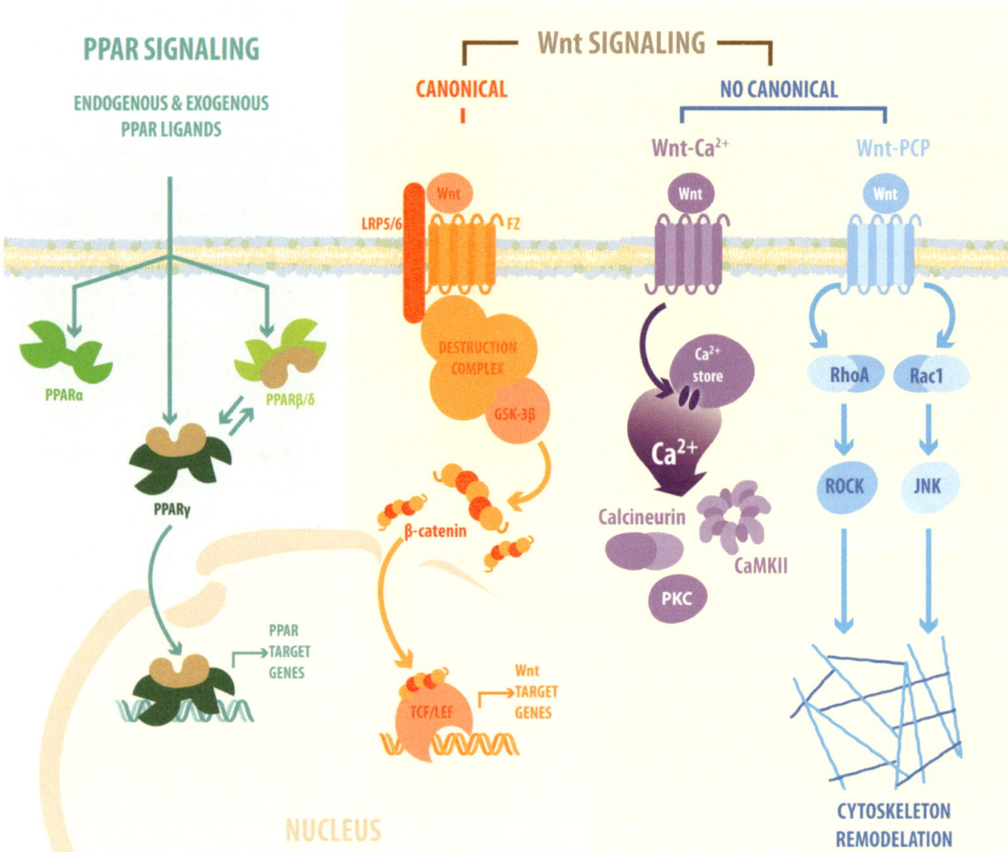

Figure 4. PPARs and Wnt pathways. The figure represents the common molecular cascades associated to PPARs and Wnt signaling. Type II nuclear receptors, such as PPARs, form heterodimers with the RXR. The PPAR/RXR dimer binds to the DNA through the consensus sequence (PPRE), inducing the expression of target genes. PPAR, peroxisome proliferator-activated receptor; PPRE, peroxisome proliferator response element. On the other hand, the Wnt signaling pathway can be divided into canonical Wnt signaling and noncanonical Wnt pathways. During activation, canonical Wnt ligands interact with the Fz-LRP5/Fz-LRP6 complex receptor, this situation leads to the disassembly of the β-catenin destruction complex, which prevents GSK3β-mediated β-catenin phosphorylation. Thus, β-catenin can translocate to the nucleus where it binds to the TCF/Lef, initiating the transcription of Wnt-related genes. The noncanonical Wnt pathway, known as Wnt/Ca^{2+}, can be triggered by noncanonical Wnt ligands. In this case, Fz will induce the release of calcium from intracellular stores, leading to the activation of calcineurin, CamKII, and PKC. In the same way, the noncanonical Wnt/PCP pathway also requires noncanonical Wnt ligands, which will interact with the Fz receptor and will activate Dvl. However, at this point, Dvl induces the activation of RhoA and Rac, which ultimately will lead to cytoskeletal rearrangement. Fz, Frizzled receptor; LRP, low-density lipoprotein receptor-related protein; GSK3β, glycogen synthase kinase 3β; TCF/Lef, T-cell factor/lymphoid enhancer factor; PCP, planar cell polarity; RhoA, Ras homolog gene family member A; ROCK, rho-associated protein kinase; Rac1, Ras-related C3 botulinum toxin substrate 1; JNK, c-Jun N-terminal kinase; PKC, protein kinase C; and CamKII, calcium/calmodulin kinase II.

enzymatic activity, increases the transcriptional activity of the PPARs mainly through the chromatin remodeling and/or stabilization of the PPAR-DNA binding. Additionally, PPARγ-coactivator 1(PGC-1α), a nonenzymatic PPAR coactivator, needs to be mentioned because it has demonstrated to be critically involved in the mitochondrial function, ther mogenesis, andenergy homeostasis. PGC-1α also requires the AF-2/LXXLL association to increase PPAR transcription. Moreover, PGC-1α-PPAR binding induces a conformational change in PGC-1α that promotes its binding to SRC-1 and CBP/p300, further enhancing the transcriptional activity. It has been proposed that in the brain, PGC-1α plays an important role in mitochondrial oxidative metabolism and in the maintenance of intracellular calcium levels [52, 53].

As pointed in previous sections, increased levels of Aβ will induce microglial and astrocyte activation and neuronal alterations and can compromise additional cells and structures, such as the BBB. As the result of such increased levels of Aβ, production of several cytokines (TNF-α, IL-1β, S100β) and chemokines (MIP-1α, MIP-1β) as well as oxidative stress-associated molecules will be enhanced. Relevantly, PPARs have demonstrated very interesting properties regarding the modulation of the inflammatory response. In this regard, the most studied isoforms are the PPARα and γ. Inhibition of activator protein 1 (AP-1) and NF-κB signaling is one of the well-known effects of PPARα and γ activation [54]. However, signal transducer and activator of transcription (STAT-1), nuclear factor of activated T cells (NFAT), early growth response protein 1 (Egr-1), and Jun and GATA-3 expression are also inhibited by PPARγ [54]. Moreover, PPARα activation also leads to reduced expression of T-box transcription factor (T-bet) and to the impairment of its binding to the DNA, limiting the expression of the pro-inflammatory cytokine IFN-γ. On the other hand, PPARα induces the expression of GATA-binding protein 3 (GATA3), a master regulator of the anti-inflammatory molecule IL-4 [55]. Because of the PPARα and γ activation, the expression of several pro-inflammatory cytokines, including IL-1, IL-4, IL-6, IL-8, IL-12, and TNF-α; vasoactive mediators, including cyclooxygenase 2 (COX-2), iNOS, and endothelin-1; expression of adhesion molecules, such as ICAM-1; chemokines, such as MCP-1, MCP-3, and INF-γ-inducible protein 10 (IP-10); and metalloproteases, such as MMP-9, are often reduced [17, 38, 55, 56]. Regarding the PPARβ/PPARδ, it is also believed that NF-κB blockade might be part of its mechanism of action, but its role against neuroinflammation is known to be related to the regulation of pro-inflammatory molecules, including C-C motif chemokine ligand 2 (CCL2), IL-6, and IL-1β [57].

An additional relevant feature of the PPARs is its ability to eventually induce an improvement in the Aβ clearance ratio from the brain ISF. It has been evidenced that increased levels of ApoE, the Aβ chaperone, can improve Aβ removal rate lowering its levels and preventing its aggregation [10]. Interestingly, ApoE is a target gene of the liver X receptor (LXR), another type II NR, which in turn is a target gene of the PPARs. Although indirectly, this genetic cross relation can explain the beneficial effects observed after PPAR agonist administration in in vivo models of AD [5, 9].

4.2. Wnt signaling pathway

The Wnt signaling constitutes a relevant molecular system related to several physiological processes, including cell proliferation and differentiation. Wnt proteins are highly conserved among different species, and beyond its physiological roles, several studies have demonstrated the involvement of this family of proteins in pathological processes of the CNS, including neurodegenerative disorders, such as AD [58].

Classically, Wnt signaling can be divided in the canonical and noncanonical Wnt pathways. In the first one, also known as the β-catenin-dependent pathway, Wnt proteins bind to the Frizzled receptor/low-density lipoprotein receptor-related protein 5/Frizzled receptor/low-density lipoprotein receptor-related protein 6 (Fz-LRP5/Fz-LRP6), inducing the activation of the disheveled protein and the interaction between LRP5 and LRP6 with Axin. This interaction causes the disassembly of the β-catenin destruction complex constituted by the adenoma polyposis coli (APC), Axin, GSK3b, and casein kinase 1 (CK1), preventing the β-catenin phosphorylation and allowing its translocation to the cell nucleus where it will bind to the T-cell factor/lymphoid enhancer factor (TCF/Lef) transcription factor to induce the expression of Wnt target genes. Without the positive input of the Wnt ligands, the destruction complex remains active inducing the β-catenin phosphorylation and the subsequent proteasomal degradation. On the other hand, the noncanonical Wnt pathway can also be divided into two additional cascades: the Wnt/planar cell polarity (Wnt/PCP) pathway, which requires the binding of Wnt ligands and signals through disheveled-Rho and Rac GTPases, inducing c-Jun N-terminal kinase (JNK) activity and leading to actin cytoskeleton modeling, and the Wnt/Ca^{2+} pathway in which the binding of Wnt ligands to the Fz receptor induces the release of Ca^{2+} from intracellular compartments, including the ER, causing the activation of several calcium-related proteins, such as protein kinase C (PKC) and calcium-/calmodulin-dependent protein kinase (Ca^{2+}/CamKII) (**Figure 4**) [20, 58].

The Wnt signaling has emerged as a very promiscuous pathway. It has been possible to identify the crosstalk between both canonical and noncanonical signals which exert a modulatory effect over its counterpart. Moreover, Wnt pathways can also interact with additional molecular pathways, including the NF-kB, fork head box O (FOXO), Notch, hypoxia-inducible factor 1a (HIF1a), and JNK [52]. Indeed, several elements of the Wnt cascade seem to constitute molecular master switches that can be accessed through diverse mechanisms. This condition is of most relevance regarding the inflammatory response. Indeed, Wnt signaling has been directly associated with the control of the inflammatory process, mainly because of its ability to modulate the NF-kB pathway. However, the complex interaction established between this pathway and the master coordinators of the inflammatory response within cells has been constantly obviated. Moreover, it is well noticed that the canonical and noncanonical pathways exert, usually, opposed actions [20, 59]. While the canonical Wnt prevents the inflammatory cascade by blocking the NF-kB pathway, interacting with RelA, the noncanonical pathway has been reported to promote the inflammatory response, actin, through the PI3K, Rac1, and MAPK, and to the subsequent release of pro inflammatory molecules. However, it must be considered that some noncanonical Wnt ligands, such as the Wnt5a, can exert an anti-inflammatory effect and vice versa [20].

We have recently suggested that in attention to the Wnt pathway-mediated NF-kB modulation, a crosstalk between the Wnt and TLR pathways seems to be evident [20]. Moreover, different authors have demonstrated that TLR activation downregulates the canonical Wnt signaling pathway. Indeed, TLR4 activation can block the Fz-LRP5/Fz-LRP6 complex inhibiting the canonical Wnt signaling [60]. Contrarily, the activation of the Wnt/Ca^{2+} induces the expression of the suppressor of cytokine signaling 1 (SOCS-1) and of protein inhibitors of activated STAT 1 (PIAS-1), causing a reduced expression of some signal transducers of the TLR cascade, such as IRAK members and MyD88. In the same way, the MyD88-mediated TLR activity results in the activation of the nemo-like kinase (NLK), which directly interacts with the nuclear β-catenin-TCF/Lef complex. On the other hand, it has recently been demonstrated that MyD88-independent TLR signaling activates the IKKe/TBK1, which can directly phosphorylate Akt, leading to GSK3β inhibition, the key β-catenin degradation-driven protein. Moreover, the blockade of the GSK3β activity prevents the binding of NF-kB with the cAMP response element-binding protein (CREB)-binding protein (CBP), suggesting that GSK3β activity modulates the TLR-dependent cytokine production [61–64].

Interestingly, lithium, a well-known canonical Wnt signaling agonist because of GSK3β inhibition, allows to further address the role of Wnt signaling in neuroinflammation. In this regard, it has been demonstrated that lithium not only reduces the expression of pro-inflammatory mediators, such as IL-6, but it also reduces TLR4 expression in astrocytes [65]. Whether these effects are mediated directly by Wnt signaling or as a part of a secondary mechanism, GSK3β seems to play a pivotal role not only in the Wnt singling itself but also as the master switch in the context of the inflammatory response.

5. Final considerations

During the recent years, the relevance of the inflammatory process in the neurodegenerative disorders, such as AD, has evolved from a consequence of such pathological events to an early sign of brain distress. Moreover, the severity and chronicity of the inflammatory response within the brain parenchyma are believed to favor the progression and spreading of these diseases across the brain.

Understanding the inflammatory cascade, triggered after Aβ exposure, and the critical nodes which allow control the process is a fundamental goal to develop new and efficient therapeutical alternatives to fight AD. In this regard, our knowledge regarding Aβ-related inflammation has increased dramatically in the last years; however, relevant questions about the molecular mechanisms involved in such response are still open, with new players appearing each day. Nuclear receptors and Wnt signaling are two of the main cellular pathways able to modulate several cellular processes. Moreover, independently each of them has proven to be involved in the Aβ-induced inflammatory response; however, little is known about its interactions as part of the inflammatory molecular network. On the other hand, one of the more recent cases of new players identified to be relevant in neuroinflammation is constituted by the TREM2 protein, which favors Aβ microglial phagocytosis. Already known, this protein and its processing have recently emerged as novel and interesting biomarker and as a target to unveil some of the questions about the neuroinflammatory process observed during AD.

Funding

This work was funded by Basal Center of Excellence in Science and Technology CONICYT PIA/BASAL PFB 12 (CONICYT-PFB12/2007) to NCI.

Author details

Juan M. Zolezzi[1] and Nibaldo C. Inestrosa[1,2,3]*

*Address all correspondence to: ninestrosa@bio.puc.cl

1 Center for Aging and Regeneration (CARE Chile UC), Department of Cellular and Molecular Biology, Faculty of Biological Sciences, P. Catholic University of Chile, Santiago, Chile

2 Centre for Healthy Brain Ageing, School of Psychiatry, Faculty of Medicine, University of New South Wales, Sydney, Australia

3 Center for Excellence in Biomedicine of Magellan (CEBIMA), University of Magallanes, Punta Arenas, Chile

References

[1] Alzheimer's Disease International. World Alzheimer Report. 2016. Available from: https://www.alz.co.uk/research/world-report [Accessed 2017-03-15]

[2] Bird TD. Early-onset familial Alzheimer disease. In: Pagon RA, Adam MP, Ardinger HH, et al., editors. Genes Reviews [Internet]. Seattle (WA): University of Washington, Seattle: 1993-2017

[3] Selkoe DJ. Alzheimer's disease. Cold Spring Harbor Perspectives in Biology. 2011;**3**:a004457. DOI: 10.1101/cshperspect.a004457

[4] Selkoe DJ, Hardy J. The amyloid hypothesis of Alzheimer's disease at 25 years. EMBO Molecular Medicine. 2016;**8**:595-608. DOI: 10.15252/emmm.201606210

[5] Zolezzi JM, Inestrosa NC. Peroxisome proliferator-activated receptors and Alzheimer's disease: Hitting the blood–brain barrier. Molecular Neurobiology. 2013;**48**:438-451. DOI: 10.1007/s12035-013-8435-5

[6] Zlokovic BV. Neurovascular pathways to neurodegeneration in Alzheimer's disease and other disorders. Nature Reviews. Neuroscience. 2011;**12**:723-738. DOI: 10.1038/nrn3114

[7] Abbott NJ, Patabendige AA, Dolman DE, Yusof SR, Begley DJ. Structure and function of the blood-brain barrier. Neurobiology of Disease. 2010;**37**:13-25. DOI: 10.1016/j.nbd.2009.07.030

[8] Carvajal FJ, Inestrosa NC. Interactions of AChE with Aβ aggregates in Alzheimer's brain: Therapeutic relevance of IDN 5706. Frontiers in Molecular Neuroscience. 2011;**4**:19. DOI: 10.3389/fnmol.2011.00019

[9] Zolezzi JM, Bastías-Candia S, Santos MJ, Inestrosa NC. Alzheimer's disease: Relevant molecular and physiopathological events affecting amyloid-β brain balance and the putative role of PPARs. Frontiers in Aging Neuroscience. 2014;**6**:176. DOI: 10.3389/fnagi.2014.00176

[10] Cramer PE, Cirrito JR, Wesson DW, Lee CY, Karlo JC, Zinn AE, et al. ApoE-directed therapeutics rapidly clear β-amyloid and reverse deficits in AD mouse models. Science. 2012;**335**:1503-1506. DOI: 10.1126/science.1217697

[11] Singh I, Sagare AP, Coma M, Perlmutter D, Gelein R, Bell RD, et al. Low levels of copper disrupt brain amyloid-β homeostasis by altering its production and clearance. Proceedings of the National Academy of Sciences of the United States of America. 2013;**110**:14771-14776. DOI: 10.1073/pnas.1302212110

[12] Yan R, Vassar R. Targeting the β secretase BACE1 for Alzheimer's disease therapy. Lancet Neurology. 2014;**13**:319-329. DOI: 10.1016/S1474-4422(13) 70276-X

[13] Ben Halima S, Rajendran L. Membrane anchored and lipid raft targeted β-secretase inhibitors for Alzheimer's disease therapy. Journal of Alzheimer's Disease. 2011;**24**: 143-152. DOI: 10.3233/JAD-2011-110269

[14] Larner AJ. Presenilin-1 mutations in Alzheimer's disease: An update on genotype-phenotype relationship. Journal of Alzheimer's Disease. 2013;**37**:653-659. DOI: 10.3233/JAD-130746

[15] Mok KY, Jones EL, Hanney M, Harold D, Sims R, Williams J, et al. Polymorphisms in BACE2 may affect the age of onset Alzheimer's dementia in down syndrome. Neurobiology of Aging. 2013;**35**:1513.e1-1513.e5. DOI: 10.1016/j.neurobiolaging.2013.12.022

[16] Natunen T, Parrado AR, Helisalmi S, Pursiheimo JP, Sarajärvi T, Mäkinen P, et al. Elucidation of the BACE1 regulating factor GGA3 in Alzheimer's disease. Journal of Alzheimer's Disease. 2013;**37**:217-232. DOI: 10.3233/JAD-130104

[17] Bastías-Candia S, Garrido NA, Zolezzi JM, Inestrosa NC. Recent advances in neuroinflammation therapeutics: PPARs/LXR as neuroinflammatory modulators. Current Pharmaceutical Design. 2016;**22**:1312-1323. DOI: 10.2174/1381612822666151223103038

[18] Mirza Z, Beg MA. Possible molecular interactions of bexarotene—A retinoid drug and Alzheimer's Aβ peptide: A docking study. Current Alzheimer Research. 2017;**14**:327-334. DOI: 10.2174/1567205013666161114115344

[19] Heneka MT, Golenbock DT, Latz E. Innate immunity in Alzheimer's disease. Nature Immunology. 2015;**16**:229-236. DOI: 10.1038/ni.3102

[20] Zolezzi JM, Inestrosa NC. Wnt/TLR dialog in neuroinflammation, relevance in Alzheimer's disease. Frontiers in Immunology. 2017;**8**:187. DOI: 10.3389/fimmu.2017.00187

[21] Heneka MT, Carson MJ, El Khoury J, Landreth GE, Brosseron F, Feinstein DL, et al. Neuroinflammation in Alzheimer's disease. Lancet Neurology. 2015;**14**:388-405. DOI: 10.1016/S1474-4422(15)70016-5

[22] Malipiero U, Koedel U, Pfister HW, Levéen P, Bürki K, Reith W, Fontana A. TGFbeta receptor II gene deletion in leucocytes prevents cerebral vasculitis in bacterial meningitis. Brain. 2006;**129**:2404-2415. DOI: 10.1093/brain/awl192

[23] Strle K, Zhou JH, Shen WH, Broussard SR, Johnson RW, Freund GG, Dantzer R, Kelley KW. Interleukin-10 in the brain. Critical Reviews in Immunology. 2001;**21**:427-449. DOI: 10.1615/CritRevImmunol.v21.i5.20

[24] Ransohoff R, Brown M. Innate immunity in the central nervous system. Journal of Clinical Investigation. 2012;**122**:1164-1171. DOI: 10.1172/JCI58644

[25] Andreasson KI, Bachstetter AD, Colonna M, Ginhoux F, Holmes C, Lamb B, Landreth G, et al. Targetin innate immunity for neurodegenerative disorders of the central nervous system. Journal of Neurochemistry. 2016;138:653-693. DOI: 10.1111/jnc.13667

[26] Landreth G, Reed-Geaghan E. Toll-like receptors in Alzheimer's disease. Current Topics in Microbiology and Immunology. 2009;**336**:137-153. DOI: 10.1007/978-3-642-00549-7_8

[27] Hanke M, Kielian T. Toll-like receptors in health and disease in the brain: Mechanisms and therapeutic potential. Clinical Science (London, England : 1979). 2011;**121**:367-387. DOI: 10.1042/CS20110164

[28] Mishra BB, Mishra PK, Teale JM. Expression and distribution of toll-like receptors in the brain during murine neurocysticercosis. Journal of Neuroimmunology. 2006;**181**:46-56. DOI: 10.1016/j.jneuroim.2006.07.019

[29] Atmaca HT, Kul O, Karakus E, Terzi OS, Canpolat S, Anteplioglu T. Astrocytes, microglia/macrophages, and neurons expressing toll-like receptor 11 contribute to innate immunity against encephalitic *Toxoplasma gondii* infection. Neuroscience. 2014;**269**:184-191. DOI: 10.1016/j.neuroscience.2014.03.049

[30] Reed-Geaghan EG, Savage JC, Hise AG, Landreth GE. CD14 and toll-like receptors 2 and 4 are required for fibrillar Ab-stimulated microglial activation. Journal of Neuroscience. 2009;**29**:11982-11992. DOI: 10.1523/JNEUROSCI.3158-09.2009

[31] Dursun E, Gezen-Ak D, Hanağası H, Bilgiç B, Lohmann E, Ertan S, Atasoy İL, et al. The interleukin 1 alpha, interleukin 1 beta, interleukin 6 and alpha-2-macroglobulin serum levels in patients with early or late onset Alzheimer's disease, mild cognitive impairment or Parkinson's disease. Journal of Neuroimmunology. 2015;**283**:50-57. DOI: 10.1016/j.jneuroim.2015.04.014

[32] Aktas O, Ullrich O, Infante-Duarte C, Nitsch R, Zipp F. Neuronal damage in brain inflammation. Archives of Neurology. 2007;**64**:185-189. DOI: 10.1001/archneur.64.2.185

[33] Little AR, Benkovic SA, Miller DB, O'Callaghan JP. Chemically induced neuronal damage and gliosis: Enhanced expression of the proinflammatory chemokine, monocyte chemoattractant protein (MCP)-1, without a corresponding increase in proinflammatory cytokines. Neuroscience. 2002;**115**:307-320. DOI: 10.1016/S0306-4522(02)00359-7

[34] Patel NS, Paris D, Mathura V, Quadros AN, Crawford FC, Mullan MJ. Inflammatory cytokine levels correlate with amyloid load in transgenic mouse models of Alzheimer's disease. Journal of Neuroinflammation. 2005;**2**:9. DOI: 10.1186/1742-2094-2-9

[35] Farina C, Aloisi F, Meinl E. Astrocytes are active players in cerebral innate immunity. Trends in Immunology. 2007;**28**:138-145. DOI: 10.1016/j.it.2007.01.005

[36] Morales I, Rodriguez M. Self-induced accumulation of glutamate in striatal astrocytes and basal ganglia excitotoxicity. Glia. 2012;**60**:1481-1494. DOI: 10.1002/glia.22368

[37] Ambrosini E, Aloisi F. Chemokines and glial cells: A complex network in the central nervous system. Neurochemical Research. 2004;**29**:1017-1038. DOI: 10.1023/B:NERE.0000021246.96864.89

[38] Cameron B, Landreth GE. Inflammation, microglia, and Alzheimer's disease. Neurobiology of Disease. 2010;**37**:503-509. DOI: 10.1016/j.nbd.2009.10.006

[39] Wake H, Moorhouse AJ, Miyamoto A, Nabekura J. Microglia: Actively surveying and shaping neuronal circuit structure and function. Trends in Neurosciences. 2013;**36**:209-217. DOI: 10.1016/j.tins.2012.11.007

[40] Crehan J, Hardy J, Pocock J. Blockage of CR1 prevents activation of rodent microglia. Neurobiology of Disease. 2013;**54**:139-149. DOI: 10.1016/j.nbd.2013.02.003

[41] Griciuc A, Serrano-Pozo A, Parrado AR, Lesinski AN, Asselin CN, Mullin K, Hooli B, et al. Alzheimer's disease risk gene CD33 inhibits microglial uptake of amyloid beta. Neuron. 2013;**78**:631-643. DOI: 10.1016/j.neuron.2013.04.014

[42] Wang Y, Cella M, Mallinson KJ, Ulrich JD, Young KL, Robinette ML, Gilfillan S, et al. TREM2 lipid sensing sustains the microglial response in an Alzheimer's disease model. Cell. 2015;**160**:1061-1071. DOI: 10.1016/j.cell.2015.01.049

[43] Guerreiro R, Wojtas A, Bras J, Carrasquillo M, Rogaeva E, Majounie E, Cruchaga C, et al. TREM2 variants in Alzheimer's disease. New England Journal of Medicine. 2013;**368**: 117-127. DOI: 10.1056/NEJMoa1211851

[44] Cai Q, Tammineni P. Mitochondrial aspects of synaptic dysfunction in Alzheimer's disease. Journal of Alzheimer's Disease. 2017;**57**:1087-1103. DOI: 10.3233/JAD-160726

[45] Kerr JS, Adriaanse BA, Greig NH, Mattson MP, Cader MZ, Bohr VA, Fang EF. Mitophagy and Alzheimer's disease: Cellular and molecular mechanisms. Trends in Neurosciences. 2017;**40**:151-166. DOI: 10.1016/j.tins.2017.01.002

[46] Godoy JA, Lindsay CB, Quintanilla RA, Carvajal FJ, Cerpa W, Inestrosa NC. Quercetin exerts differential neuroprotective effects against H_2O_2 and Aβ aggregates in hippocampal neurons: The role of mitochondria. Molecular Neurobiology. DOI: 10.1007/s12035-016-0203-x

[47] Arrázola MS, Ramos-Fernández E, Cisternas P, Ordenes D, Inestrosa NC. Wnt signaling prevents the Aβ oligomer-induced mitochondrial permeability transition pore opening preserving mitochondrial structure in hippocampal neurons. PLoS ONE. 2017;**12**:e0168840. DOI: 10.1371/journal.pone.0168840

[48] Sáez PJ, Lange S, Pérez-Acle T, Owen GI. Nuclear receptor genes: Evolution. In: Encyclopedia of Life Sciences. Chichester: John Wiley & Sons, Ltd.; 2010. DOI: 10.1002/9780470015902.a0006145.pub3

[49] Zolezzi JM, Santos MJ, Bastías-Candia S, Pinto C, Godoy JA, Inestrosa NC. PPARs in the central nervous system: Roles in neurodegeneration and neuroinflammation. Biological Reviews of the Cambridge Philosophical Society. DOI: 10.1111/brv.12320

[50] Inestrosa NC, Godoy JA, Quintanilla RA, Koenig CS, Bronfman M. Peroxisome proliferator-activated receptor gamma is expressed in hippocampal neurons and its activation prevents beta-amyloid neurodegeneration: Role of Wnt signaling. Experimental Cell Research. 2005;**304**:91-104. DOI: 10.1016/j.yexcr.2004.09.032

[51] Kim TH, Kim MY, Jo SH, Park JM, Ahn YH. Modulation of the transcriptional activity of peroxisome proliferator-activated receptor gamma by protein-protein interactions and post-translational modifications. Yonsei Medical Journal. 2013;**54**:545-559. DOI: 10.3349/ymj.2013.54.3.545

[52] Zolezzi JM, Silva-Alvarez C, Ordenes D, Godoy JA, Carvajal FJ, Santos MJ, Inestrosa NC. Peroxisome proliferator-activated receptor (PPAR) γ and PPARα agonists modulate mitochondrial fusion-fission dynamics: Relevance to reactive oxygen species (ROS)-related neurodegenerative disorders? PLoS ONE. 2013;**8**:e64019. DOI: 10.1371/journal.pone.0064019

[53] Qi Y, Yin X, Wang S, Jiang H, Wang X, Ren M, Su XP, Lei S, Feng H. PGC-1α silencing compounds the perturbation of mitochondrial function caused by mutant SOD1 in skeletal muscle of ALS mouse model. Frontiers in Aging Neuroscience. 2015;**7**:204. DOI: 10.3389/fnagi.2015.00204

[54] Skerrett R, Malm T, Landreth G. Nuclear receptors in neurodegenerative diseases. Neurobiology of Disease. 2014;**72**:104-116. DOI: 10.1016/j.nbd.2014.05.019

[55] Dasgupta S, Roy A, Jana M, Hartley DM, Pahan K. Gemfibrozil ameliorates relapsing-remitting experimental autoimmune encephalomyelitis independent of peroxisome proliferator-activated receptor-alpha. Molecular Pharmacology. 2007;**72**:934-946. DOI: 10.1124/mol.106.033787

[56] Paterniti I, Impellizzeri D, Crupi R, Morabito R, Campolo M, Esposito E, Cuzzocrea S. Molecular evidence for the involvement of PPAR-δ and PPAR-γ in anti-inflammatory and neuroprotective activities of palmitoylethanolamide after spinal cord trauma. Journal of Neuroinflammation. 2013;**10**:20. DOI: 10.1186/1742-2094-10-20

[57] Malm T, Mariani M, Donovan LJ, Neilson L, Landreth GE. Activation of the nuclear receptor PPARdelta is neuroprotective in transgenic mouse model of Alzheimer's disease through inhibition of inflammation. Journal of Neuroinflammation. 2015;**12**:7. DOI: 10.1186/s12974 014 0229 9

[58] Lambert C, Cisternas P, Inestrosa NC. Role of Wnt signaling in central nervous system injury. Molecular Neurobiology. 2016;**53**:2297-2311. DOI: 10.1007/s12035-015-9138-x

[59] Godoy JA, Rios JA, Zolezzi JM, Braidy N, Inestrosa NC. Signaling pathway cross talk in Alzheimer's disease. Cell Communication and Signaling: CCS. 2014;**12**:23. DOI: 10.1186/1478-811X-12-23

[60] Yi H, Patel AK, Sodhi CP, Hackam DJ, Hackam AS. Novel role for the innate immune receptor Toll-like receptor 4 (TLR4) in the regulation of the Wnt signaling pathway and photoreceptor apoptosis. PLoS ONE. 2012;**7**:e36560. DOI: 10.1371/journal.pone.0036560

[61] Trinath J, Holla S, Mahadik K, Prakhar P, Singh V, Balaji KN. The WNT signaling pathway contributes to dectin-1-dependent inhibition of Toll-like receptor-induced inflammatory signature. Molecular and Cellular Biology. 2014;**34**:4301-4314. DOI: 10.1128/MCB.00641-14

[62] Ishitani T. Context-dependent dual and opposite roles of nemo-like kinase in the Wnt/β-catenin signaling. Cell Cycle. 2012;**11**:1743-1745. DOI: 10.4161/cc.20183

[63] Ishitani T, Kishida S, Hyodo-Miura J, Ueno N, Yasuda J, Waterman M, Shibuya H, et al. The TAK1-NLK mitogen-activated protein kinase cascade functions in the Wnt-5a/Ca(2+) pathway to antagonize Wnt/beta-catenin signaling. Molecular and Cellular Biology. 2003;**23**:131-139. DOI: 10.1128/MCB.23.1.131-139.2003

[64] Xie X, Zhang D, Zhao B, Lu MK, You M, Condorelli G, Wang CY, Guan KL. IkappaB kinase epsilon and TANK-binding kinase 1 activate AKT by direct phosphorylation. Proceedings of the National Academy of Sciences of the United States of America. 2011;**108**:6474-6479. DOI: 10.1073/pnas.1016132108

[65] Li N, Zhang X, Dong H, Zhang S, Sun J, Qian Y. Lithium ameliorates LPS-induced astrocytes activation partly via inhibition of Toll-like receptor 4 expression. Cellular Physiology and Biochemistry. 2016;**38**:714-725. DOI: 10.1159/000443028

Chapter 4

Neuroimmune Dynamics in Alzheimer's Disease Progression

Víctor Andrade, Leonardo Guzmán-Martínez,
Katiana Vergara-Pulgar and Ricardo B. Maccioni

Additional information is available at the end of the chapter

http://dx.doi.org/10.5772/intechopen.68941

Abstract

Alzheimer's disease (AD) is a neurodegenerative disease, the most common cause of dementia in senile population. According to the World Health Organization, AD represents around 12% of people over 65 worldwide. Due to its etiological agents, neurofibrillary tangles (NFT) and amyloid plaques (AP), several attempts to explain the genesis and progression of AD have been proposed. Pathological variants of tau protein, are the main precursor for AD onset, with a molecular mechanism based on neuroinflammatory processes in the context of the neuroimmunomodulation theory. Microglial cells play preponderant roles in innate immunity and are the main source of proinflammatory factors in the central nervous system (CNS), the links between microglia and neurons are the main focus on AD pathogenesis. Depending on these factors, either a neuroprotective or a proinflammatory effect could be triggered. In AD, a persistently active microglial condition generates neuronal damage and death, causing the release of pathological tau toward the extracellular environment. This causes the activation of microglia, **promoting a feedback mechanism** and generating a continuous cellular damage. After activation of microglia, generation of NF-kB occurs, thus promoting the expression and release of pro-inflammatory cytokines. As a consequence, short-lived cytotoxic factors, such as O2, NO and other reactive oxygen species, are released. In normal physiological conditions, tau's kinases play a role in regulating normal tau functions in neurons. Glycogen synthase kinase 3-beta (GSK3β)-mediated tau phosphorylation promotes N-methyl-D aspartate receptor (NMDAr)-mediated long-term depression. The increase of proinflammatory cytokines during AD by microglia leads to an increase in kinase expression and activity of cyclin-dependent kinase 5 (Cdk-5) and GSK3-β. On the other hand, TNF-α and IL-8 increase expression and activity of Cdk5, whereas IL-1β hyperactivates GSK3-β, leading to tau hyperphosphorylation and impairing its normal function. Tau hyperphosphorylation results in microtubule destabilization, impaired axonal transport, NMDAr-mediated neurotoxicity, synaptic dysfunction and cell death. Finally, the previously summarized mechanisms could explain the onset and progression of AD, opening a new projection to focus research on therapeutic agents that could modulate the interactions between tau and microglial cells. The neuroimmunomodulation mechanism has been the conceptual framework for the search of therapeutic approaches for AD and other neurodegenerative disorders.

Keywords: Alzheimer's disease, natural compounds, molecular networks, molecular functions, prevalent neurological disorders, neuroimmunomodulation, inflammation

---

1. Introduction

1.1. Alzheimer's disease

Alzheimer's disease (AD) is the most common type of brain dementia in senile population (over 60 years old) [1], which gradually affects learning and memory, displaying a prevalence and impact in constant expansion according to the World Health Organization (WHO). This expansive and epidemic behavior is concerning medical and public health opinion focusing efforts on its prevention and treatment. On its biological context, two main etiological effectors have been reported: (i) NFT, composed by accumulation of the hyperphosphorylated protein tau, inside the neuron, and assembled in oligomerical structures denominated paired helical filaments (PHF) [2–5] (ii) Senile plaques, composed by deposits of the amyloid-β (Aβ) peptide of 39–42 aminoacidic residues, generated by the proteolytic excision of the amyloid precursor protein (APP) by the enzymes β and γ secretases, in the extracellular space, both promoting loss of synaptic processes and neuronal death [1, 6]. Among the novel clinical studies to control progression of this pathology, new strategies are being implemented to prevent this brain impairment based on dietary changes and nutritional supplements, functional foods and nutraceuticals. We proposed earlier that the onset of AD is a consequence of the response of microglial cells to "damage signals" or tau oligomers, which triggers a neuroinflammatory response, promoting the misfolding of the cytoskeleton structure [4, 7, 8]. Innovative treatments are essential to improve the life quality of affected subjects. Pharmaceutical industry has failed to developed new drugs of efficacy to control it. In this context, major attention has been given to nutraceuticals and novel bioactive compounds, such as the Andean Compound, obtained from areas in the north of Chilean mountains [9, 10]. We hope that this compound be effective in order to control the disease or serve as a coadjuvant for an effective treatment. Intensive work toward elucidation of the molecular mechanisms involved in the action of these compounds is being carried out. In addition, an advanced second phase clinical trial is actually being developed.

1.2. Neuroinflammation and neurological diseases

Neuroinflammation is defined as the response of the CNS against exogenous and/or endogenous agents, which can interfere with the normal homeostatic processes in the cell. This inflammatory response is usually triggered from a secondary signaling cascade after a trauma or infection. Nevertheless, this mechanism has been characterized as one of the central axis during the progression in neurodegeneration. Probably, during this secondary response, there will be an important loss of neurons, in contrast with the first damage [11]. The previous effect is also involved in every neurological disease, including developmental pathologies, traumatic, ischemic, metabolic, infectious, toxic ones, neoplasic and neurodegenerative disorders. Inflammation plays one of the main roles in triggering a number of different neuropathologies, such as AD, Parkinson's or amyotrophic lateral sclerosis, among others [12]. In AD, a continuously active inflammatory condition could promote neural damage, consequently, neuronal cells death, which as a consequence induce the release of pathological forms of the protein tau into the extracellular environment. Since it has been reported that certain tau oligomers are able to activate microglial cells, they subsequently trigger a positive feedback mechanism, generating a constant damage to cells [7, 13, 14]. Moreover, an overexpression of inflammatory mediators has been reported in the vicinity of Aβ and the paired helical filaments (PHF) in AD, which, at the meantime, are associated with highly affected zones in the pathology [15].

Chronic metabolic diseases as hypertension, diabetes, clinical depression, dementia or traumatic lesions in the brain are considered as a silent contribution to neuroinflammation [16]. In the same context, other risk factors causing impairment or even death in the CNS tissue are strokes and atherosclerosis. Moreover, during normal aging, there is a natural chronic activation of proinflammatory signals in the same areas, contributing to an even higher vulnerability for neuropsychiatric disorders [17]. Finally, proinflammatory agents, IL-6, IL-8, C-reactive protein and adipokines are correlated with clinical depression and anxiety symptoms [16, 18].

Over activation of the immune response in the CNS compromises the generation of neurotropic factors and releases of cytotoxic agents to the microglial cell [7]. Since the microglia have an important role in the immune system of the brain and it is widely distributed in every region of the CNS, especially in the hippocampal region and the substantia nigra [19], the effect of this positive feedback gives insights of the genesis and progression in neurodegenerative diseases.

1.3. Microglial cells role on neuroinflammation

Microglial cells have an irregular morphology, with an enlarged nucleus and represent between 5 and 20% of the total glial cell population in the CNS. They are able to produce phagocytosis, releasing cytotoxic factors and behaving as antigen presentation cells [20]. These cells are derived from macrophages produced during the hematopoietic processes in the primitive yolk sac [21], migrating to the neural tube during development [22]. Their physiological functions are essential for the control of the normal homeostasis in the CNS, even in altered conditions, such as the presence of disease [15]. They are capable of sensing different damage signals which could represent a possible impairment for the CNS, some of them are: (i) microorganisms, (ii) abnormal endogenous proteins, (iii) complement factors, (iv) antibodies and (v) citoquines, chemoquines, among others. These impairment agents are able to interact with receptors such as toll-like ones (TLR), inducing the cellular activation of the microglia [19, 23]. Under the previous conditions, microglial cells control the expression of different surface markers, for example, the major histocompatibility complex II (CMH-II) and pattern of molecular recognition receptors (PRRs). After these interactions, the production of proinflammatory cytoquines is triggered, among them: interleukin I beta (IL-1β), interleukin 6 (IL-6), interleukin 8 (IL-8), interleukin 12 (IL-12), interferon gamma (IFN-γ) and the tumor necrosis factor-alpha (TNF-α) [15]. At the same time, there are synthesis and release of cytotoxic factors with a low biological half-life as superoxide radicals (O_2^-), NO and other ROS [24, 25]. During brain development, microglial cells play the specific role in apoptotic cells elimination. In the cerebellum, they regulate phagocytosis of Purkinje neurons after cell death mediated by caspase-3. Therefore, microglia have been implicated with synapse removal during development after birth [26]. Finally, the activation process for these cells will be related to the intensity, context and kind of stimulus generated and, depending on these factors, the microglia could trigger a neuroprotector or neuroinflammatory effect. Precisely, it is the equilibrium between neurotoxicity and neuroprotection, which will determine the microglia functional effect in neurological diseases or/and specific condition [15].

As we said previously, microglial cells mediate the immune response in the CNS. In order to accomplish this task, the microglia will turn into a functional polarized state, being able to carry out a specific effector program. This brain cellular type exhibits two polarized forms: one of them develops the classical proinflammatory response, being the most common phenotype. The alternative form generates an anti-inflammatory effect directed to heal an affected zone by an acute injury [27].

Additionally, microglial cells are characterized by the expression of several receptors in the membrane surface and also, by the release of different soluble factors. The activated cell, with the proinflammatory phenotype, promotes the regulation of Fc receptors as CD16, CD32, CD64, CD86, IL-1b, IL-6, IL-12, IL-23, TNF-α, inducible nitric oxide synthase (iNOS) and chemokines; meanwhile, the alternative anti-inflammatory phenotype regulates positive arginase-1 (Arg-1), the mannose receptor (CD206), insulin growth factor-1 (IGF-1), the triggering receptor expressed in myeloid cells 2 (TREM1), chitinase 3-like 3 (Ym-1), among others. All previous proteins contribute the active microglia in order to produce additional cytokines and inflammatory mediators which could direct the neurons to apoptotic mechanisms in multiple neurodegenerative pathologies [12]. Although microorganisms and their related secreted proteins (LPS among them) are recognized by the Toll receptors family, neurons suffering apoptosis are sensed by different receptor systems, such as asialoglycoproteins, vitronectin and phosphatidylserine mediated ones [28].

Recent reports have demonstrated that after the microglial cells are activated, they overexpress several receptors and ligands belonging to the main chemokines families (CC, CXC and CX3C). Some of these are also expressed in astrocytes, which suggest that chemokines may serve as communication signals between them and microglia. It has been proposed that CX3CR1 and its ligand, fractaline (CX3CL1), which are expressed in neurons too, play a paramount role in neuronal signaling with the microglial cells [29]. There are diverse factors regulating the phagocytic activity of microglial cells, one of them is the chloride intracellular channel (CLIC1). The pharmacological inhibition of this channel or its negative regulation of its expression at transcriptional level, by an interference RNA, alters the normal phagocytic activity of the microglia. On the other hand, it has been reported that the ciliary neurotrophic factor (CNTF) promotes the phagocytosis in a way mediated by Ca^{2+} [30]. In conclusion, microglial cells can receive stimulus by environmental agents or endogenous proteins, which triggers an over activated state, releasing proinflammatory factors, ROS, reactive nitrogen species (RNS) and, evoking toxicity in the vicinity of neuronal population [31].

1.4. Astrocytes and their role in neuroinflammation

Another cellular type implicated with neuroinflammation is the astrocyte, which is the most widely and heterogeneously distributed glial class cell in the CNS. Their morphology can change depending on the development, sub-type and localization of the CNS [32]. This kind of cells has been considered as the support in the brain; nowadays, it is known that they display several functions in the CNS and that they are seriously implicated with neurodegenerative diseases. Astrocytes do not generate action potentials, although are excitable cells with the properties of communication with themselves or with neurons. Their activation is mediated by inner and/or external signals, sending specific messages to their neighbor cells. This process is called "gliotransmission" [33]. During the astrocyte/cells communication, there is a transitory increase in the intracellular calcium concentration. These variations are responsible for this cross-talking, and they occur in two different ways: (i) as intrinsic oscillations resulting after the release of intracellular calcium (spontaneous excitability) and (ii) induced by neurotransmitters. In the last case, neurons release ATP or glutamate [34], activating protein G receptors, driving to the increase of inositol trisphosphate, which will direct the calcium release from the endoplasmatic reticulum to the extracellular space [35]. Some other gliotransmitters are D-serine, a co-agonist, as glutamate, for the NMDA receptor (Panatier et al., 2006), growth factors and cytokines, which promote stronger and long-term effects over synapses, polyunsaturated fatty acids and steroids as estradiol and progesterone and other neuroactive metabolites with affinity to $GABA_A$ receptors [36].

As the microglia, astrocytes are reactive to endogenous and/or exogenous injuries affecting the CNS, by a process called astrogliosis. This phenomenon triggers molecular, cellular and functional changes in cells, as a response to damage and CNS diseases. The undergone changes in astrocytes will be different according to the injury severity and will be regulated in order to modify the astrocytic activity, gaining or losing functionality, which could have an effect over circundante cells [37]. There are three severity levels: (i) mild to moderate, (ii) severe diffuse and (iii) severe reactive with compact glial scar. The first one increases the glial fibrillary acidic protein (GFAP) expression in astrocytes and triggers hypertrophy in the cell body and their astrocytic processes. The second does the same but the astrocyte processes are more pronunciated, and there is an astrocyte overlap with a proliferation increase. These changes are able to conduct a long-term tissue reorganization. Finally, on the third case, there is formation of a glial scar preventing the axonal regeneration and cellular migration, but at the same time, protecting the tissue from infectious or proinflammatory agents [38–41]. After astrocytes activation, the transcription factor NF-κB, which controls chemokines and adhesion molecules, is also overactivated, promoting the periferic lymphocytes infiltration and the improvement in the inflammatory response, which could lead to neurodegeneration. It has been demonstrated that blocking the transcriptional function of

NF-κB in astrocytes severely reduce the inflammation, which suggest that the inhibition of NF-κB in astrocytes could be a potential therapy for brain pathologies, such as AD [42]. Astrocytes also protect the CNS by glutamate hijack which could be potentially cytotoxic [43], glutathione (GSH) release in order to counteract the oxidative stress [44], Aβ peptide degradation (Koistinaho et al., 2004), blood-brain barrier reconstitution [38], synaptogenesis promotion and dynamic modulation of synaptic transmission and neural plasticity, enhancing the metabolic trafficking [45].

Another evidence linking the astroglial activation with the development of neurodegenerative processes makes allusion to the nuclear magnetic resonance spectroscopy, because this technique has allowed the discovery of consistent evidence related with a significant raise of myoinositol (characteristic marker of astroglial cells) in neurodegenerative diseases. This has been observed in the brains of patients with mild cognitive impairment (MCI) and patients with AD, and according to some studies, this raise is correlated with the progression of this pathology [12].

It has been possible to associate neurodegenerative diseases of the CNS with neuroinflammatory events based on the appearance of high levels of proinflammatory cytoquines during disease progression, like in AD, Parkinson's disease, Huntington's disease, multiple sclerosis, amyotrophic lateral sclerosis and others [13]. For all of these diseases, neuropathological and neuroradiological studies have been carried out, providing evidence that neuroinflammatory responses could appear before the loss of neuronal cells. In this issue, robust evidence has been obtained about the role of certain cytokines in the direct activation of the cell cascade leading to neurodegeneration and AD. In world population terms, AD is the most common form of dementia and it generally affects people older than 65 years old. The anomalous tau structures, PHF and NFT, cause a loss of synaptic function ending in neuronal death [46]. This neurodegeneration process is automatically amplified when the tau aggregates are released to the extranuclear medium. At the meantime, in AD, an increase of the microglial activity in the first stages of the disease has been observed, which could be indicative of the microglia attempts to eliminate the noxious elements involved in AD such as the Aβ plaques. In later stages, when the microglial cells are chronically exposed to injuries, they could lead to a chronic neuroinflammatory response, which is almost always harmful to the nervous tissue. Thus, the progressive deposition of Aβ [47] and the liberation of pathogenic tau protein to the extracellular medium could trigger a constant microglia activation [13]. Also, the neuronal loss, characteristic to this disease, contributes even more to the generation of residues that are liberated by these degenerating neurons, which could keep the microglia in a long term activation condition. Thus, the activated glial cells respond with an overproduction of proinflammatory cytokines like TNF-α, IL-1β and IL-6, which are considerably increased in AD. In conclusion, neuroinflammation is a fundamental stage in the development of this disease, because it implicates different etiological factors for AD.

1.5. Alzheimer disease and synapse

In AD, degradation can be located in several sections of the brain, such as the entorhinal cortex, amygdala, cerebral cortex, forebrain and hippocampus, among others [48, 49]. Furthermore, there is evidence of serious changes in glutamatergic neurons present in certain sections of the hippocampus, as well as frontal, temporal and parietal cortexes. These areas of the brain are essential for the generation of new memories and for learning processes, which is a major function compromised in this disease [50, 51].

The glutamatergic system works by transforming electric neural impulses with chemical stimuli, which allows for control of glutamate neurotransmitter in the synapse process. In the presynaptic neuron, vesicular transporters VGLUT1 and VGLUT2 are in charge of maintaining glutamate in the vesicle [52] for its release on the synaptic cleft following a depolarization, where the neurotransmitter interacts with the glutamatergic receptors in the postsynaptic membrane [53–55]. Two families of these receptors are present in the neural membrane, the iGluR (ionotropic) and mGluR (metabotropic). The first group can be divided in three classes: NMDA, which are permeable for Ca^{2+} ions, the AMPA (**α-amino-3-hydroxy-5-methyl-4-isoxazolepropionic acid**) and the kainite, which are permeable for Na^{+} and K^{+} ions. On the other hand, there are eight metabotropic glutamate receptors associated with G-Protein, which are then divided in three more groups [55]. Contrary to the ionotropic receptors, which are primarily found in the postsynaptic membrane for rapid modulation of excitatory impulses, metabotropic receptors are found in several membrane compartments on glial and neural cells [56]. Functionally, it has been suggested that group 1 of these receptors mediates inhibitory effects on a presynaptic level, group 2 would be activated in the presence of the released glutamate and group 3 would serve as autoreceptors [56, 57].

In a synaptic context, plasticity regulation is negatively affected by the Aβ peptide. Previous experiments show that soluble oligomers of the peptide are capable of blocking the long-term potentiation (LTP) generation in the hippocampus, establishing in electrophysiological terms the relation of this compound with memory and learning processes [58–61]. At a molecular level, previous reports support the effect of AD on components that play roles in the glutamatergic synapse. Lee et al. experiments in 2004 detected a non-regulated overexpression of the metabotropic receptor 2 (Group 2) in patients with Alzheimer's disease, which through ERK (extracellular signal-regulated kinases) receptors affect the abnormal hyperphosphorylation of tau protein observed in the disease. Through the same methods, mRNA levels of AMPA receptor subunits were measured, and thus, their differential expression in the hippocampus of *postmortem* brains with the disease was evaluated [62]. In a different point of view, Shao et al. in 2011 [63] utilized two transgenic mice models (5XFAD and JNPL3) to observe, at different periods of time, a correlation between the development of the disease and the decrease of PSD-95 protein on excitatory synapses, where AD is mediated by Aβ deposition or hyperphosphorylated tau protein. PSD-95 protein has a structural role within the postsynaptic density (or PSD), where it interacts with a complex of scaffolding proteins, along which are NMDA ionotropic receptors that participate in synaptic transmission. The postsynaptic density is considered an organized structure with mainly glutamatergic receptors associated along with other signaling proteins and cytoskeleton elements, which work together with scaffold proteins in the postsynaptic membrane [63, 64]. Specifically, it has also been indicated that PSD-related gene products could be impaired during this pathology [65]. On that regard, reports also show that the expression of several genes involved in PSD, including genes of glutamate receptors, varies on different stages during growth, which would imply its relation to synapse development [66]. Finally, since there is evidence of the role of pro inflammatory microglial agents in synaptic impairment, an overview of their possible molecular effects on synapses is paramount in the study of new treatments.

1.6. Physiological function of cytokine-regulated tau kinases

In neurons, there are several kinases that phosphorylates tau protein under physiological conditions and during AD, being Cdk5, GSK3-β, C-Jun-N-terminal kinase (JNK) regulated by cytokines released by astrocytes and glia. Cdk5 is a proline-directed serine threonine kinase, this is, phosphorylate serine and threonine residues, particularly serine 202 (Ser202) and threonine 205 (Thr205) residues of tau protein, also found in PHFs. Cdk5 activity is regulated by p35 and p39, which has a short mid-life and phosphorylates Cdk5 at its T-loop, and translocates to cellular membrane. This activation and translocation of Cdk5 have important biological roles in cortex layer formation, neurite outgrowth, migration and differentiation of neurons, synapse formation and cognitive processes. Cdk5 also regulates mitochondrial morphology and cell survival to stress [67–69]. GSK3-β is also a serine threonine, which phosphorylates tau at threonine 221 (thr221), and its kinase activity is upregulated by phosphorylation of tyrosine 216 (Tyr216) and tyrosine 279 (Tyr279) residues; meanwhile, Akt-mediated phosphorylation of Ser9 and Ser21 residues inactivates its activity. GSK3-β regulates memory processes by induction of LTD and inhibition of LTP, being these effects reversed by GSK3-β inactivation by insulin and Wnt. Also, GSK3-β promotes assembly of actin to form filaments and of tubulin, leading to microtubule formation, thus regulating the reorganization of synaptic architecture [70–72]. Finally, JNK phosphorylates tau at serine 396 (Ser396) and threonine 221 (Thr221). This kinase has three isoforms that participate in brain development, immune modulation, induction of LTP, neurite formation and JNK3 in particular induces cell death by apoptosis [67].

1.7. Physiological function of cytokine-releasing cells: microglia and astrocytes

Microglia are the principal component of innate immune response in the brain, and the first line of defense of central nervous system from pathogen aggressions. Microglia phagocytes pathogens, and releases proinflammatory cytokines, ROS and RNS to eradicate infections. Microglia also participate in neurogenesis by the release of brain-derived neurotrophic factor (BDNF), and in remodeling of brain tissue during embryonic development and in adult brain by inducing apoptosis mediated by release of cytokines (TNF-α, IL-1β), neurotrophic factors (NGF) and NO, and subsequently phagocytizing apoptotic neurons, thus allowing the maturation of surviving cells and posterior memory and learning processes. Additionally, microglia play a paramount role in synaptic plasticity, regulating presynaptic and postsynaptic processes according to their fuction [73]. Astrocytes are antigen presenting cells (APC) of brain where their functions are scaffolding and guidance of developing neurons, formation of synapses and promoting of phagocytosis of synapses by microglia, by inducing the expression of complement system that tags synapses for their elimination by microglia. Also, regulates the diameter of brain vessels, the blood flow to neurons in relation with synaptic activity and synaptic interstitial fluid homeostasis. Astrocytes also participate and regulate synaptic activity by releasing vesicles that uptake neurotransmitters of synaptic interspace for their posterior recycling and releasing neurotransmitters, as we said previously [74].

1.8. Dysfunction of astrocytes, microglia and tau kinases hyperactivation by proinflammatory cytokines in AD

During AD, Aβ oligomers are, on first instance, uptaken and degraded by microglia, apparently in an attempt to maintain neuronal environment homeostasis and functionality during early stages of disease. Aβ is able to induce the expression of complement system and microglia activation at two levels: activating CR1 transmembrane receptor, which initiates the activation cascade of complement system, associated to cytokines and ROS release. On the other hand, Aβ also induces its own phagocytosis by activating Fc receptor and C3 factor of complement system, being the last one capable of activating microglia and induce microglial-mediated free radicals release. Proinflammatory molecule C5 is downstream of activation cascade and binds CD88 receptor, inducing the release of IL-1Beta and IL-6, two proinflammatory cytokines [75]. Also, fibrillar Aβ binds to CD14 coreceptor of Toll-like receptor 4 (TLR4), which recruits and transport TLR4 to lipid rafts, followed by recruitment of coreceptor of myeloid differentiation factor 2 (MID-2) which bind to CD14/TLR4 heterodimer to form a heterotrimer CD14/TLR4/MID-2, that is phagocytized by the cell to cytoplasm. Thus, TLR4 binds to the myeloid differentiation primary response protein 88 (MyD88) and recruits IL-1 receptor-associated kinase (IRAK4) which in turn dissociates from MyD88 and binds to and activates tumor necrosis factor associated receptor factor 6 (TRAF6) forming the complex 1. The later dissociates from TLR4 and forms complex 2 by recruiting of transforming growth factor alpha-related kinase (TAK-1) and TAK-1 binding protein (TAB), then IRAK4 phosphorylates TAK-1 which in turn phosphorylates and activates the inhibitor of kappa beta kinases complex which phosphorylates kappa beta inhibitor of NF (Ikβ). This targets to degradation by proteasome, and releasing NF-κB for its translocation to the nucleus where binds to its NF transcription factor promoter in DNA, leading to expression of coding genes of IL-1β, IL-6 and TNF-α proinflammatory cytokines [76, 77]. This signaling pathway is also activated by binding of Aβ to TLR-2, but this receptor does not need a coreceptor for signal transduction [77].

Astrocytes, as well as microglia, uptake Aβ, since transplanted astrocytes in hippocampal cells of mice, carrying the Swedish mutation of amyloid precursor protein (APPSwe) together with a mutation of presenilin 1 (Psen), were able to internalize Aβ oligomers deposition characteristic of these mice [78]. The phagocytosis of Aβ is mediated by CD36, CD47 and RAGE receptors present in cellular membrane, which subsequently activates astrocytes, promotes their proliferation, and induces the activation of NF-κB signaling pathway. These receptors have affinity for this molecular hallmark of AD and promote its degradation by astrocytic lysosomes [79–83]. Unlike microglia, astrocytes do not need to be activated for its Aβ clearance ability that depends on the apolipoprotein E (ApoE)-induced formation of cell aggregates around Aβ deposits, since astrocytes of mouse lacking the ApoE gene were unable to aggregate around AP [84]. Another response of astrocytes to Aβ oligomers is the increase of expression of glutamate transporters GLT and GLAST whose physiological function is to prevent excitotoxicity and promote the survival of mouse [85]. Since Aβ is able to trigger excitotoxicity by the hyperactivation of NMDAr, the augment of expression of astrocytic glutamate transporters in the presence of Aβ could be a mechanism to counteract this effect [86].

During AD progression, astrogliosis and microgliosis appear before the formation of NFT and AP [87]. The exposition of astrocytes to Aβ oligomers triggers their activation, revealed by a change in astrocytic morphology from stellate to a swelling morphology with more processes than inactive astrocytes. The previous effect induces cellular aggregation around Aβ oligomers and also triggers calcium influx into astrocytes, activating the nicotinamide adenine dinucleotide phosphate (NADPH) oxidase. The subsequent release of ROS and activation of IL-6 induce APP processing and a major Aβ production, together with the induction of Cdk5-p35-mediated tau hyperphosphorylation at Ser203 and Thr205 [88, 89]. Another astrocytic response to Aβ oligomers is the activation of GSK3-β which in turn activates NMDAr present in membrane of these cells, triggering CREB binding protein mediated (CPB) translocation of NF-κB transcription factor from cytoplasm to nucleus, where it binds to its promoter and induces the expression of proinflammatory cytokines like IL-1β and TNF-α [90–92]. IL-1β and IL-6 will contribute with the processing of APP and subsequent Aβ overproduction. IL-6 and IL-1 beta trigger a positive feedback that increases Aβ and proinflammatory cytokine overproduction [88]. IL-1β is able to trigger chronic activation of NF-κB signaling pathway by binding to type 1 IL-1 receptor (IL-1R1), which recruits IL-1 receptor accessory protein (IL-1RAcP)—a co-receptor for signal transduction—forming a trimer that later recruits and assembles MyD88 and IRAK4. This last one phosphorylated by itself and induced to phosphorylate IRAK1 and IRAK2, subsequently recruits TRAF6 which in turn bind to E2 ligase complex, thus promoting ubiquitination of TAK-1 and its binding with TRAF6 and mitogen-activated protein kinase kinase kinase (MAPKKK), forming a complex which activates NF-κB signaling pathway by phosphorylation of its inhibitor Ikβ, with subsequent activation of JNK and COX-2 expression [93]. Furthermore, IL-1β induces the cleavage of tau at Asp421 in neurons by the exacerbation of caspase 3 activation, together with the hyperphosphorylation of tau in Ser199, Thr221, Ser396 and Ser413 due to induction of GSK3-β activation that reduces the production of anti-inflammatory cytokine IL-10, known to inhibit NF-κB pathway [88, 94–96]. TNF-α expression activates NF-κB and c-Jun kinase signaling pathways, inducing cell proliferation and migration [88]. Both IL-1β and TNF-α bind to its respective receptors IL-1R and TNFR, respectively, and lead to MAP kinase kinases 3 and 6-mediated activation of p38-mitogen-activated-protein-kinase (p38 MAPK) by dual phosphorylation of Thr and Tyr residues in its kinase activation loop, leading to p38 MAPK hyperphosphorylation of tau at residue 356 and, to a reduction of synaptophysin expression, thus affecting synaptic activity [97]. These two cytokines also induce phospholipase A-mediated production of arachidonic acid (AA), together with the NF-κB-mediated expression of cyclooxygenase 2 gene (COX-2) which dioxygenates AA to produce prostaglandins (PG's) like PGE2, whose binding to its EP3 receptor leads to a reduction of adenylyl cyclase monophosphate (cAMP) activity and, to subsequent reduction of LTP [94, 98–100]. On the other hand, IL-18 release promotes BACE and Ps1 mediated APP processing, caspase-1, mediated IL-1β activation and, tau hyperphosphorylation, mediated by activation of Cdk-5/p35 [89, 101]. Finally, IL-6 induces JAK/STAT and MAPK signaling pathways, triggering Cdk5/P35 deregulation and subsequent tau hyperphosphorylation at Ser202 and Thr205 [102].

Microglia, as the same as astrocytes, are activated by Aβ, turning its morphology from a cell with a soma and processes to an ameboid active form [73], and its activation leads to the expression of cytokines by astrocytes in AD, thus activated astrocytes and glia act together in Aβ overproduction, tau cleavage and its hyperphosphorylation. Both, **hyperphosphorylation and caspase cleavage of tau are early events of AD that make this protein more prone to aggregate**, disassembling from microtubules, impairing microtubule stabilization, axonal transport and vesicle release. This leads to synaptic dysfunction, axonal degeneration and formation of tau oligomers, PHF and NFTs and finally to cell death [103–106]. Also, it has been demonstrated that tau oligomers are able to activate astrocytes and glia, triggering its uptake by these cells [107].

It has been demonstrated that age-related senescence of astrocytes and microglia with aging diminish their Aβ phagocytic capability and that the exposure to increasing concentrations of a neurotoxic compound reduces glial capability to protect neurons from damage. This may lead to progressive Aβ accumulation and subsequent inflammation in brain tissue during AD. This, in turn, triggers a chronic inflammatory environment mediated by astrocytes and glia, changing their initial neuroprotective response to neurodegeneration mediated by proinflammatory cytokines which, induces AP formation and accumulation of NFTs. This effect results in activation of signaling pathways that activates the expression and release of proinflammatory cytokines, in a vicious circle that finally leads to synaptic dysfunction, neurodegeneration and cell death [108, 109].

1.9. Proposed new targets and therapies for AD in the neuroimmunemodulation context

On the same autoneuroimmune context, several new targets attempt to control Alzheimer's disease by modulation of the inflammatory signals (**Table 1**), among them, some are based on inhibitors of acetylcholinesterase like rivastigmine to improve cholinergic synapses which are severely diminished in AD, and inhibitors of N-methyl-D-aspartate receptor, which are hyperactivated in AD and exerts excitotoxicity, however these drugs only delay the progress of disease [110]. As mentioned above, neuroinflammation is an early event of AD, even earlier than NFT and Aβ plaques formation, which makes the modulation of inflammation an attractive target for development of new drugs for treatment and prevention of AD. One alternative is non-steroidal anti-inflammatories (NSAID's)—such as ibuprofen, paracetamol, aspirin and sulindac—commonly used for treatment of other illness whose symptoms are inflammation (e.g., infections, headache), which appear to reduce the risk of AD onset in patients who were in treatment for a long period [111]. One of the mechanisms of action that has been proposed to explain the preventive capability of AD of these drugs is the inhibition of NF-κB signaling pathway by inhibiting the phosphorylation IκBα subunit of inhibitor of kappa beta kinases complex, thus impairing NF-κB release for its translocation to the nucleus and so the induction of expression of proinflammatory cytokines [46]. Another mechanism consists of inhibition of enzymatic activity of cyclooxygenases, preventing the production of prostaglandins [112]. NSAIDs also activate the peroxisome proliferator-activated receptor gamma (PPARγ) signaling pathway which induces expression of anti-inflammatory substances, and direct Aβ processing and reduction of its release, impairing the formation of plaques. These anti-inflammatory drugs also act

Drug/Active agent	Mechanism	Reference
Rivastigmine	Inhibition of AchE	[110]
Memantine	Inhibition of NMDAr	
Non-steroidal anti-inflammatories	Inhibition of NF-κB signaling pathway	[112]
	Inhibition of cyclooxygenase enzymatic activity	
	Activation of PPARγ receptor	
Cannabinoids	Impairment of aperture of ion channels of astrocytes	[115]
	Inhibits tau hyperphosphorylation and inflammation	[119]
Quercetin	Reduction of levels of IL-6 and TNF-α	[120]
Apigenin	Reduction of expression of COX and iNOS	[118]
Curcumin	Reduction of the expression of COX-2, iNOS	
	Impairment of IL-6, NF-κB and MAPK signaling pathways	
Magnesium	Inhibits GSK3-β	[121]
Lithium	Inhibits GSK3-β	[122]
Dihydropyridines	Reduce all type of tau levels	[123]
Nobiletin	Reduce tau hyperphosphorylation and oxidative stress	[124]
Brain–Up10®	Reduces tau aggregation and increases neuritogenesis	[9]

Table 1. Drugs or active compounds for neuroimmunomodulation therapies.

inhibiting microglial and astroglial activation, thus impairing NFT and AP formation mediated by chronic inflammation induced by these cells [113]. However, these drugs does not work in patients who are already suffering of AD with cognitive impairment, and thus for the effective use of NSAID's, there is necessary an early diagnosis, when inflammatory process is in course but prior to inflammation-induced formation of NFT and Aβ plaque deposition [108]. Another approach is the use of biological active molecules of polyunsaturated fatty acids as agonists of PPARγ transcription factor, which inhibits the expression of proinflammatory cytokines and turn response of immune cells to anti-inflammatory [114]. Another challenge to overcome for these approaches is tissue specificity, since these compounds inhibit signaling pathways which are ubiquitously expressed, which means that their use as therapy for AD would be detrimental for immune response against pathogens aggressions. A recent study targets ionic hemichannels

http://dx.doi.org/10.5772/intechopen.68941

of astrocytes by using cannabinoids to impair the aperture of astrocytic hemichannels triggered by proinflammatory cytokines released upon Aβ stimulation, thus impairing the activation of astrocytes, the release of more proinflammatory cytokines and cell death [115]. Also, the use of stem cells has been proposed as treatment of AD, since administration of mesenchymal stem cells reduces plaque formation, promotes Aβ degradation and reduces levels of proinflammatory cytokines, thus reducing microglial proliferation and general neuroinflammation, and so did the treatment with soluble factors, which means that stem cells could release anti-inflammatory cytokines, and more interesting, when these cells are injected intravenously, they migrate to brain [116]. A disadvantage of this approach is the invasiveness of this possible treatment. Lately, efforts have been made to find natural compounds for effective and non-invasive treatment against AD, like quercetin, which is a flavonoid is able to reduce astrocyte activation, thus reducing neuroinflammation and improving learning and memory in SAMP8 accelerated senescence mice which were treated with an oral formulation of quercetin nanoencapsulated in zein nanoparticles [117]. Another flavonoid compound with AD treatment potential is apigenin, which can be found, between other sources, in flowers of chamomile and grapefruit. This compound is able to inhibit microglia-mediated release of IL-6 and TNF-α, the prostaglandin and NO production by inhibiting COX-2 and iNOS enzymatic activities, respectively, and also inhibits the NF-κB signaling pathway [118]. However, the most promising natural compound for anti-inflammatory treatment of AD is a compound called curcumin, a polyphenol isolated from rhizomes of curcuma which reduces the expression of COX-2 and iNOS, impairs IL-6, NF-κB and MAPK signaling pathways, reduces astroglial activation and also prevents and reverts tau aggregation *in vitro*, which could mean that this compound could be used in AD patients with cognitive impairment, if it demonstrates that also have these effects in animal models and human, so more studies have to be made, not only for this compound but also to find or develop new natural or synthetic anti-inflammatory and anti-aggregant compounds to treat AD [118].

2. Conclusion

Alzheimer's disease cases are growing faster every year, not even in senile population, yet also with early onset cases. We have studied different issues related with the beginning and progression of neurodegenerative pathologies. Since in a biological context, the neuroimmuneinflammatory response theory could be the new focus for possible treatments, the research efforts to follow-up should be focused in the control of neuroinflammatory processes.

Microglia seem to be the main brain cells in the pathological pathway of damage signals in the neuronal population of neurodegenerative diseases. The positive feedback cycle, between microglia and neurons, is started by tau oligomers released in the extracellular space after neuron degeneration, triggering the microglia activation (**Figure 1**). Different clinical trials on pharmacological agents attempted to stop the progress of AD or revert its consequences, but only a few ones, are promising. On the other hand, natural compounds have received special attention, because of their benefits in neuritogenesis or possible applications to control the progression of the inflammatory process in AD. Such is the case of "Andean Compound," which we present as an alternative treatment for this pathology (**Figure 1**).

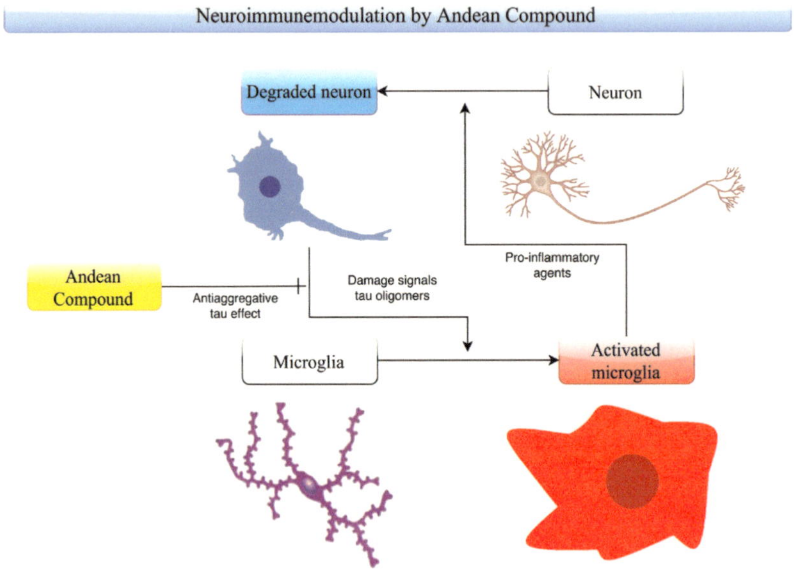

Figure 1. Model of neuroinflammation and neurodegeneration cycle modulated by the "Andean Compound." Non-activated microglial cells are susceptible to different damage signals as aggregated forms of the tau protein, leading to its activation. After activation, several pro-inflammatory agents are release into the extracellular media, being able to promote neuronal damage and degeneration. While neurons are degraded, different tau forms are released, causing a positive feedback in this neurodegenerative pro-inflammatory cycle, triggering the onset and progression of pathologies such as AD. The Andean Compound displays and anti-aggregation effect on tau oligomers, diminishing damage signals and, at the same time, it promotes neuritogenesis processes, featuring itself as an excellent target for the treatment of AD.

We encourage researchers to set their aim in new neuroprotective and anti-neuroinflammatory drugs or nutraceuticals, projecting the answers for neurodegenerative diseases on the basis of the neuroimmunemodulation theory, as the most valuable and useful tools for AD treatment.

Acknowledgements

We are grateful of Corfo Project on High Technology and to the International Center for Biomedicine (ICC) for generous financial support to carry out this research. We also acknowledge Constanza Maccioni for his help in this research process.

Author details

Víctor Andrade, Leonardo Guzmán-Martínez, Katiana Vergara-Pulgar and Ricardo B. Maccioni*

*Address all correspondence to: rmaccion@manquehue.net

Laboratory of Neurosciences, International Center for Biomedicine (ICC) and Faculty of Sciences, University of Chile, Ñuñoa, Santiago, Chile

References

[1] Bettens K, Sleegers K, Van Broeckhoven C. Current status on Alzheimer disease molecular genetics: From past, to present, to future. Human Molecular Genetics. 15 Apr 2010;**19**(R1):R4-R11

[2] Maccioni RB. Introductory remarks. Molecular, biological and clinical aspects of Alzheimer's disease. Archives of Medical Research. Nov 2012;**43**(8):593-594

[3] Maccioni RB, Munoz JP, Barbeito L. The molecular bases of Alzheimer's disease and other neurodegenerative disorders. Archives of Medical Research. Sep–Oct 2001;**32**(5):367-381

[4] Farias G, Cornejo A, Jimenez J, Guzman L, Maccioni RB. Mechanisms of tau self-aggregation and neurotoxicity. Current Alzheimer Research. Sep 2011;**8**(6):608-614

[5] Guzman-Martinez L, Farias GA, Maccioni RB. Tau Oligomers as potential targets for Alzheimer's diagnosis and novel drugs. Frontiers in Neurology 2013;**4**:167

[6] Lambert JC, Schraen-Maschke S, Richard F, Fievet N, Rouaud O, Berr C, et al. Association of plasma amyloid beta with risk of dementia: The prospective three-City study. Neurology. Sep 15 2009;**73**(11):847-853

[7] Maccioni RB, Rojo LE, Fernandez JA, Kuljis RO. The role of neuroimmunomodulation in Alzheimer's disease. Annals of the New York Academy of Sciences. Feb 2009;**1153**:240-246

[8] Fernandez JA, Rojo L, Kuljis RO, Maccioni RB. The damage signals hypothesis of Alzheimer's disease pathogenesis. Journal of Alzheimer's Disease. Jul 2008;**14**(3):329-333

[9] Carrasco-Gallardo C, Farias GA, Fuentes P, Crespo F, Maccioni RB. Can nutraceuticals prevent Alzheimer's disease? Potential therapeutic role of a formulation containing shilajit and complex B vitamins. Archives of Medical Research. Nov 2012;**43**(8):699-704

[10] Carrasco-Gallardo C, Guzman L, Maccioni RB. Shilajit: A natural phytocomplex with potential procognitive activity. International Journal of Alzheimer's Disease. 2012;**2012**:674142

[11] Akiyama H, Barger S, Barnum S, Bradt B, Bauer J, Cole GM, et al. Inflammation and Alzheimer's disease. Neurobiology of Aging. May–Jun 2000;**21**(3):383-421

[12] Morales I, Farias GA, Cortes N, Maccioni RB. Neuroinflammation and Neurodegeneration. Update on Dementia. Rijeka: InTech; 2017. p. Ch. 0

[13] Morales I, Jimenez JM, Mancilla M, Maccioni RB. Tau oligomers and fibrils induce activation of microglial cells. Journal of Alzheimer's Disease. 1 Jan 2013;**37**(4):849-856

[14] Morales I, Guzman-Martinez L, Cerda-Troncoso C, Farias GA, Maccioni RB. Neuroinflammation in the pathogenesis of Alzheimer's disease. A rational framework for the search of novel therapeutic approaches. Frontier Cell Neuroscience. 2014;**8**:112

[15] Morales I, Farias G, Maccioni RB. Neuroimmunomodulation in the pathogenesis of Alzheimer's disease. Neuroimmunomodulation 2010;**17**(3):202-204

[16] Chen WW, Zhang X, Huang WJ. Role of neuroinflammation in neurodegenerative diseases (Review). Molecular Medicine Reports. Apr 2016;**13**(4):3391-3396

[17] Capuron L, Su S, Miller AH, Bremner JD, Goldberg J, Vogt GJ, et al. Depressive symptoms and metabolic syndrome: Is inflammation the underlying link? Biological Psychiatry. 15 Nov 2008;**64**(10):896-900

[18] Ouchi N, Parker JL, Lugus JJ, Walsh K. Adipokines in inflammation and metabolic disease. Nature Reviews Immunology. Feb 2011;**11**(2):85-97

[19] Venneti S, Wiley CA, Kofler J. Imaging microglial activation during neuroinflammation and Alzheimer's disease. Journal of NeuroImmune Pharmacology. Jun 2009;**4**(2):227-243

[20] Perry VH. A revised view of the central nervous system microenvironment and major histocompatibility complex class II antigen presentation. Journal of Neuroimmunology. 1 Oct 1998;**90**(2):113-121

[21] Alliot F, Godin I, Pessac B. Microglia derive from progenitors, originating from the yolk sac, and which proliferate in the brain. Developmental Brain Research 18 Nov 1999;**117**(2):145-152

[22] Ginhoux F, Lim S, Hoeffel G, Low D, Huber T. Origin and differentiation of microglia. Frontiers in Cellular Neuroscience. 2013;**7**:45

[23] Streit WJ, Miller KR, Lopes KO, Njie E. Microglial degeneration in the aging brain—bad news for neurons? Frontiers in Bioscience. 2008;**13**:3423-3438

[24] Meda L, Baron P, Scarlato G. Glial activation in Alzheimer's disease: The role of Abeta and its associated proteins. Neurobiology of Aging. Nov-Dec 2001;**22**(6):885-893

[25] Colton C, Wilcock DM. Assessing activation states in microglia. CNS & Neurological Disorders—Drug Targets. Apr 2010;**9**(2):174-191

[26] Kettenmann H, Hanisch UK, Noda M, Verkhratsky A. Physiology of microglia. Physiological Reviews. Apr 2011;**91**(2):461-553

[27] Jha MK, Lee WH, Suk K. Functional polarization of neuroglia: Implications in neuroinflammation and neurological disorders. Biochemical Pharmacology. 01 Mar 2016;103:1-16

[28] Witting A, Muller P, Herrmann A, Kettenmann H, Nolte C. Phagocytic clearance of apoptotic neurons by Microglia/Brain macrophages in vitro: Involvement of lectin-, integrin-, and phosphatidylserine-mediated recognition. Journal of Neurochemistry. Sep 2000;**75**(3):1060-1070

[29] Rock RB, Gekker G, Hu S, Sheng WS, Cheeran M, Lokensgard JR, et al. Role of microglia in central nervous system infections. Clinical Microbiology Reviews. Oct 2004;**17**(4):942-964, table of contents

[30] Lee TI, Yang CS, Fang KM, Tzeng SF. Role of ciliary neurotrophic factor in microglial phagocytosis. Neurochemical Research. Jan 2009;**34**(1):109-117

[31] Innamorato NG, Lastres-Becker I, Cuadrado A. Role of microglial redox balance in modulation of neuroinflammation. Current Opinion in Neurology. Jun 2009;**22**(3):308-314

[32] Steardo L, Jr., Bronzuoli MR, Iacomino A, Esposito G, Steardo L, Scuderi C. Does neuroinflammation turn on the flame in Alzheimer's disease? Focus on astrocytes. Frontiers in Neuroscience. 2015;**9**:259

[33] Volterra A, Meldolesi J. Astrocytes, from brain glue to communication elements: the revolution continues. Nature Reviews Neuroscience. Aug 2005;**6**(8):626-640

[34] Paukert M, Bergles DE. Synaptic communication between neurons and NG2+ cells. Current Opinion in Neurobiology. Oct 2006;**16**(5):515-521

[35] Agulhon C, Petravicz J, McMullen AB, Sweger EJ, Minton SK, Taves SR, et al. What is the role of astrocyte calcium in neurophysiology? Neuron. 25 Sep 2008;**59**(6):932-946

[36] Garcia-Segura LM, Melcangi RC. Steroids and glial cell function. Glia. Nov 01 2006;**54**(6): 485-498

[37] Sofroniew MV. Molecular dissection of reactive astrogliosis and glial scar formation. Trends in Neurosciences. Dec 2009;**32**(12):638-647

[38] Bush TG, Puvanachandra N, Horner CH, Polito A, Ostenfeld T, Svendsen CN, et al. Leukocyte infiltration, neuronal degeneration, and neurite outgrowth after ablation of scar-forming, reactive astrocytes in adult transgenic mice. Neuron Jun 1999;**23**(2):297-308

[39] Faulkner JR, Herrmann JE, Woo MJ, Tansey KE, Doan NB, Sofroniew MV. Reactive astrocytes protect tissue and preserve function after spinal cord injury. Journal of Neuroscience. 03 Mar 2004;**24**(9):2143-2155

[40] Silver J, Miller JH. Regeneration beyond the glial scar. Nature Reviews Neuroscience. Feb 2004;**5**(2):146-156

[41] Voskuhl RR, Peterson RS, Song B, Ao Y, Morales LB, Tiwari-Woodruff S, et al. Reactive astrocytes form scar-like perivascular barriers to leukocytes during adaptive immune inflammation of the CNS. Journal of Neuroscience. 16 Sep 2009;**29**(37):11511-11522

[42] Medeiros R, LaFerla FM. Astrocytes: Conductors of the Alzheimer disease neuroinflammatory symphony. Experimental Neurology. Jan 2013;**239**:133-138

[43] Rothstein JD, Dykes-Hoberg M, Pardo CA, Bristol LA, Jin L, Kuncl RW, et al. Knockout of glutamate transporters reveals a major role for astroglial transport in excitotoxicity and clearance of glutamate. Neuron. Mar 1996;**16**(3):675-686

[44] Shih AY, Johnson DA, Wong G, Kraft AD, Jiang L, Erb H, et al. Coordinate regulation of glutathione biosynthesis and release by Nrf2-expressing glia potently protects neurons from oxidative stress. Journal of Neuroscience. 15 Apr 2003;**23**(8):3394-3406

[45] Perea G, Navarrete M, Araque A. Tripartite synapses: astrocytes process and control synaptic information. Trends in Neurosciences. Aug 2009;**32**(8):421-431

[46] Giannakopoulos P, Herrmann FR, Bussiere T, Bouras C, Kovari E, Perl DP, et al. Tangle and neuron numbers, but not amyloid load, predict cognitive status in Alzheimer's disease. Neurology. 13 May 2003;**60**(9):1495-1500

[47] Krause DL, Muller N. Neuroinflammation, microglia and implications for anti-inflammatory treatment in Alzheimer's disease. International Journal of Alzheimer's Disease. 14 Jun 2010;**2010**

[48] DeKosky ST, Scheff SW, Styren SD. Structural correlates of cognition in dementia: Quantification and assessment of synapse change. Neurodegeneration. Dec 1996;**5**(4): 417-421

[49] Selkoe DJ, Schenk D. Alzheimer's disease: Molecular understanding predicts amyloid-based therapeutics. Annual Review of Pharmacology and Toxicology. 2003;**43**:545-584

[50] Braak H, Braak E. Evolution of neuronal changes in the course of Alzheimer's disease. Journal of Neural Transmission. Supplementa. 1998;**53**:127-140

[51] Francis PT. Glutamatergic systems in Alzheimer's disease. International Journal of Geriatric Psychiatry. Sep 2003;**18**(Suppl 1):S15–S21

[52] Fremeau RT, Jr, Troyer MD, Pahner I, Nygaard GO, Tran CH, Reimer RJ, et al. The expression of vesicular glutamate transporters defines two classes of excitatory synapse. Neuron. 02 Aug 2001;**31**(2):247-260

[53] Ozawa S, Kamiya H, Tsuzuki K. Glutamate receptors in the mammalian central nervous system. Progress in Neurobiology. Apr 1998;**54**(5):581-618

[54] Danbolt NC. Glutamate uptake. Progress in Neurobiology. Sep 2001;**65**(1):1-105

[55] Kew JN, Kemp JA. Ionotropic and metabotropic glutamate receptor structure and pharmacology. Psychopharmacology (Berl). Apr 2005;**179**(1):4-29

[56] Ferraguti F, Shigemoto R. Metabotropic glutamate receptors. Cell and Tissue Research. Nov 2006;**326**(2):483-504

[57] Vogt KE, Nicoll RA. Glutamate and gamma-aminobutyric acid mediate a heterosynaptic depression at mossy fiber synapses in the hippocampus. PNAS, Proceedings of the National Academy of Sciences. 02 Feb 1999;**96**(3):1118-1122

[58] Shankar GM, Li S, Mehta TH, Garcia-Munoz A, Shepardson NE, Smith I, et al. Amyloid-beta protein dimers isolated directly from Alzheimer's brains impair synaptic plasticity and memory. Nature Medicine. Aug 2008;**14**(8):837-842

[59] Klyubin I, Wang Q, Reed MN, Irving EA, Upton N, Hofmeister J, et al. Protection against Abeta-mediated rapid disruption of synaptic plasticity and memory by memantine. Neurobiology of Aging. Apr 2009;**32**(4):614-623

[60] Li S, Hong S, Shepardson NE, Walsh DM, Shankar GM, Selkoe D. Soluble oligomers of amyloid Beta protein facilitate hippocampal long-term depression by disrupting neuronal glutamate uptake. Neuron. 25 Jun 2009;**62**(6):788-801

[61] Palop JJ, Mucke L. Amyloid-beta-induced neuronal dysfunction in Alzheimer's disease: from synapses toward neural networks. Nature Reviews Neuroscience. Jul 2010;**13**(7):812-818

[62] Pellegrini-Giampietro DE, Bennett MV, Zukin RS. AMPA/kainate receptor gene expression in normal and Alzheimer's disease hippocampus. Neuroscience. Jul 1994;**61**(1):41-49

[63] Shao CY, Mirra SS, Sait HB, Sacktor TC, Sigurdsson EM. Postsynaptic degeneration as revealed by PSD-95 reduction occurs after advanced Abeta and tau pathology in transgenic mouse models of Alzheimer's disease. Acta Neuropathologica. Sep 2011;**122**(3):285-292

[64] Revett TJ, Baker GB, Jhamandas J, Kar S. Glutamate system, amyloid ss peptides and tau protein: Functional interrelationships and relevance to Alzheimer disease pathology. Journal of Psychiatry & Neuroscience. Jan 2012;**38**(1):6-23

[65] Sheng M, Hoogenraad CC. The postsynaptic architecture of excitatory synapses: a more quantitative view. Annual Review of Biochemistry 2007;**76**:823-847

[66] Petralia RS, Sans N, Wang YX, Wenthold RJ. Ontogeny of postsynaptic density proteins at glutamatergic synapses. Molecular and Cellular Neuroscience. Jul 2005;**29**(3):436-452

[67] Martin L, Latypova X, Wilson CM, Magnaudeix A, Perrin ML, Yardin C, et al. Tau protein kinases: involvement in Alzheimer's disease. Ageing Research Reviews. Jan 2013;**12**(1):289-309

[68] Liu SL, Wang C, Jiang T, Tan L, Xing A, Yu JT. The Role of Cdk5 in Alzheimer's Disease. Molecular Neurobiology. Sep 2016;**53**(7):4328-4342

[69] Jin X, Sasamoto K, Nagai J, Yamazaki Y, Saito K, Goshima Y, et al. Phosphorylation of CRMP2 by Cdk5 Regulates Dendritic Spine Development of Cortical Neuron in the Mouse Hippocampus. Neural Plasticity. 2016;**2016**:6790743

[70] Hanger DP, Noble W. Functional implications of glycogen synthase kinase-3-mediated tau phosphorylation. International Journal of Alzheimer's Disease. 2011;**2011**:352805

[71] Meunier CN, Cancela JM, Fossier P. Lack of GSK3beta activation and modulation of synaptic plasticity by dopamine in 5-HT1A-receptor KO mice. Neuropharmacology. Feb 2017;**113**(Pt A):124-136

[72] Maixner DW, Weng HR. The Role of Glycogen Synthase Kinase 3 Beta in Neuroinflammation and Pain. Journal of Pharmacy and Pharmacology (Los Angel). 2013;**1**(1):001

[73] Wake H, Moorhouse AJ, Nabekura J. Functions of microglia in the central nervous system--beyond the immune response. Neuron Glia Biology. Feb 2011;**7**(1):47-53

[74] Sofroniew MV, Vinters HV. Astrocytes: biology and pathology. Acta Neuropathologica. Jan 2010;**119**(1):7-35

[75] Doens D, Fernandez PL. Microglia receptors and their implications in the response to amyloid beta for Alzheimer's disease pathogenesis. Journal of Neuroinflammation. 13 Mar 2014;**11**:48

[76] Rahimifard M, Maqbool F, Moeini-Nodeh S, Niaz K, Abdollahi M, Braidy N, et al. Targeting the TLR4 signaling pathway by polyphenols: A novel therapeutic strategy for neuroinflammation. Ageing Research Reviews. 21 Feb 2017;**36**:11-19

[77] Landreth GE, Reed-Geaghan EG. Toll-like receptors in Alzheimer's disease. In: Kielian T, editor. Toll-like Receptors: Roles in Infection and Neuropathology. Berlin, Heidelberg: Springer Berlin Heidelberg; 2009. pp. 137-153

[78] Pihlaja R, Koistinaho J, Malm T, Sikkila H, Vainio S, Koistinaho M. Transplanted astrocytes internalize deposited beta-amyloid peptides in a transgenic mouse model of Alzheimer's disease. Glia. 15 Jan 2008;**56**(2):154-163

[79] Baker RG, Hayden MS, Ghosh S. NF-kappaB, inflammation, and metabolic disease. Cell Metabolism. 05 Jan 2011;**13**(1):11-22

[80] Yi B, Luye Q, Eunhee K, Sangram B, Hengchang G, Maria F, et al. CD36 is involved in astrocyte activation and astroglial scar formation. Journal of Cerebral Blood Flow & Metabolism. 2012;**32**(8):1567-1577

[81] Jones RS, Minogue AM, Connor TJ, Lynch MA. Amyloid-beta-induced astrocytic phagocytosis is mediated by CD36, CD47 and RAGE. Journal of NeuroImmune Pharmacology. Mar 2013;**8**(1):301-311

[82] Kim J, Waldvogel HJ, Faull RL, Curtis MA, Nicholson LF. The RAGE receptor and its ligands are highly expressed in astrocytes in a grade-dependant manner in the striatum and subependymal layer in Huntington's disease. Journal of Neurochemistry. Sep 2015;**134**(5):927-942

[83] Sick E, Boukhari A, Deramaudt T, Ronde P, Bucher B, Andre P, et al. Activation of CD47 receptors causes proliferation of human astrocytoma but not normal astrocytes via an Akt-dependent pathway. Glia. Feb 2011;**59**(2):308-319

[84] Koistinaho M, Lin S, Wu X, Esterman M, Koger D, Hanson J, et al. Apolipoprotein E promotes astrocyte colocalization and degradation of deposited amyloid-beta peptides. Nature Medicine. Jul 2004;**10**(7):719-726

[85] Petr GT, Sun Y, Frederick NM, Zhou Y, Dhamne SC, Hameed MQ, et al. Conditional deletion of the glutamate transporter GLT-1 reveals that astrocytic GLT-1 protects against fatal epilepsy while neuronal GLT-1 contributes significantly to glutamate uptake into synaptosomes. Journal of Neuroscience. 01 Apr 2015;**35**(13):5187-5201

[86] Alberdi E, Sanchez-Gomez MV, Cavaliere F, Perez-Samartin A, Zugaza JL, Trullas R, et al. Amyloid beta oligomers induce Ca2+ dysregulation and neuronal death through activation of ionotropic glutamate receptors. Cell Calcium. Mar 2010;**47**(3):264-272

[87] Schwab C, Klegeris A, McGeer PL. Inflammation in transgenic mouse models of neurodegenerative disorders. Biochimica et Biophysica Acta. Oct 2010;**1802**(10):889-902

[88] Narayan P, Holmstrom KM, Kim DH, Whitcomb DJ, Wilson MR, St George-Hyslop P, et al. Rare individual amyloid-beta oligomers act on astrocytes to initiate neuronal damage. Biochemistry. 22 Apr 2014 ;53(15):2442-2253

[89] Wang WY, Tan MS, Yu JT, Tan L. Role of pro-inflammatory cytokines released from microglia in Alzheimer's disease. Annals of Translational Medicine. Jun 2015;**3**(10):136

[90] Becher B, Spath S, Goverman J. Cytokine networks in neuroinflammation. Nature Reviews Immunology. Jan 2017;**17**(1):49-59

[91] Kawamoto EM, Lepsch LB, Boaventura MF, Munhoz CD, Lima LS, Yshii LM, et al. Amyloid beta-peptide activates nuclear factor-kappaB through an N-methyl-D-aspartate signaling pathway in cultured cerebellar cells. Journal of Neuroscience Research. Mar 2008;**86**(4):845-860

[92] Shih RH, Wang CY, Yang CM. NF-kappaB signaling pathways in neurological inflammation: A mini review. Frontiers in Molecular Neuroscience. 2015;**8**:77

[93] Weber A, Wasiliew P, Kracht M. Interleukin-1 (IL-1) pathway. Science Signaling. 19 Jan 2010;**3**(105):cm1

[94] Garwood CJ, Pooler AM, Atherton J, Hanger DP, Noble W. Astrocytes are important mediators of Abeta-induced neurotoxicity and tau phosphorylation in primary culture. Cell Death & Disease. 02 Jun 2011;**2**:e167

[95] Llorens-Martin M, Jurado J, Hernandez F, Avila J. GSK-3beta, a pivotal kinase in Alzheimer disease. Frontiers in Molecular Neuroscience. 2014;**7**:46

[96] Grunnet LG, Aikin R, Tonnesen MF, Paraskevas S, Blaabjerg L, Storling J, et al. Proinflammatory cytokines activate the intrinsic apoptotic pathway in beta-cells. Diabetes. Aug 2009;**58**(8):1807-1815

[97] Correa SA, Eales KL. The role of p38 MAPK and its substrates in neuronal plasticity and neurodegenerative disease. Journal of Signal Transduction. 2012;**2012**:649079

[98] Kuwata H, Nakatani Y, Murakami M, Kudo I. Cytosolic phospholipase A2 is required for cytokine-induced expression of type IIA secretory phospholipase A2 that mediates optimal cyclooxygenase-2-dependent delayed prostaglandin E2 generation in rat 3Y1 fibroblasts. The Journal of Biological Chemistry. 16 Jan 1998;**273**(3):1733-1740

[99] Aid S, Bosetti F. Targeting cyclooxygenases-1 and -2 in neuroinflammation: Therapeutic implications. Biochimie. Jan 2011;**93**(1):46-51

[100] Maingret V, Barthet G, Deforges S, Jiang N, Mulle C, Amedee T. PGE2-EP3 signaling pathway impairs hippocampal presynaptic long-term plasticity in a mouse model of Alzheimer's disease. Neurobiology of Aging. Feb 2017;**50**:13-24

[101] Ojala JO, Sutinen EM, Salminen A, Pirttila T. Interleukin-18 increases expression of kinases involved in tau phosphorylation in SH-SY5Y neuroblastoma cells. Journal of Neuroimmunology. 15 Dec 2008;**205**(1-2):86-93

[102] Quintanilla RA, Orellana DI, Gonzalez-Billault C, Maccioni RB. Interleukin-6 induces Alzheimer-type phosphorylation of tau protein by deregulating the cdk5/p35 pathway. Experimental Cell Research. 15 Apr 2004;**295**(1):245-257

[103] Ding H, Matthews TA, Johnson GV. Site-specific phosphorylation and caspase cleavage differentially impact tau-microtubule interactions and tau aggregation. The Journal of Biological Chemistry. 14 Jul 2006;**281**(28):19107-19114

[104] Zempel H, Thies E, Mandelkow E, Mandelkow EM. Abeta oligomers cause localized Ca(2+) elevation, missorting of endogenous Tau into dendrites, Tau phosphorylation, and destruction of microtubules and spines. Journal of Neuroscience. 08 Sep 2010;**30**(36):11938-11950

[105] Yoshiyama Y, Higuchi M, Zhang B, Huang SM, Iwata N, Saido TC, et al. Synapse loss and microglial activation precede tangles in a P301S tauopathy mouse model. Neuron. 1 Feb 2007;**53**(3):337-351

[106] Cho YE, Lee MH, Song BJ. Neuronal cell death and degeneration through increased nitroxidative stress and tau phosphorylation in HIV-1 transgenic rats. PLoS One 2017;**12**(1):e0169945

[107] Nilson AN, English KC, Gerson JE, Barton Whittle T, Nicolas Crain C, Xue J, et al. Tau oligomers associate with inflammation in the brain and retina of tauopathy mice and in neurodegenerative diseases. Journal of Alzheimer's Disease. 2017;**55**(3):1083-1099

[108] Breitner JC, Baker LD, Montine TJ, Meinert CL, Lyketsos CG, Ashe KH, et al. Extended results of the Alzheimer's disease anti-inflammatory prevention trial. Alzheimer's & Dementia. Jul 2011;**7**(4):402-411

[109] Efremova L, Chovancova P, Adam M, Gutbier S, Schildknecht S, Leist M. Switching from astrocytic neuroprotection to neurodegeneration by cytokine stimulation. Archives of Toxicology. Jan 2017;**91**(1):231-246

[110] Tan CC, Yu JT, Wang HF, Tan MS, Meng XF, Wang C, et al. Efficacy and safety of donepezil, galantamine, rivastigmine, and memantine for the treatment of Alzheimer's disease: A systematic review and meta-analysis. Journal of Alzheimer's Disease. 2014;**41**(2):615-631

[111] Gupta SC, Sundaram C, Reuter S, Aggarwal BB. Inhibiting NF-kappaB activation by small molecules as a therapeutic strategy. Biochimica et Biophysica Acta. Oct-Dec 2010;**1799**(10-12):775-787

[112] Ajmone-Cat MA, Bernardo A, Greco A, Minghetti L. Non-steroidal anti-inflammatory drugs and brain inflammation: Effects on microglial functions. Pharmaceuticals (Basel). 14 Jun 2010;**3**(6):1949-1965

[113] Imbimbo BP, Solfrizzi V, Panza F. Are NSAIDs useful to treat Alzheimer's disease or mild cognitive impairment?. Frontiers in Aging Neuroscience. 2010;**2**

[114] Martin H. Role of PPAR-gamma in inflammation. Prospects for therapeutic intervention by food components. Mutation Research. 07 Aug 2010;690(1-2):57-63

[115] Gajardo-Gomez R, Labra VC, Maturana CJ, Shoji KF, Santibanez CA, Saez JC, et al. Cannabinoids prevent the amyloid beta-induced activation of astroglial hemichannels: A neuroprotective mechanism. Glia. Jan 2017;**65**(1):122-137

[116] Harach T, Jammes F, Muller C, Duthilleul N, Cheatham V, Zufferey V, et al. Administrations of human adult ischemia-tolerant mesenchymal stem cells and factors reduce amyloid beta pathology in a mouse model of Alzheimer's disease. Neurobiology of Aging. Mar 2017;**51**:83-96

[117] Moreno LC, Puerta E, Suarez-Santiago JE, Santos-Magalhaes NS, Ramirez MJ, Irache JM. Effect of the oral administration of nanoencapsulated quercetin on a mouse model of Alzheimer's disease. International Journal of Pharmaceutics. 30 Jan 2017;**517**(1-2):50-57

[118] Venigalla M, Gyengesi E, Munch G. Curcumin and apigenin - novel and promising therapeutics against chronic neuroinflammation in Alzheimer's disease. Neural Regeneration Research. Aug 2015;**10**(8):1181-1185

[119] Bedse G, Romano A, Lavecchia AM, Cassano T, Gaetani S. The role of endocannabinoid signaling in the molecular mechanisms of neurodegeneration in Alzheimer's disease. Journal of Alzheimer's Disease. 2015;**43**(4):1115-1136

[120] Rinwa P, Kumar A. Quercetin suppress microglial neuroinflammatory response and induce antidepressent-like effect in olfactory bulbectomized rats. Neuroscience 2013; **255**:86-98

[121] Xu ZP, Li L, Bao J, Wang ZH, Zeng J, Liu EJ, et al. Magnesium protects cognitive functions and synaptic plasticity in streptozotocin-induced sporadic Alzheimer's model. PLoS One 2014;**9**(9):e108645

[122] Klein PS, Melton DA. A molecular mechanism for the effect of lithium on development. PNAS, Proceedings of the National Academy of Sciences U S A. 06 Aug 1996;**93**(16):8455-8459

[123] Huang Y, Mucke L. Alzheimer mechanisms and therapeutic strategies. Cell. 16 Mar 2012 ;**148**(6):1204-1222

[124] Nakajima A, Ohizumi Y, Yamada K. Anti-dementia Activity of Nobiletin, a Citrus Flavonoid: A Review of Animal Studies. Clinical Psychopharmacology and Neuroscience. Aug 2014;**12**(2):75-82

Chapter 5

Interleukin 1 Receptor and Alzheimer's Disease-Related Neuroinflammation

Huanhuan Wang and Xizhen Wang

Additional information is available at the end of the chapter

http://dx.doi.org/10.5772/intechopen.69067

Abstract

Neuroinflammation as one of the pathogenic mechanisms concerning to the development of Alzheimer's disease (AD) has aroused more attention since last decades. Amyloid beta (Aβ) peptide generation is supposed to be the initial event in AD progress, followed by neuronal impairment, neuroinflammation, and severe substantial neuronal dysfunction. Interleukin-1 receptor (IL-1R) as one of the most prevalent inflammatory mediated surface receptors, participates not only in peripheral inflammation but also in AD-related neuroinflammation. In microglia, IL-1R activation triggers the downstream signaling and the production of proinflammatory cytokines and chemokines. IL-1R signaling also participates in AD-related Aβ-induced inflammasome activation. Besides, IL-1R activation in neurons may increase APP non-amyloid pathway by modulation of APP α-secretase activity, which may prevent neurotoxic Aβ generation. Thus, the exact role of IL-1R signaling in AD development and neuronal functions is somehow tricky.

Keywords: interleukin 1 receptor, Alzheimer's disease, neuroinflammation

1. Introduction

Alzheimer's disease (AD) is kind of neurodegenerative disease, which affects elder's health and living quality. There are some hypotheses raised up for the pathogenesis of the disease, such as amyloid cascade and tau hyperphosphorylation. Besides, neuroinflammation induced by neurotoxic amyloid β (Aβ) peptide is also considered contribute to the development of AD. Inteleukin-1 receptor (IL-1R) is one of the inflammation-related surface receptors that are distributed widely in various tissues and cells in the body. Evidence has been shown that IL-1R-mediated neuroinflammation may be closely related to pathogenesis and development of AD. In the current chapter, AD-related neuroinflammation and the participation of IL-1R in such progress would be reviewed and discussed in detail.

2. Alzheimer's disease

As a kind of chronic neurodegenerative disease, AD usually starts slowly and gets worse over comparatively longer time. The initial symptoms of AD are often mistaken with normal aging. The most common early symptom for AD is the difficulty in remembering recent events (short-term memory loss). As the disease advances, symptoms may include problems with language, disorientation (easily getting lost), mood swings, loss of motivation, not managing self-care, and behavioral issues. AD patients may suffer from the disease symptoms for years and especially at the later stage of the progress.

AD is currently supposed to be the cause of approximately 60–70% of total dementia cases. There is a large amount of data about potential risk factors for AD, including age [1], genetics [2], and injury [3]. Many treatable medical conditions are also associated with an increased risk of AD, including stroke [4], diabetes [5], midlife hypertension [6], and hypercholesterolemia [7, 8].

The early identification of molecular pathological description of AD was the functional reduction of cholinergic nerve system in the cerebral cortex, like the remarkable reduction in choline acetyltransferase (ChAT) [9]. Later, senile plaques and neurofibrillary tangles (NFTs), two typical protein depositions, were confirmed related to AD [10]. The main component of senile plaques is Aβ peptide; while NFTs are made from abnormal tau proteins [11]. A 42-amino acid long form of Aβ (Aβ42) was found as the main content in fibrillar Aβ peptides [12]. Aβ40, which is also found in the plaque, although is normally more abundantly produced by cells, contributes to the lower portion of the plaque [13]. Compared to Aβ40, Aβ42 is the more hydrophobic form that aggregates more easily and quickly [14]. NFTs are formed by hyperphosphorylated tau protein. As the raise of Aβ concentration, tau protein happens to be more easily phosphorylated, leading to an imbalance of various kinases and phosphatases [15]. Consequently, mass transport and impaired impulse occurs in neurons, followed by severe neuronal dysfunction.

Thus, the amyloid hypothesis puts Aβ accumulation at the core of AD pathogenesis. Aβ is the sequential proteolytic product of its precursor amyloid precursor protein (APP). APP is a type I transmembrane protein, consisted of a large N-terminal ectodomain, a transmembrane domain, and a short cytoplasmic domain. The Aβ peptide generation is supposed to be influenced by the pattern of cleavage from APP by α, β, and γ-secretases [16]. APP can be processed in two different pathways, the amyloid, and non-amyloid pathway. In the amyloid pathway, APP can be cleaved by β-secretase (BACE1), releasing the soluble APP β fragment (sAPPβ); and the C-terminal fragment (CTF) is still in the membrane and can be cleaved by γ-secretase (presenilin1, PS1) to release Aβ [17]. This process leads to Aβ generation, aggregation, and deposit. In the other non-amyloid pathway, APP can be cleaved by α-secretase (ADAM10/17), releasing soluble APP α fragment (sAPPα). The cleavage site of α-secretase is between the sites of β- and γ-secretase. So the non-amyloid pathway can reduce the damage induced by Aβ on neurons.

Consider to the crucial role of Aβ in the amyloid cascade, therapeutic approaches related to APP metabolic pathways were always under careful and detail research and develop [18]. Those therapeutic approaches include inhibition of Aβ monomers developing into toxic oligomers or enhancement of clearance and disaggregation of fibrillar aggregates from cerebral cortex [19]; modulation of the fate and toxicity of Aβ using antibodies against Aβ [20]. However, the only clinical effective therapeutic approach so far is the treatment and enhancement of the functions of cholinergic neurons. Acetylcholinesterase (AChE) inhibitors, galantamine, and rivastigmine were thought to improve cognition and indirectly help function and behavior in patients with AD [21–23]. Such treatments for AD have been widely available since the mid-1990s, but these drugs do not treat the underlying mechanism, so the effects are limited.

3. AD-related neuroinflammation

As described above, the amyloid hypothesis was raised up as the most popular and acceptable pathogenesis mechanism for AD. The initial changes of the cascade happen to Aβ metabolism. The Aβ balance in favor of Aβ42 followed by the formation of diffuse plaques can induce the toxic effect to neurons to different extends. The diffuse Aβ plaques can then convert to more toxic Aβ deposit fibrillars. Aβ triggers the activation of the cellular signaling cascade, the induction of inflammatory enzyme systems in a vicious cycle and finally the expression and secretion of proinflammatory cytokines. The activation of microglial and astrocyte, together with the corresponding inflammatory reactions, is another important event in AD pathogenesis. Both aggregated amyloid fibrils and inflammatory mediators secreted by microglia contribute to neuronal dystrophy. NFTs occur under such condition, which enhances neuronal dysfunction and death. The widespread neuronal dysfunction is regarded as the immediate cause of the disease [18, 24]. On the basis of these observations, Aβ has become a major pharmacological target for the treatment of the disease. However, such trails of treatment have not reached a satisfactory outcome. Thus, the AD-related neuroinflammation starts to sneak into current research attention.

In parallel, neuroinflammation has been implicated in contributing to the etiology of AD. Epidemiological and prospective population-based studies show an association between suppression of inflammation and reduced risk for AD [25, 26]. The protective effects of nonsteroidal anti-inflammatory drugs (NSAIDs) against AD development [27] further support the neuroinflammation hypothesis. In animals, the beneficial effects of NSAIDs have also been confirmed, including behavioral improvement and reductions in glial activation, Aβ levels, and plaque size [28]. Inflammatory responses to amyloidosis have also been observed in animal models overexpressing Aβ [29, 30]. Proinflammatory cytokines, such as (interleukin-1) IL-1, IL-6, and tumor necrosis factor α (TNFα), are elevated in the plasma, brains, and cerebrospinal fluid of patients with AD or mild cognitive impairment, whereas anti-inflammatory cytokines are decreased [31, 32]. Besides, inhibition of TNFα signaling has been shown to attenuate AD-like pathology and cognitive impairments in transgenic mouse models, as well as in AD patients [33, 34].

Inflammation is a complex cellular and molecular response to insults (stress, injury or infection), an attempt to defend against these insults. AD-associated inflammation is generally considered as a secondary response to the pathological lesions evoked by Aβ [35, 36]. AD-related inflammatory response is supposed to be driven mainly by activated microglia [37, 38].

The activation of migrolia has been reported in both AD patients and animal models [39], accompanied by increased levels of specific chemokines and cytokines [40]. Microglia surrounding plaques stain positive for activation markers and proinflammatory mediators, including cyclooxygenase-2 (Cox-2), monocyte chemotactic protein 1 (MCP-1), TNFα, transforming growth factor-β (TGFβ), IL-1α, IL-1β, and IL-6 [41–43]. Aβ and its fibrils can induce self-defense, inflammatory responses via pattern recognition receptors (PRRs), such as toll-like receptors (TLRs) [44, 45]. Aβ aggregates interact with microglial receptors like TLR4, CD14, CD36, CD47, the receptor for advanced glycation end products (RAGE), and some integrins [46–50]. More recently, it has been reported that Aβ activates microglia through its interaction with the APP present in the membrane of these cells [51], which defines a novel function of APP in microglial regulation of the inflammatory response in AD.

Microglial activation seems to be the comparative early event in AD pathological development. Imaging study results showed that reactive microglia can be detected at the very early clinical stage of the disease [39]. In AD mouse model, microglial activation was observed before amyloid plaque formation [52]. Once activated, microglia can produce several proinflammatory signal molecules, including cytokines, growth factors, chemokines, and cell adhesion molecules. Besides, Microglia may also play a role in plaque evolution by phagocytosing and/or degrade deposited Aβ. Many different laboratories have shown that microglia, both *in vivo* and in culture, phagocytose exogenous fibrillar Aβ [53, 54].

4. Interleukin 1 receptor

IL-1R family belongs to one category of TIR domain-containing receptor superfamily. The TIR domain-containing receptors are a large family of molecules involved in the activation of innate immunity [55]. The TIR superfamily can be broadly divided into two main groups: the immunoglobulin (Ig) domain-bearing receptors and the receptors with a leucine-rich repeat (LRR) domain [56, 57]. The Ig domain subgroup of TIR receptors includes 10 members of the IL-1R family, whereas the LRR group includes the toll-like receptors (TLR). When an agonist IL-1 family cytokine binds to its specific TIR-containing receptor, the initiation of IL-1R activation signaling occurs [56]. The signaling pathway involves the recruitment of adapter molecule MyD88 and kinase IRAK, followed by interaction with TRAF6. The final step is the phosphorylation of the inhibitory molecule IκB by IκB kinase complex leading to relocalization of transcription factor NF-κB. NF-κB is translocated into the nucleus and intermediates inflammatory immune response [58]. NF-κB is a major inflammatory switch that comprises a family of transcription factors that regulate expression of various proinflammatory cytokines (IL-1, IL-6, IL-8 and TNFα), chemokines, antiapoptotic factors and stress factors [59].

IL-1 family is the typical ligands for IL-1R and its activation. IL-1 family includes a set of cytokines, some of which have been demonstrated to play a critical role in host responses to pathogens and other noxious agents [60]. IL-1α and IL-1β are two most prevalent ligands that are supposed to trigger the activation of IL-1R. IL-1α/β are endogenous pyrogens with activities similar to lipopolysaccharides (LPS), which are the major molecular components of the outer membrane of Gram-negative bacteria [61].

One of IL-1R ligand cytokine IL-1β appears to play an important role in AD. IL-1β level was confirmed obviously in and around the area of Aβ deposit [62, 63]. The inhibition of IL-1 signaling by IL-1R knockout could significantly relief the Aβ burden in transgenic AD mice [64]. And the protective impact by IL-1R knockout was believed to be dependent on attenuated AD-related neuroinflammation [65]. Besides, the inflammation- or IL-1β-induced pathological tau development has also been well documented [66–68]. The inhibition of IL-1 signaling significantly suppressed the activation of cdk5/p25, GSK-3β, and p38-MAPK, all major kinases that phosphorylate tau in neurons. Another study demonstrated a direct effect of IL-1β secreted by microglia on neurons and subsequent activation of p38-MAPK and accumulation of tau phosphorylation [69]. NSAIDs could be repurposed as NLRP3 inflammasome inhibitors that provide neuroprotective impact against AD [70].

5. IL-1R signaling and inflammasome

Inflammasomes are responsible for the maturation of pro-inflammatory cytokines such as interleukin IL-1, IL-18, and IL-33 and activation of inflammatory cell death, pyroptosis [71]. The inflammasome is a multiprotein oligomer consisting of caspase 1, PYCARD, NALP, and sometimes caspase 5 (also known as caspase 11 or ICH-3). It is expressed in myeloid cells and is a component of the innate immune system. Analogous to the apoptosome, which activates apoptotic cascades, the inflammasome activates an inflammatory cascade. Once active, the inflammasome binds to pro-caspase-1 (the precursor molecule of caspase-1), either homotypically via its own caspase activation and recruitment domain (CARD) or via the adaptor protein ASC. Caspase-1 then assembles into its active form which obtains the peptidase activity. The metabolic process performed by caspase-1 includes the proteolytic cleavage of pro-IL-1β at Asp116 into IL-1β [72] and cleavage of pro-IL-18 into IL-18 to induce IFN-γ secretion and natural killer cell activation [73]. Thus, the inflammasome promotes the maturation of the inflammatory cytokines, interleukin 1β (IL-1β) and interleukin 18 (IL-18) [72]. Thus, IL-1R signaling is considered to play a crucial role in inflammasome activation-induced inflammation.

Nucleotide oligomerization domain (NOD)-like receptor family, pyrin domain 3 (NLRP3) containing inflammasome is an intracellular multiprotein complex, which has been verified to participate in Aβ-induced neuroinflammation [74]. Halle et al. demonstrated that the phagocytosis of fibrillar Aβ activates NALP3 inflammasomes in mouse microglia. The activation of NALP3 was dependent on lysosomal damage and cathepsin B release, as was observed earlier in the crystal-induced NALP3 activation [75, 76]. Then, more evidence was supportive for that Aβ activate the NLRP3 inflammasome in microglial cells *in vitro* and *in vivo* [77–79]. NLRP3 inflammasome inhibitor treatment in AD mice led to decreased levels of Aβ deposition and decreased levels of soluble and insoluble Aβ42 in the brain [80]. NLRP3 or caspase-1 knockout could significantly suppress amyloidosis and neuropathology, as well as improve cognition-associated parameters in AD mice model [77].

The possible roles of the NLRP3 inflammasome in AD pathogenesis discussed above open a novel investigation of inflammasome signaling pathway for understanding AD. Designing agents for critically controlling the activation of NLRP3 inflammasome at the molecular level might offer considerable promise to tackle neuroinflammation and slow AD progression.

6. IL-1R signaling in neurons

IL-1R is widely distributed in the central nerves system (CNS). Early evidence revealed that IL-1R was detected in high density in the dentate gyrus of the hippocampus, choroid plexus, meninges, and anterior pituitary and is low expressed in the frontoparietal cortex. Both neurons and glial cells were shown to express IL-1R [81]. Later, a pile of data demonstrated that IL-1R could be activated in various cell types in CNS. In cultured human microglia, numerous proinflammatory cytokines such as IL-1, IL-6, and TNFα are produced after IL-1 stimulation. In cultured rat astrocytes, IL-1 could stimulate astrocytes to release nerve growth factor which can mediate neuroprotective effects [82]. In addition, administration of IL-1 in the cerebral ventricle induced COX-2 exclusively in endothelial cells comprising brain blood vessels [83]. As we described in the previous paragraph, IL-1R plays an important role in glial activation-induced neuroinflammation, the participation of IL-1R in neuronal function has not been carefully discussed.

IL-1β has been reported to increase the expression of APP in neuronal culture [69]. The amyloid precursor protein (APP), via stimulation of amyloidogenic processing, undergoes sequential proteolytic cleavage by β-secretase and γ-secretase to generate Aβ. Alternatively, a non-amyloidogenic pathway involving α-secretase activation could reduce Aβ generation, which competitively inhibits activation of the detrimental amyloidogenic pathway. Also, sAPPα is proven to possess neuroprotective and memory-enhancing properties, often being compared to cerebral growth stimulants. Thus, the non-amyloidogenic pathway is supposed to be a suitable therapeutic target for AD.

The identity of α-secretase of APP has been verified to be ADAM10 (a disintegrin and metalloprotease 10) constitutively and ADAM17 regulatively [84]. Different kinds of stimuli have been suggested to increase the secretion of sAPPα under certain conditions via ADAM17, including various cytokine, chemokines, adhesion molecules and growth factors [85]. The two most important ligands for IL-1R, IL-1α [86] and IL-1β [87, 88] were proved to enhance ADAM17 activity in neurons. The detail mechanism research concerning to IL-1 signaling and APP proteolysis revealed that the GC-rich APP mRNA 5′UTR-stem loop structure bears an amyloid-specific CAGA sequence, IL-1 responsive element, and an iron responsive element.

IL-1 binding to its responsive element significantly impacts the functioning of APP 5′UTR that affects APP metabolism and thus sAPPα release [89]. Besides, p38/ERK/JNK pathway and PI3K/AKT pathway are believed to participate in IL-1 signaling mediated activity regulation of APP α-secretase ADAM17 [90, 91].

Thus, IL-1R is considered play an important and distinct role in different aspects in the process of AD development. The exact relationship of IL-1R signaling activation between microglial activation-induced neuroinflammation and APP α-shedding in neurons is somehow tricky. The cytokines and growth factors from reactive microglia induced by neurotoxic Aβ may enhance ADAM17 activity in nearby neurons (paracrine), which provides a possible self-protection against Ab-induced neuronal dystrophy.

7. Conclusion

IL-1R participates in AD-related neuroinflammation by microglial activation and the secretion of various pro-inflammatory cytokines and chemokines. The anti-inflammation treatment has been raised up, including IL-1R antagonist as a potential AD therapeutic approach. However, IL-1R activation in neurons, where exactly APP proteolysis takes place, may enhance the activity of neuroprotective α-secretase. The safety of novel promising therapeutic approaches targeting IL-1R activity regulation has to be evaluated carefully to avoid unexpected side effects.

Acknowledgements

This work was financially supported by National Natural Science Foundation of China (81302781).

Author details

Huanhuan Wang[1]* and Xizhen Wang[2]

*Address all correspondence to: huanval@hznu.edu.cn

1 School of Medicine, Hangzhou Normal University, Hangzhou, China

2 Vastec Medical LTD, Hong Kong, China

References

[1] Ferri CP, Prince M, Brayne C, Brodaty H, Fratiglioni L, Ganguli M, Hall K, Hasegawa K, Hendrie H, Huang Y, Jorm A, Mathers C, Menezes PR, Rimmer E, Scazufca M. Global prevalence of dementia: A Delphi consensus study. Lancet. 2005;**366**(9503):2112-2117

[2] Goate A. Segregation of a missense mutation in the amyloid beta-protein precursor gene with familial Alzheimer's disease. Journal of Alzheimer's Disease. 2006;**9**(3 Suppl):341-347

[3] Sundstrom A, Nilsson LG, Cruts M, Adolfsson R, Van Broeckhoven C, Nyberg L. Increased risk of dementia following mild head injury for carriers but not for non-carriers of the APOE epsilon4 allele. International Psychogeriatrics. 2007;**19**(1):159-165

[4] Savva GM, Stephan BC. Epidemiological studies of the effect of stroke on incident dementia: A systematic review. Stroke. 2010;**41**(1):e41–e46

[5] Lu FP, Lin KP, Kuo HK. Diabetes and the risk of multi-system aging phenotypes: A systematic review and meta-analysis. PLoS One. 2009;**4**(1):e4144

[6] Qiu C, Winblad B, Fratiglioni L. The age-dependent relation of blood pressure to cognitive function and dementia. The Lancet Neurology. 2005;**4**(8):487-499

[7] Anstey KJ, Lipnicki DM, Low LF. Cholesterol as a risk factor for dementia and cognitive decline: A systematic review of prospective studies with meta-analysis. The American Journal of Geriatric Psychiatry. 2008;**16**(5):343-354

[8] McGuinness B, Craig D, Bullock R, Passmore P. Statins for the prevention of dementia. The Cochrane Database of Systematic Reviews. 2016;**1**:CD003160

[9] Selkoe DJ, Schenk D. Alzheimer's disease: Molecular understanding predicts amyloid-based therapeutics. Annual Review of Pharmacology and Toxicology. 2003;**43**:545-584

[10] Ballard C, Gauthier S, Corbett A, Brayne C, Aarsland D, Jones E. Alzheimer's disease Lancet. 2011;**377**(9770):1019-1031

[11] Scheltens P, Blennow K, Breteler MM, de Strooper B, Frisoni GB, Salloway S, Van der Flier WM. Alzheimer's disease. Lancet. 2016;**388**(10043):505-517

[12] Iwatsubo T, Odaka A, Suzuki N, Mizusawa H, Nukina N, Ihara Y. Visualization of A beta 42(43) and A beta 40 in senile plaques with end-specific A beta monoclonals: Evidence that an initially deposited species is A beta **42**(43). Neuron. 1994;**13**(1):45-53

[13] Selkoe DJ. Translating cell biology into therapeutic advances in Alzheimer's disease. Nature. 1999;**399**(6738 Suppl):A23–A31

[14] Harper JD, Lansbury PT Jr. Models of amyloid seeding in Alzheimer's disease and scrapie: Mechanistic truths and physiological consequences of the time-dependent solubility of amyloid proteins. Annual Review of Biochemistry. 1997;**66**:385-407

[15] Selkoe DJ. Alzheimer's disease: Genes, proteins, and therapy. Physiological Reviews. 2001;**81**(2):741-766

[16] Hardy J. Has the amyloid cascade hypothesis for Alzheimer's disease been proved? Current Alzheimer Research. 2006;**3**(1):71-73

[17] Vassar R, Bennett BD, Babu-Khan S, Kahn S, Mendiaz EA, Denis P, Teplow DB, Ross S, Amarante P, Loeloff R, Luo Y, Fisher S, Fuller J, Edenson S, Lile J, Jarosinski MA, Biere

AL, Curran E, Burgess T, Louis JC, Collins F, Treanor J, Rogers G, Citron M. Beta-secretase cleavage of Alzheimer's amyloid precursor protein by the transmembrane aspartic protease BACE. Science. 1999;**286**(5440):735-741

[18] Sisodia SS, St George-Hyslop PH. gamma-Secretase, Notch, Abeta and Alzheimer's disease: Where do the presenilins fit in? Nature Reviews Neuroscience. 2002;**3**(4):281-290

[19] Fraser PE, Darabie AA, McLaurin JA. Amyloid-beta interactions with chondroitin sulfate-derived monosaccharides and disaccharides: Implications for drug development. The Journal of Biological Chemistry. 2001;**276**(9):6412-6419

[20] Bard F, Cannon C, Barbour R, Burke RL, Games D, Grajeda H, Guido T, Hu K, Huang J, Johnson-Wood K, Khan K, Kholodenko D, Lee M, Lieberburg I, Motter R, Nguyen M, Soriano F, Vasquez N, Weiss K, Welch B, Seubert P, Schenk D, Yednock T. Peripherally administered antibodies against amyloid beta-peptide enter the central nervous system and reduce pathology in a mouse model of Alzheimer disease. Nature Medicine. 2000;**6**(8):916-919

[21] Birks J, Harvey RJ. Donepezil for dementia due to Alzheimer's disease. The Cochrane Database of Systematic Reviews. 2006;**1**:CD001190

[22] Loy C, Schneider L. Galantamine for Alzheimer's disease and mild cognitive impairment. The Cochrane Database of Systematic Reviews. 2006;**1**:CD001747

[23] Birks JS, Chong LY, Grimley Evans J. Rivastigmine for Alzheimer's disease. The Cochrane Database of Systematic Reviews. 2015;**9**:CD001191

[24] Hardy J, Selkoe DJ. The amyloid hypothesis of Alzheimer's disease: progress and problems on the road to therapeutics. Science. 2002;**297**(5580):353-356

[25] McGeer PL, Schulzer M, McGeer EG. Arthritis and anti-inflammatory agents as possible protective factors for Alzheimer's disease: A review of 17 epidemiologic studies. Neurology. 1996;**47**(2):425-432

[26] Breitner JC, Zandi PP. Do nonsteroidal antiinflammatory drugs reduce the risk of Alzheimer's disease? The New England Journal of Medicine. 2001;**345**(21):1567-1568

[27] Vlad SC, Miller DR, Kowall NW, Felson DT. Protective effects of NSAIDs on the development of Alzheimer disease. Neurology. 2008;**70**(19):1672-1677

[28] Lin X, Koelsch G, Wu S, Downs D, Dashti A, Tang J. Human aspartic protease memapsin 2 cleaves the beta-secretase site of beta-amyloid precursor protein. Proceedings of the National Academy of Sciences of United States of America. 2000;**97**(4):1456-1460

[29] Matsuoka Y, Picciano M, Malester B, LaFrancois J, Zehr C, Daeschner JM, Olschowka JA, Fonseca MI, O'Banion MK, Tenner AJ, Lemere CA, Duff K. Inflammatory responses to amyloidosis in a transgenic mouse model of Alzheimer's disease. American Journal of Pathology. 2001;**158**(4):1345-1354

[30] Wirz KT, Bossers K, Stargardt A, Kamphuis W, Swaab DF, Hol EM, Verhaagen J. Cortical beta amyloid protein triggers an immune response, but no synaptic changes

in the APPswe/PS1dE9 Alzheimer's disease mouse model. Neurobiology of Aging. 2013;**34**(5):1328-1342

[31] Galimberti D, Fenoglio C, Lovati C, Venturelli E, Guidi I, Corra B, Scalabrini D, Clerici F, Mariani C, Bresolin N, Scarpini E. Serum MCP-1 levels are increased in mild cognitive impairment and mild Alzheimer's disease. Neurobiology of Aging. 2006;**27**(12): 1763-1768

[32] Forlenza OV, Diniz BS, Talib LL, Mendonca VA, Ojopi EB, Gattaz WF, Teixeira AL. Increased serum IL-1beta level in Alzheimer's disease and mild cognitive impairment. Dementia and Geriatric Cognitive Disorders. 2009;**28**(6):507-512

[33] Giuliani F, Vernay A, Leuba G, Schenk F. Decreased behavioral impairments in an Alzheimer mice model by interfering with TNF-alpha metabolism. Brain Research Bulletin. 2009;**80**(4-5):302-308

[34] McAlpine FE, Lee JK, Harms AS, Ruhn KA, Blurton-Jones M, Hong J, Das P, Golde TE, LaFerla FM, Oddo S, Blesch A, Tansey MG. Inhibition of soluble TNF signaling in a mouse model of Alzheimer's disease prevents pre-plaque amyloid-associated neuropathology. Neurobiology of Disease. 2009;**34**(1):163-177

[35] Eikelenboom P, Veerhuis R, Scheper W, Rozemuller AJ, van Gool WA, Hoozemans JJ. The significance of neuroinflammation in understanding Alzheimer's disease. Journal of Neural Transmission (Vienna). 2006;**113**(11):1685-1695

[36] Heneka MT, O'Banion MK. Inflammatory processes in Alzheimer's disease. Journal of Neuroimmunology. 2007;**184**(1-2):69-91

[37] Das S, Basu A. Inflammation: A new candidate in modulating adult neurogenesis. Journal of Neuroscience Research. 2008;**86**(6):1199-1208

[38] Bolos M, Perea JR, Avila J. Alzheimer's disease as an inflammatory disease. Biomolecular Concepts. 2017;**8**(1):37-43.

[39] Cagnin A, Brooks DJ, Kennedy AM, Gunn RN, Myers R, Turkheimer FE, Jones T, Banati RB. In-vivo measurement of activated microglia in dementia. Lancet. 2001;**358**(9280):461-467

[40] Swardfager W, Lanctot K, Rothenburg L, Wong A, Cappell J, Herrmann N. A meta-analysis of cytokines in Alzheimer's disease. Biological Psychiatry. 2010;**68**(10):930-941

[41] Akiyama H, Barger S, Barnum S, Bradt B, Bauer J, Cole GM, Cooper NR, Eikelenboom P, Emmerling M, Fiebich BL, Finch CE, Frautschy S, Griffin WS, Hampel H, Hull M, Landreth G, Lue L, Mrak R, Mackenzie IR, McGeer PL, O'Banion MK, Pachter J, Pasinetti G, Plata-Salaman C, Rogers J, Rydel R, Shen Y, Streit W, Strohmeyer R, Tooyoma I, Van Muiswinkel FL, Veerhuis R, Walker D, Webster S, Wegrzyniak B, Wenk G, Wyss-Coray T. Inflammation and Alzheimer's disease. Neurobiology of Aging. 2000;**21**(3):383-421

[42] Cartier L, Hartley O, Dubois-Dauphin M, Krause KH. Chemokine receptors in the central nervous system: role in brain inflammation and neurodegenerative diseases. Brain Research. Brain Research Reviews. 2005;**48**(1):16-42

[43] Glass CK, Saijo K, Winner B, Marchetto MC, Gage FH. Mechanisms underlying inflammation in neurodegeneration. Cell. 2010;**140**(6):918-934

[44] Walter S, Letiembre M, Liu Y, Heine H, Penke B, Hao W, Bode B, Manietta N, Walter J, Schulz-Schuffer W, Fassbender K. Role of the toll-like receptor 4 in neuroinflammation in Alzheimer's disease. Cellular Physiology and Biochemistry. 2007;**20**(6):947-956

[45] Udan ML, Ajit D, Crouse NR, Nichols MR. Toll-like receptors 2 and 4 mediate Abeta(1-42) activation of the innate immune response in a human monocytic cell line. Journal of Neurochemistry. 2008;**104**(2):524-533

[46] Fassbender K, Walter S, Kuhl S, Landmann R, Ishii K, Bertsch T, Stalder AK, Muehlhauser F, Liu Y, Ulmer AJ, Rivest S, Lentschat A, Gulbins E, Jucker M, Staufenbiel M, Brechtel K, Walter J, Multhaup G, Penke B, Adachi Y, Hartmann T, Beyreuther K. The LPS receptor (CD14) links innate immunity with Alzheimer's disease. The FASEB Journal. 2004;**18**(1):203-205

[47] Koenigsknecht J, Landreth G. Microglial phagocytosis of fibrillar beta-amyloid through a beta1 integrin-dependent mechanism. Journal of Neuroscience. 2004;**24**(44):9838-9846

[48] Stewart CR, Stuart LM, Wilkinson K, van Gils JM, Deng J, Halle A, Rayner KJ, Boyer L, Zhong R, Frazier WA, Lacy-Hulbert A, El Khoury J, Golenbock DT, Moore KJ. CD36 ligands promote sterile inflammation through assembly of a Toll-like receptor 4 and 6 heterodimer. Nature Immunology. 2010;**11**(2):155-161

[49] Hines DJ, Choi HB, Hines RM, Phillips AG, MacVicar BA. Prevention of LPS-induced microglia activation, cytokine production and sickness behavior with TLR4 receptor interfering peptides. PLoS One. 2013;**8**(3):e60388

[50] Go M, Kou J, Lim JE, Yang J, Fukuchi KI. Microglial response to LPS increases in wild-type mice during aging but diminishes in an Alzheimer's mouse model: Implication of TLR4 signaling in disease progression. Biochemical and Biophysical Research Communications. 2016;**479**(2):331-337

[51] Manocha GD, Floden AM, Rausch K, Kulas JA, McGregor BA, Rojanathammanee L, Puig KR, Puig KL, Karki S, Nichols MR, Darland DC, Porter JE, Combs CK. APP Regulates Microglial Phenotype in a Mouse Model of Alzheimer's Disease. Journal of Neuroscience. 2016;**36**(32):8471-8486

[52] Heneka MT, Sastre M, Dumitrescu-Ozimek L, Dewachter I, Walter J, Klockgether T, Van Leuven F. Focal glial activation coincides with increased BACE1 activation and precedes amyloid plaque deposition in APP[V717I] transgenic mice. Journal of Neuroinflammation. 2005;**2**:22

[53] Cui YH, Le Y, Zhang X, Gong W, Abe K, Sun R, Van Damme J, Proost P, Wang JM. Up-regulation of FPR2, a chemotactic receptor for amyloid beta 1-42 (A beta 42), in murine microglial cells by TNF alpha. Neurobiology of Disease. 2002;**10**(3):366-377

[54] Neher JJ, Neniskyte U, Brown GC. Primary phagocytosis of neurons by inflamed microglia: potential roles in neurodegeneration. Frontiers in Pharmacology. 2012;**3**:27

[55] Boraschi D, Tagliabue A. The interleukin-1 receptor family. Vitamins and Hormones. 2006;**74**:229-254

[56] O'Neill LA. The interleukin-1 receptor/Toll-like receptor superfamily: 10 years of progress. Immunological Reviews. 2008;**226**:10-18

[57] Casanova JL, Abel L, Quintana-Murci L. Human TLRs and IL-1Rs in host defense: Natural insights from evolutionary, epidemiological, and clinical genetics. Annual Review of Immunology. 2011;**29**:447-491

[58] Martin MU, Wesche H. Summary and comparison of the signaling mechanisms of the Toll/interleukin-1 receptor family. Biochimica et Biophysica Acta. 2002;**1592**(3):265-280

[59] Li Q, Verma IM. NF-kappaB regulation in the immune system. Nature Reviews Immunology. 2002;**2**(10):725-734

[60] Palomo J, Dietrich D, Martin P, Palmer G, Gabay C. The interleukin (IL)-1 cytokine family—Balance between agonists and antagonists in inflammatory diseases. Cytokine. 2015;**76**(1):25-37

[61] Kwak A, Lee Y, Kim H, Kim S. Intracellular interleukin (IL)-1 family cytokine processing enzyme. Archives of Pharmacal Research. 2016;**39**(11):1556-1564

[62] Benzing WC, Wujek JR, Ward EK, Shaffer D, Ashe KH, Younkin SG, Brunden KR. Evidence for glial-mediated inflammation in aged APP(SW) transgenic mice. Neurobiology of Aging. 1999;**20**(6):581-589

[63] Holmes C, El-Okl M, Williams AL, Cunningham C, Wilcockson D, Perry VH. Systemic infection, interleukin 1beta, and cognitive decline in Alzheimer's disease. Journal of Neurology, Neurosurgery, and Psychiatry. 2003;**74**(6):788-789

[64] Williamson LL, Sholar PW, Mistry RS, Smith SH, Bilbo SD. Microglia and memory: Modulation by early-life infection. Journal of Neuroscience. 2011;**31**(43):15511-15521

[65] Barrientos RM, Hein AM, Frank MG, Watkins LR, Maier SF. Intracisternal interleukin-1 receptor antagonist prevents postoperative cognitive decline and neuroinflammatory response in aged rats. Journal of Neuroscience. 2012;**32**(42):14641-144648

[66] Yoshiyama Y, Higuchi M, Zhang B, Huang SM, Iwata N, Saido TC, Maeda J, Suhara T, Trojanowski JQ, Lee VM. Synapse loss and microglial activation precede tangles in a P301S tauopathy mouse model. Neuron. 2007;**53**(3):337-351

[67] Li Y, Liu L, Barger SW, Griffin WS. Interleukin-1 mediates pathological effects of microglia on tau phosphorylation and on synaptophysin synthesis in cortical neurons through a p38-MAPK pathway. Journal of Neuroscience. 2003;**23**(5):1605-1611

[68] Kitazawa M, Oddo S, Yamasaki TR, Green KN, LaFerla FM. Lipopolysaccharide-induced inflammation exacerbates tau pathology by a cyclin-dependent kinase 5-mediated pathway in a transgenic model of Alzheimer's disease. Journal of Neuroscience. 2005;**25**(39):8843-8853

[69] Kitazawa M, Cheng D, Tsukamoto MR, Koike MA, Wes PD, Vasilevko V, Cribbs DH, LaFerla FM. Blocking IL-1 signaling rescues cognition, attenuates tau pathology, and restores neuronal beta-catenin pathway function in an Alzheimer's disease model. The Journal of Immunology. 2011;**187**(12):6539-6549

[70] Daniels MJ, Rivers-Auty J, Schilling T, Spencer NG, Watremez W, Fasolino V, Booth SJ, White CS, Baldwin AG, Freeman S, Wong R, Latta C, Yu S, Jackson J, Fischer N, Koziel V, Pillot T, Bagnall J, Allan SM, Paszek P, Galea J, Harte MK, Eder C, Lawrence CB, Brough D. Fenamate NSAIDs inhibit the NLRP3 inflammasome and protect against Alzheimer's disease in rodent models. Nature Communications. 2016;**7**:12504

[71] Fink SL, Cookson BT. Apoptosis, pyroptosis, and necrosis: Mechanistic description of dead and dying eukaryotic cells. Infection and Immunity. 2005;**73**(4):1907-1916

[72] Martinon F, Burns K, Tschopp J. The inflammasome: A molecular platform triggering activation of inflammatory caspases and processing of proIL-beta. Molecular Cell. 2002;**10**(2):417-426

[73] Gu Y, Kuida K, Tsutsui H, Ku G, Hsiao K, Fleming MA, Hayashi N, Higashino K, Okamura H, Nakanishi K, Kurimoto M, Tanimoto T, Flavell RA, Sato V, Harding MW, Livingston DJ, Su MS. Activation of interferon-gamma inducing factor mediated by interleukin-1beta converting enzyme. Science. 1997;**275**(5297):206-209

[74] Wang K, Yao Y, Zhu X, Zhang K, Zhou F, Zhu L. Amyloid beta induces NLRP3 inflammasome activation in retinal pigment epithelial cells via NADPH oxidase- and mitochondria-dependent ROS production. Journal of Biochemical and Molecular Toxicology. 2016; Epub.

[75] Halle A, Hornung V, Petzold GC, Stewart CR, Monks BG, Reinheckel T, Fitzgerald KA, Latz E, Moore KJ, Golenbock DT. The NALP3 inflammasome is involved in the innate immune response to amyloid-beta. Nature Immunology. 2008;**9**(8):857-865

[76] Gustin A, Kirchmeyer M, Koncina E, Felten P, Losciuto S, Heurtaux T, Tardivel A, Heuschling P, Dostert C. NLRP3 inflammasome is expressed and functional in mouse brain microglia but not in astrocytes. PLoS One. 2015;**10**(6):e0130624

[77] Heneka MT, Kummer MP, Stutz A, Delekate A, Schwartz S, Vieira-Saecker A, Griep A, Axt D, Remus A, Tzeng TC, Gelpi E, Halle A, Korte M, Latz E, Golenbock DT. NLRP3 is

activated in Alzheimer's disease and contributes to pathology in APP/PS1 mice. Nature. 2013;**493**(7434):674-678

[78] Sheedy FJ, Grebe A, Rayner KJ, Kalantari P, Ramkhelawon B, Carpenter SB, Becker CE, Ediriweera HN, Mullick AE, Golenbock DT, Stuart LM, Latz E, Fitzgerald KA, Moore KJ. CD36 coordinates NLRP3 inflammasome activation by facilitating intracellular nucleation of soluble ligands into particulate ligands in sterile inflammation. Nature Immunology. 2013;**14**(8):812-820

[79] Gold M, El Khoury J. beta-Amyloid, microglia, and the inflammasome in Alzheimer's disease. Seminars in Immunopathology. 2015;**37**(6):607-611

[80] Yin J, Zhao F, Chojnacki JE, Fulp J, Klein WL, Zhang S, Zhu X. NLRP3 inflammasome inhibitor ameliorates amyloid pathology in a mouse model of Alzheimer's disease. Molecular Neurobiology. 2017; Epub.

[81] Ban EM. Interleukin-1 receptors in the brain: Characterization by quantitative in situ autoradiography. ImmunoMethods. 1994;**5**(1):31-40

[82] Gadient RA, Cron KC, Otten U. Interleukin-1 beta and tumor necrosis factor-alpha synergistically stimulate nerve growth factor (NGF) release from cultured rat astrocytes. Neuroscience Letters. 1990;**117**(3):335-340

[83] Cao C, Matsumura K, Shirakawa N, Maeda M, Jikihara I, Kobayashi S, Watanabe Y. Pyrogenic cytokines injected into the rat cerebral ventricle induce cyclooxygenase-2 in brain endothelial cells and also upregulate their receptors. European Journal of Neuroscience. 2001;**13**(9):1781-1790

[84] Kuhn PH, Wang H, Dislich B, Colombo A, Zeitschel U, Ellwart JW, Kremmer E, Rossner S, Lichtenthaler SF. ADAM10 is the physiologically relevant, constitutive alpha-secretase of the amyloid precursor protein in primary neurons. The EMBO Journal. 2010;**29**(17):3020-3032

[85] Qian M, Shen X, Wang H. The distinct role of ADAM17 in APP proteolysis and microglial activation related to Alzheimer's disease. Cellular and Molecular Neurobiology. 2016;**36**(4):471-482

[86] Bandyopadhyay S, Hartley DM, Cahill CM, Lahiri DK, Chattopadhyay N, Rogers JT. Interleukin 1alpha stimulates non-amyloidogenic pathway by alpha-secretase (ADAM-10 and ADAM-17) cleavage of APP in human astrocytic cells involving p38 MAP kinase. Journal of Neuroscience Research. 2006;**84**(1):106-118

[87] Tachida Y, Nakagawa K, Saito T, Saido TC, Honda T, Saito Y, Murayama S, Endo T, Sakaguchi G, Kato A, Kitazume S, Hashimoto Y. Interleukin-1 beta up-regulates TACE to enhance alpha-cleavage of APP in neurons: resulting decrease in Abeta production. Journal of Neurochemistry. 2008;**104**(5):1387-1393

[88] Kong Q, Peterson TS, Baker O, Stanley E, Camden J, Seye CI, Erb L, Simonyi A, Wood WG, Sun GY, Weisman GA. Interleukin-1beta enhances nucleotide-induced and alpha-secretase-dependent amyloid precursor protein processing in rat primary cortical neurons via up-regulation of the P2Y(2) receptor. Journal of Neurochemistry. 2009;**109**(5):1300-1310

[89] Wang YQ, Qu DH, Wang K. Therapeutic approaches to Alzheimer's disease through stimulating of non-amyloidogenic processing of amyloid precursor protein. European Review for Medical and Pharmacological Sciences. 2016;**20**(11):2389-2403

[90] Mudher A, Chapman S, Richardson J, Asuni A, Gibb G, Pollard C, Killick R, Iqbal T, Raymond L, Varndell I, Sheppard P, Makoff A, Gower E, Soden PE, Lewis P, Murphy M, Golde TE, Rupniak HT, Anderton BH, Lovestone S. Dishevelled regulates the metabolism of amyloid precursor protein via protein kinase C/mitogen-activated protein kinase and c-Jun terminal kinase. Journal of Neuroscience. 2001;**21**(14):4987-4995

[91] Ma G, Chen S, Wang X, Ba M, Yang H, Lu G. Short-term interleukin-1(beta) increases the release of secreted APP(alpha) via MEK1/2-dependent and JNK-dependent alpha-secretase cleavage in neuroglioma U251 cells. Journal of Neuroscience Research. 2005;**80**(5):683-692

Section 3

Neuroinflammation and Therapeutic Research

Chapter 6

A Review of Neuroinflammatory Mechanisms in Ischemic Stroke: Background and Therapeutic Approaches

Attila Sas, László Horváth, Csaba Oláh and
Attila Valikovics

Additional information is available at the end of the chapter

http://dx.doi.org/10.5772/intechopen.69234

Abstract

In this review, we will discuss the relevant clinical details of acute ischemic stroke and its currently very limited therapeutic opportunities, sequentially emphasizing its populational and economical burden. Based on our increasing knowledge in molecular and cell biology of immunological mechanisms of ischemic stroke, we will introduce the main processes in the background of arterial vessel occlusion, ensuing tissue damage and following reparation. After that, we will compare the obtained results from animal models with clinical studies and thus the possible causes of foregoing failures. Following this, we will demonstrate the most important drugs tested and/or being tested in human or animal studies from the field of neuroprotection. Finally, we raise possible opportunities that can be considered in development or clinical applications of neuroprotectants.

Keywords: acute ischemic stroke, stroke induced immunodepression, neuro-inflammation, neuroprotection, future perspectives

1. Introduction

In 2013, the Stroke Council of the American Heart Association/American Stroke Association laid an up-to-date definition of ischemic stroke. According to this, it is defined as brain, spinal cord or retinal cell death attributable to ischemia, based on neuropathological, neuroimaging and/or clinical evidence of permanent injury. In a clinical spectrum, it can be accompanied by symptoms or can be asymptomatic. Transient ischemic attack (TIA) is defined as a transient episode of neurological dysfunction caused by focal brain, spinal cord or retinal ischemia, without acute infarction [1].

Estimates from the Global Burden of Diseases, Injuries, and Risk Factors Study (GBD 2010) ranked stroke as the second most common cause of death [2] and the third most common cause of disability-adjusted life-years (DALYs) [3] worldwide in 2010. Expressed by numbers, roughly 10% of the 52,769,700 deaths [2] and about 4% of the 2,490,385,000 DALYs [3] worldwide were due to stroke. Further analysis of the GBD study showed that although stroke mortality rates and mortality-to-incidence ratios have decreased in the past two decades, the global burden of stroke in terms of the absolute number of people affected every year, stroke survivors, related deaths, and DALYs lost are great and increasing, with most of the burden in low-income and middle-income countries. If these trends in stroke incidence, mortality, and DALYs continue, by 2030, there will be almost 12 million stroke deaths, 70 million stroke survivors, and more than 200 million DALYs lost globally [4]. Furthermore, stroke changes the lives not only of those who experience a stroke but also of their family and other caregivers [5].

We can classify the stroke subtypes by aetiology. According to this, 80–85% of all stroke events are ischemic, the other 15–20% are of haemorrhagic origin [6]. The theme of our review is about ischemic stroke, so from now on, we will discuss only this subtype—means, that if 'stroke' is written, it refers to ischemic stroke automatically.

The ischemic stroke has its well-known risk factors, some of them are the common vascular risk factors. Among these, we can find so called non-modifiable ones: genetics, age, ethnicity/race, and low birth weight. Fortunately an international case-control study of 6000 individuals found that 10 potentially modifiable risk factors explained 90% of the risk of stroke [7]. These are—with no purpose of detailed description—physical inactivity with or without diet and nutrition failure (containing dyslipidaemia, obesity and body fat distribution, metabolic syndrome, diabetes mellitus) hypertension, cigarette smoking, atrial fibrillation and other cardiac conditions, carotid artery stenosis, sickle cell disease, migraine, alcohol consumption, drug abuse, sleep-disordered breathing [8].

Despite the intensive populational stroke education of these methods of primary prevention, the number of stroke patients increases to date.

After so many years of unsuccessful therapeutic approaches, recombinant tissue plasminogen activator (rtPA) was approved by the U.S. Food and Drug Administration (FDA) in 1996 for the treatment of acute ischemic stroke [9]. Since then, scores of stroke patients have been treated worldwide with this drug, managed by comprehensive stroke centres.

In a selected patient population (see detailed inclusion and exclusion criteria as per applied protocol), intravenous or intra-arterial thrombolysis can be a reliable choice. With this method of recanalisation, the treatment physician must calculate certain complications and a relatively poor outcome in several cases [10].

Most of these severely disabled stroke patients have intra- or extra-cranial large arterial vessel occlusion. In the past decade, a new form of acute revascularisation treatment, the endovascular stroke treatment (EST), appeared. After the failure of the first 'unhappy' trials with first-generation devices; in the past few years, smashing successes were achieved with the newer stent retrievers. These results—especially combined with iv thrombolysis—were comparably better than iv thrombolysis alone, and patient safety with risk/benefit ratio is also very promising [11].

Although several patients can benefit from the above mentioned methods of acute stroke treatment, they still have a few significant weak spots, above all, the narrow therapeutic time window.

Even in the countries with the best achievements, just like Austria with about 10% of stroke patients, can receive either or other treatment, the others, with wider stroke onset-to-treatment time have no or minimal chance of revascularisation, thus of good clinical outcome.

There is an urgent need to aim this enormous patient population with an effective treatment.

Neuroprotection would be a promising choice for this group, but until now, controversial results came to light in this field.

Hereinafter, we will introduce the main known reactions, immune responses in the brain following acute arterial vessel occlusion and potential therapeutic targets in this process.

2. Immunological background of acute stroke

2.1. First processes that appear immediately after arterial occlusion

The brain is highly dependent on continuous delivery of oxygen and glucose through blood flow, and the permanent interruption of this supply leads to irretrievable brain damage [12]. Cascade of cellular and molecular events caused by sudden lack of blood flow ends in ischemic cell death via necrosis or apoptosis. Among cells traceable in the brain, the neurons are more vulnerable than glia and vascular cells, and suffering from hypoxia-ischemia, these are the first ones to become dysfunctional and die [13]. Neurons can further be divided particularly into sensitive ones by location: the caudate body, putamen, insular ribbon, paracentral lobule, precentral-, middle- and inferior-frontal gyri [14].

In clinical practice, one of the most common types of severe stroke is the occlusion of the middle cerebral artery (MCA). This is also the one that provides a basis for animal models, as will be discussed later. After MCA occlusion, the ischemic damage will be more rapid and severe in the centre of the infracted territory—named the ischemic core— where the blood flow is the lowest. The periphery of the core is a region, the so called penumbra, where neuronal damage develops more slowly, because blood flow from adjacent vascular territories (collateral flow) provides a barely acceptable cerebral perfusion, that is enough to avoid immediate cell death [12]. In the core, a bioenergetic failure develops after a few seconds of arterial occlusion. Without oxygen and glucose, neurons cannot produce ATP needed to fuel the ionic pumps—most of all Na/K ATPase—that maintain the ionic gradient across neuronal membrane. This process results in accumulation of Na and Ca ions and efflux of K contributing to a widespread anoxic depolarisation in the membranes of neurons and glial cells, to swelling (cytotoxic oedema), degeneration of the cell organelles, loss of membrane integrity and finally the necrotic cell death [13, 15–17]. In contrast with the core, the flow reduction in the penumbra is not sufficient to cause energy failure, and the neurons remain viable for a prolonged period of time [12].

The before-mentioned reduced ATP production also contributes to reduced reuptake of glutamate, the main excitatory neurotransmitter. The resulting over activation of the NMDA type glutamate receptors leads to further cytoplasmatic accumulation of Ca ions. Because of the elevated intracellular Ca level, mitochondrial failure sets in, and Ca-dependent enzymes activate mainly in neurons, rather than astrocytes, such as proteases calpain and caspase and enzymes producing nitric oxide, free radicals (reactive oxygen species: ROS) and arachidonic acid metabolites [13, 18]. Besides these steps, the constant arterial occlusion results in a critical reduction of pO_2 and concomitant elevation of pCO_2 that leads to hypercapnia and falling of tissue pH. This process ends in lactate acidosis and irreversible cell injury mediated by Ca^- permeable acid-sensing ion channels [19–21]. Altogether, these steps lead to necrosis or apoptosis depending on the intensity of the insult and the metabolic state of the neurons.

2.2. Inflammatory mechanisms in the ischemic brain

Cerebral ischemia contributes to both, first the innate and then, the adaptive immunity, the two main branches of human immune system [22]. The innate immunity is germline-coded, rapidly activated and consists of low-affinity receptors to gain wide-range target recognition. In contrast, the adaptive immune system is based on high-affinity receptors (like immunoglobulins and T-cell receptors), that are randomly generated by somatic mutations. The adaptive branch needs several days for activation because of antigen-driven clonal cell expansion, but it retains a memory of this certain antigen exposure [22].

Immediately after vessel occlusion, post-ischemic inflammation begins in the vascular compartment. With appearance of ROS, the procoagulant state increases that means platelet, complement and endothelial cell activation [23, 24]. Besides this effect, ROS—that are produced by NADPH oxidase and iNOS, traceable in almost all inflammatory cells, and the synthesized peroxynitrite and its hydroxyl radical derivates are highly cytotoxic—alters cellular proteins, lipids, RNA, leading to cell dysfunction or death [25]. Blood brain barrier (BBB) breakdown starts—secondary to the pericyte death—as its permeability increases by oxidative stress and inflammatory mediators, impairing the neurovascular unit, that consists of endothelial cells, astrocytes and neurons. Along this process, extravasation of proteins and activation of macrophages initiates [26, 27].

Injured and dying cells play a key role in post-ischemic inflammation by releasing danger signals, the so-called damage-associated molecular patterns (DAMPs). These molecules activate macrophages via pattern recognition receptors (PRR, i.e. toll like receptors—TLR) and inflammasomes. The first pathway involves such pro-inflammatory factors that get released by nuclear gene expression mediated by transcriptional mediators, activated by TLR.

Studies highlighted importance of these TLRs in mediation of inflammation. In transgenic mice, lacking TLR2 and TLR4, much smaller brain infarcts were observed [28, 29]. In a clinical trial, patients, who exhibited reduced expression of TLR 4, had a better outcome [30].

The second mechanism means caspase-1 activation that results in pro-inflammatory IL-1, IL-6 and IL-18 activation [31, 32]. Besides macrophage activation and thus pro-inflammatory cytokines release, this process also results in mast cells releasing vasoactive mediators, proteases and tumour necrosis factor (TNF).

As part of the innate immune system, complement system is also involved in cerebral ischemic tissue changes. Mannose-binding lectin (MBL) and MBL-associated serine proteases initiate lectin pathway of complement activation. Animal experiment with transgenic mice lacking MBL showed reduced infarct size. Clinical observation showed that patients with low MBL genotype expressed lower levels of C3-C4 complement and C-reactive protein (CRP), showing better functional outcome [33–35].

Monocytes also take part in the regulation of inflammation and tissue repair. They can be found early in the infarcted area shortly after vessel occlusion [36, 37]. In acute stroke, these cells increase in number in peripheral blood and show such phenotypic changes as reduced expressions of antigen presenting molecules, and low production of pro-inflammatory TNF, and unchanged production of anti-inflammatory IL-10 [38, 39]. These cells will differentiate into two sub-types. M1 macrophages promote strong T-helper1 (Th1), while M2 macrophages support Th2 response, playing a part in the resolution of inflammation [36]. Macrophages also play a great role in clearance of debris and damaged cells at later stages as a regenerative process [36].

Immune cell extravasation is initiated by interaction of adhesion molecules and selectins that contributes to a rolling mechanism of leukocytes on endothelium followed by adhesion and to subsequent transmigration to the brain parenchyma (leukocyte infiltration).

In response to ischemia, glial cells develop an inflammatory phenotype and release such mediators that attract neutrophils, monocytes and lymphocytes.

The increasing number of these cells and the produced pro-inflammatory mediators by them, rapidly results in a progrediation of inflammation and thus ischemic tissue damage. The before-mentioned DAMPs induced release of interleukins by macrophages and microglia, leading to further leukocyte infiltration and activation of antigen presentation between dendritic cells (DC) with MHC II receptors and T-cells [40, 41].

These infiltrating T-cells are the main source of interferon gamma that is responsible for delayed neurotoxic effect of the brain tissue [42]. Blockage of lymphocyte invasion of the brain by FTY720 improved stroke outcome in animal models, but was not verified by other study [43]. Gamma-delta T-cell sub-population and IL-17, IL-23 have a crucial role of damage progression. These cells are activated by infiltrating macrophages and DAMPs, produce pro-inflammatory IFN gamma and IL-17. Depletion of these cells or pharmacological blockade of IL-17 and IL-23 pathways suppressed brain damage in a mouse model [44]. Depletion of CD4 and CD8 T cells and ablation of perforin that mediates cytotoxicity of CD8 T cells also reduced infarct size and improved stroke outcome in experimental stroke model [42].

Cell damage and disruption lead to exposition of such brain epitopes that were previously hidden from the immune system. The antigen presenting cells (APCs) recognise these epitopes and take part in lymphocyte priming and auto-reactive activation. These auto-reactive lymphocytes worsen the local inflammation resulting in poor outcome. In clinical experiments, neuronal and myelin epitopes were found in cervical lymph nodes and palatine tonsils of acute stroke patients. Relative neuronal predominance of these epitopes was associated with poorer clinical outcome [45].

2.3. Cytoprotective effects and reparation of damaged tissue

Besides so many damaging effects of the immune system, there are cytoprotective ones as well.

In animal models, T-cells that are specific to myelin antigens can reduce secondary neuro-degeneration, enhance neurogenesis and promote recovery after stroke [46]. Local immune suppression can be achieved with tolerized lymphocytes to CNS antigens. In rodent model, immunisation with intra-nasal or oral administration of MBP or MOG weeks before induced stroke showed better outcome [47]. According to these studies, patients with a history of stroke may benefit of CNS antigen immunisation, and we could prevent a recurrent stroke, but recent studies raised concerns on this. We can induce a deleterious auto-immune process against the brain by such drugs [48, 49].

T reg cells are the main protectors of the brain after ischemia. They can exert anti-inflammatory effects by either direct cell-cell interaction or secretion of tumour growth factor beta (TGF-β) and IL-10 as well [50]. Depletion of these cells in mice increased infarct size [42] and enhanced activation of invading pro-inflammatory T-cells [51].

Regulatory B-cells are also reported as beneficial ones after experimental models. Lack of these cells resulted in increased inflammatory cell infiltration and conversely, transfer of these cells reduced infarct size and pro-inflammatory cytokine production of T-cells [52].

The immunological processes following brain ischemia is self limiting, and numerous factors play a role in the immunosuppressive activity. The first mechanism in the reparative phase is performed by microglia and macrophages. These phagocytes remove the dead cells and accompanying immunoregulatory cytokines can facilitate tissue repair. Concomitant growth factors (like TGF-β and insulin like growth factor) released by neurons and astrocytes help in cell sprouting, neurogenesis, angiogenesis and matrix reorganisation as well. Angiogenesis also required the concomitant action of vascular endothelial growth factor (VEGF) and neutrophil matrix metallo-proteases (MMPs) [53–55].

2.4. Stroke-induced immunodepression and related post stroke infections

Acute stroke can result a stroke-induced immune depression syndrome (SIID) [56, 57].

The central nervous system has multiple pathways to modulate the systemic immunity. Among these are hypothalamic-pituitary-adrenerg axis, the vagus nerve, and the sympathetic nervous system. Complex functional reactions between these systems together suppress the peripheral release of inflammatory cytokines from T-cells, monocytes and macrophages and promote the release of anti-inflammatory IL-10. The released noradrenalin from nerve terminals and adrenal medulla induces an anti-inflammatory type of lymphocytes, monocytes and macrophages. These mechanisms together reduce the inflammation in the infarcted brain area, but parallel to this, suppress the systemic immune responses, giving a chance for post-stroke infections.

An unknown proportion of patients are affected by this condition, because there is no commonly accepted definition for this, and representative investigations in large stroke patient population are missing. It can only be estimated, as about 30% post-stroke infections were reported [56].

It was confirmed in a meta-analysis of 87 studies involving more than 130,000 patients, published in 2011, that the overall infection rate was 30%, most commonly pneumonia and urinary tract infections [58]. According to a multicenter retrospective cohort study including consecutive patients with ischemic stroke admitted to Regional Stroke Centers participating in the Registry of Canadian Stroke Network in July 2003-March 2007 pneumonia increased 30 days and 1 year mortality as well [59]. Statistical analysis showed that half of the pneumonia cases occurred in the first two days after stroke onset, but almost all cases occurred in the first week [60]. The most susceptible patients for aquiring pneumonia as a concomitant disease, are the ones who have dysphagia, even with aspiration, are of older age, and the male sex, stroke severity, chronic obstructive pulmonary disease, coronary artery disease and pre-stroke dependency (greater than 2 points in modified ranking scale mRS) are also independent risk factors for pneumonia [61, 62].

According to urinary tract infections, a study showed 16% prevalence in stroke patients mostly in the first two weeks after stroke onset [63].

A few trials detected correlation between the locations of infarction in the brain, resulting in a higher risk for post-stroke infection. Affection of the anterior MCA cortex, and the insula caused more infections; however, other study found that the extent of the infarcted brain tissue is a better prognostic factor for this [64–66].

Many clinical studies were conducted to evaluate the benefit of prophylactic use of antibiotics in stroke patients, but according to the latest AHA/ASA guideline for secondary stroke prevention [10], routine use of prophylactic antibiotics has not been shown to be beneficial (class III, level B recommendation).However in selected patient population, it can be considered.

3. Challenges in neuroprotection

Neuroprotection can be defined as a therapy that enhances the brain's resilience to ischemia to improve the clinical outcome of affected patients. It aims not only the neurons but also is equally applicable to other brain constituents like cells of vessels and glia. A neuroprotective drug is designed to target one or more components of ischemic cascade. The disappointing results of the neuroprotective trials to date raise the question that successes in pre-clinical animal models can even translate in clinical practice [67–69].

4. Reasons why neuroprotective agents have failed in human stroke trials

It is almost impossible to create a true, representative model for human acute ischemic stroke (AIS). In laboratory, scientists work with animals. They are mostly rats, or other rodents, in that several physiological processes differ from ones in human. In addition, these animals are basically healthy and not suffering from such civilisational concomitant diseases, like hypertonia, diabetes and dyslipidemia. They are not exposed to smoke, and not influenced by other unhealthy conditions, just to emphasize some factors.

As a basic of stroke, patients usually develop atherosclerotic disease over decades, causing decaying cerebral autoregulation, poorer collateral system, etc. while in laboratory, animals are tested as a sudden occlusion of the MCA on the ground, besides healthy vessel system. Many patients take medications, prescribed for cardiovascular (CV) risk factors, that affect the ischemic process and that can interact with the investigational neuroprotective drugs [70–73].

Last but not the least, a few more practical factors to consider.

- Clinical trials have real life difficulties like time window (pre-clinical studies usually using such short time window that are unfeasible in real life).
- The optimal duration of neuroprotectant administration is unknown (only the start of administration seems to be clear as early as possible).
- Outcome measure is different in pre-clinical trials, where particularly infarct size is judged to evaluate efficacy of a drug, while clinical trials use clinical and functional scales, such as National Institutes of Health Stroke Scale (NIHSS), modified Rankin Scale (mRS), Barthel index, etc.
- Pre-clinical trials evaluate mainly early outcomes, while clinical ones rely on late assessments.
- In laboratory, scientists use just a very few stroke models, most widespread are the transient and permanent middle cerebral artery occlusion models (tMCAO and pMCAO), while in human studies, patients develop a broad pathophysiological heterogenity of stroke in duration, extent, location and severity [74].

In spite of all these difficulties, there is still a massive trend of drug development in this field. In the course of past unsuccessful trials, we have become more and more aware of each molecular or cellular step of the ischemic cascade, and the knowledge gained from these experiments helped us to understand the immunological processes beyond tissue damage after stroke.

5. Therapeutic approaches in the field of neuroprotection

In pre-clinical phase of studies, over a thousand of potential neuroprotective agents have been investigated to date and many of them seemed to be promising. They aimed one or more steps of the above mentioned ischemic cascade to minimize the tissue injury. Different therapeutic approaches, tried on animals and/or in clinical trials will be discussed below sorted by mechanism of action [73, 74].

As discussed before, immediately after ischemia onset, a few processes lead to excessive activation of excitatory amino acid receptors, accumulation of intra-cellular calcium and release of toxic products that all results in cell damage.

5.1. NMDA antagonists

The most widely studied neuroprotective agents are the N-methyl-D-aspartate (NMDA) receptor antagonists. The first neuroprotective drug applied in human trial was also a non-competitive NMDA antagonist. It was *dextrorphan*, a metabolite of the cough suppressant dextrometorpohan. Further investigation was stopped because of occurred hallucinations and hypotension as adverse events [75].

A competitive NMDA antagonist *CGS 19755 or selfotel* reduced infarct size by 50% with 40 mg/kg dose in animal studies [76], but in a phase III trial, with a total of 567 enrolled patients, a higher mortality rate was observed than in the placebo group, so it was terminated [77, 78].

Two non-competitive NMDA antagonists were tested in placebo controlled trials (*MK801 or dizocilpine and aptiganel HCL-Cerestat*) but they were terminated because of poor risk-benefit ratio and hallucination [79, 80]. These frightening adverse reactions mimic those seen with phencyclidine which binds at a similar site.

This recognition led to development of indirect NMDA antagonists that connects with the glycine site of the NMDA receptor and thus has fewer side effects [81]. Prominent representative of this glycine antagonist group was *GV150526*, which was well tolerated and reported as safe in a trial with 1367 patients but showed no positive effect in 3-month outcome measures, so no further investigations were planned [82].

In a recent pre-clinical study, investigating NMDA modulation with post-synaptic density-95 (PSD-95) protein inhibitor *NA-1* that uncouple PSD-95 from neurotoxic signalling pathways in neurons, showed promising result. This trial was conducted not with rodents, but primate class cynomolgus macaques, in which animals have closer genetic, anatomic and behavioural relationship with humans. They found reduced infarct volumes and significantly better neurological function in neuro-behavioural tests in the NA-1 treated group [83]. NA-1 was also tested in patients, who underwent endovascular aneurysm coiling, to prevent small embolic strokes, that can occur during such procedure (evaluating neuroprotection in aneurysm coiling therapy [ENACT]). It was a multicentre, double-blind, placebo-controlled, randomized trial, with 185 participants. They received either a single dose of NA-1 infusion or saline at the termination of the coiling procedure and were evaluated with MRI and neuro-psychological tests in a 30-day follow-up period. The subjects, who received NA-1, developed fewer emollitions, and by patients with ruptured aneurysms, NA-1 reduced the number of stroke events, volume of tissue damage and improved neurological outcome in 30 days [84].

5.2. Free-radical scavengers and antioxidants

In a murine model of stroke, animals treated with *carnosine*, a naturally occurring dipeptide with several neuroprotective properties, developed significantly decreased infarct size when administered both before and after induction of ischemia. This neuroprotective effect was related to decreased level of reactive oxygen species, preserved glutathione levels and attenuated matrix metallo-protease (MMP) levels and activity [85, 86].

Anthocyanins (isolated from tart cherry) are strong antioxidants and thus have anti-inflammatory effects. In a mouse model, it reduced infarct volume significantly by 27% pre-treated and by 25% in delayed treatment and was associated with better functional outcome in both pre- and post-treated group. These effects are considered to decrease level of superoxide in brain and blockage of apoptosis-inducing factor released from mitochondria [87].

Ebselen, a seleno-organic compound with antioxidant effect mediated by a glutathione peroxidase like action, was evaluated in a multicentre, double blind, placebo-controlled trial with 302 patients [88]. A positive effect was found at 1 and 3 months follow-up in functional scores. However, the final results are still not available [89].

Edaravone, another free radical scavenger was investigated in more clinical studies. Administered in 72 hours of stroke onset, better functional scores were observed compared with placebo, especially in small vessel disease [90, 91]. However, there were no significant differences in outcome after 1 year against placebo group [91].

NXY-059, also a free radical trapping agent, was found to be effective in animal models [92].

Two large trials were conducted to evaluate this drug. In SAINT I., administered in 6 hours after stroke onset, it showed controversial results in functional scales (better outcome by mRS, but not by NIHSS). Following SAINT II, NXY-059 was found safe but ineffective compared to placebo. This result was confirmed by another study by Diener et al. [93–95].

Citicoline is an intermediate in the biosynthesis of phosphatidylcholine (PtdCho) showed reduced infarct volume in animal model of stroke [96]. It enhances the synthesis of PtdCho and sphingomyelin, attenuates lipid peroxidation and restores Na/K ATP-ase activity. In ICTUS study, with 2298 patients from 2006 to 2011, it was not effective in the treatment of stroke [97]. In a clinical trial, that compared edaravone and citicoline in AIS, edaravone was more effective and showed a better neurological outcome at 3-month follow-up [98].

Cerebrolysin, a porcine brain-derived preparation of low-molecular-weight neuropeptide and free amino acids, showed improved functionality in animal models, but not in clinical trials (CASTA) [99].

Tirilazad is a non-glucocorticoid, 21-aminosteroid that inhibits lipid peroxidation. It was effective in animal models of focal ischemia, by reducing infarct volume by 29.2% and improved neuro-behavioral scores by 48.1%. However, it did not show any significant effects in clinical trials of AIS [100, 101].

5.3. Excitotoxicity and magnesium

Magnesium has a multi-pathway neuro-protective effect, as it antagonizes calcium channels, it is also a non-competitive NMDA antagonist, inhibits excitatory neurotransmitter release and relaxes vascular smooth muscles. It was observed that magnesium also antagonize the vaso-constrictive effect of endothelin 1, thus ameliorates cerebral blood flow [102, 103]. Eighty percent of acute stroke patients show a significantly decreased serum ionized magnesium level [104]. As a phase III, double blind, placebo-controlled, randomized trial, with 1700 patients, the FAST-MAG was the first of the pre-hospital administered neuroprotectant trials.

It was designed to overcome the drawback of the delayed administration of neuro-protective agents in prior clinical trials, which has demonstrated that initiation of magnesium by paramedics in the field within 2 hours of symptom onset is feasible and safe; however, it did not improve disability outcomes at 90 days [105]. Based on the somewhat positive results, a large Phase III clinical trial is ongoing [106], to investigate if magnesium is effective when administrated by emergency medical service personnel between 15 min and 2 hours after stroke onset.

5.4. GABA agonists

Clomethiazole, as a gamma-aminobutyric acid (GABA) agonist, can decrease excitatory neurotransmission by increasing activity of inhibitory pathways. It is widely used as anti-convulsant or sedative. In pre-clinical trials, clomethiazole appeared to be effective both in focal and global cerebral ischemia, at plasma concentrations known to be well-tolerated by patients [107]. In the CLASS I, randomized, double blind, multicentre, placebo-controlled trial with 1198 severe stroke patients, this drug did not improve disability, or reduced infarct volume, administered as a 24 hours intravenous infusion within 12 hours of stroke onset. As predicted, primary side effect was sedation [108].

5.5. AMPA antagonists

The α-amino-3-hydroxy-5-methyl-4-isoxazole propionic acid (AMPA) receptor is a non-NMDA-type ionotropic transmembrane receptor for glutamate that mediates fast synaptic transmission in the central nervous system (CNS).

ZK 200775 reduced infarct size in animal model of tMCAO [109]. In clinical trial, it transiently worsened the neurological condition of the stroke patients by neuronal dysfunction, glial cell toxicity and sedation [110].

YM872 pre-clinically showed reduced infarct volume in rats and was neuro-protective by restoring cortical cells and decreasing oedema in traumatic brain injury [111]. Two clinical trials were conducted, the ARTIST MRI and ARTIST+, in the second one, with combined administration of alteplase. The drug was given within 6 hours of stroke onset in a 24-hour infusion. Both of them stopped after interim analysis, but results are still not available since 2003 [112].

5.6. Ion channel blockers or modulators and chelators

More than 50% of the total synthesized ATP in the brain is for maintaining the energy-dependent ion pumps, the ones that are responsible for maintaining the ionic balance between intra- and extra-cellular compartments. In two minutes after stroke, total ATP level in the brain significantly decreases, triggering an ionic imbalance of intra-cellularly decreasing K and increasing Na ions, that results membrane depolarization [113, 114]. After this anoxic depolarization, neuronal death starts along with the opening of the voltage gated Ca channels, thus causing intra-cellular Ca overload, resulting in cell death pathways discussed earlier.

Animal studies revealed that in the penumbra, a rapid de- and re-polarisation happens, causing further neuronal damage [115].

Na channel blockers (phenytoin, carbamazepine, lamotrigine, sipatrigine (619C89) and riluzole) are believed to reduce the elevated Na influx and thus the following damaging pathways in AIS and are investigated in clinical trials. The ones with sipatrigine and fosphenytoin were terminated due to toxicity and lack of efficacy [116–120].

A drug, named lubeluzole, has effects that are not completely clear. It blocks Na channels and reduces the release of nitric oxide. Trials could not confirm its positive effects in AIS patients [121, 122].

Ca channel blockers were also strongly investigated, unfortunately without significant positive effect. A clinical trial with nimodipin (VENUS) was terminated after enrolling 439 acute stroke patients within 6 hours of symptom onset because of lack of efficacy [123]. A large meta-analysis of 22 T- and L-type Ca antagonist trials in AIS found no benefit of this family of drug. A possible explanation for this can be that such Ca antagonists caused hypotension and thus impaired auto-regulation of cerebral circulation by acute stroke patients, and this effect is known to be harmful for penumbral neurons to survive [124]. For future trials, N-type Ca channel blocker can be a promising choice with less hypotensive effect.

K channel modulators showed hopeful results in animal stroke models. However, BMS-204352 (MaxiPost), a fluorooxindole K channel opener, did not reveal significant benefit in an extensive phase III trial (POST), that enrolled 1978 AIS patients in 200 centres worldwide [125].

Zinc is neurotoxic in cerebral ischemia in an environment of impaired ionic homeosthasis. *Zinc chelator DP-b99* presented positive effect in pre-clinical and phase II trials, but not in a phase III, double blind, placebo-controlled, multicentre, randomized study (MACSI), where severe stroke patients were included within 9 hours of stroke onset, and received four dose of drug infusion in four consecutive days. Unfortunately it did not show any positive effect.

5.7. Albumin

Animal studies highlighted that albumin's neuroprotective effects are related to its antioxidant properties, preservation of microvascular integrity, decreasing endothelial cell apoptosis, hemodilution, and mobilization of free fatty acids [126]. In the ALIAS study, 82 acute stroke patients received either iv. albumin and rtPA or iv. albumin alone. Albumin-related adverse events like pulmonary oedema were mild or moderate in severity. Patients who received a higher dose of albumin presented significantly better clinical outcome than subjects treated with lower dose of the drug [127]. These findings led to ALIAS 2 trial, where albumin therapy was compared with placebo. It was terminated on the basis of interim analysis [128].

5.8. Inflammatory cascade inhibition

In ischemic stroke, tissue damage develops by processes such as endothelial activation, pro-inflammatory and pro-thrombotic interactions between endothelium and different circulating blood elements, resulting in thrombogenesis [129]. Cell adhesion is directed by different adhesion molecules. Animal stroke studies proved that administered anti-adhesion antibody can decrease infarct size [130].

Enlimomab, a mono-clonal anti-ICAM antibody, was investigated in a phase III trial (EAST) in patients with AIS. Six hundred patients within 6 hours of stroke onset received either boluses of enlimomab or placebo for five days. Unfortunately, it was associated with greater mortality, compared with the placebo group. Patients in enlimomab group often had fevers and developed an immune response to the murine antibody [131]. Humanized antibody could be a rational choice for research to avoid this adverse reaction.

Hu23F2G or LeukArrest is a humanized IgG1 antibody against CD18, thus blocking leukocyte infiltration in AIS. In a phase III trial, with patients within 12 hours of stroke onset, that allowed concomitant use of rtPA, LeukArrest had unfavourable results.

Tacroliums (FK506), a drug for prevention of organ rejection after transplantation, was confirmed to have neuro-protective effect in animal model of pMCAO administered within 4 hours of stroke onset [132].

Statins have such pleiotropic effects, besides decreasing cholesterol levels, like modulating the immune system, increasing cerebral perfusion by up-regulating angiogenesis and by activation of survival signals [133]. Lovastatin was investigated in a phase IB trial (Neu-START) and showed the drug to be safe in different doses up to 3 days after AIS [134].

5.9. Other agents

Tetracycline class of antibiotics reduces leukocyte infiltration and improves stroke outcome. In addition, minocycline proved to inhibit caspase, inducible NOS and P38 MARK and can generate hypothermia. It can penetrate to CNS, has low cost and had positive effects in animal studies, so it is a good neuroprotectant candidate. A dose finding IB study of minocycline in patients within 6 hours of stroke resulted in significantly better outcome compared with placebo group [135]. It was also safe and tolerable to administer with combination of rtPA. It can decrease matrix metallo-protease 9 (MMP 9) levels, which occurs with rtPA associated cerebral haemorrhage. Based on these result, a phase III study Neu-MAST is ongoing.

Antiplatelet antibodies inhibit platelet aggregation, thus prevent additional ischemic injury. Abciximab (ReoPro) was investigated in a phase III AIS trial (AbESTT II), but the lack of efficacy and the increased rate of symptomatic and fatal intra-cranial haemorrhage led to termination of the study [136].

Citicoline is used in membrane biosynthesis. It can stabilize membranes and decrease free radical formation. A phase II, then a few phase III trials were conducted, with somewhat promising trend, but finally no such significant positive effect was found that would led the drug to clinical practice [97, 137–139].

Fiblast, a fibroblast growth factor, can regulate neuronal healing after ischemic injury. After promising first data from clinical trials, a large study that evaluated its efficacy in stroke patients within 6 hours of stroke onset, was terminated because of poor risk-to-benefit ratio [140].

Autologous mesenchymal stem cell therapy has also promising data, additional trials are in progress [141].

GSK249320 is an anti-MAG (myelin-associated glycoprotein) antibody. MAG inhibits axon outgrowth after neuronal injury. Dose finding studies were completed till now [142].

Hypothermia showed significant pre-clinical efficacy in animal models. In stroke patients, it can be executed either by surface cooling or in an endovascular way. COAST II, CHILI, Euro-Hyp trials investigate the process in stroke patients [143, 144].

Uric Acid was evaluated in a phase III study (URICO-ICTUS). It was administered together with rtPA within 4.5 hours of stroke onset. It was finished in Oct. 2013, but no study results are available yet [145].

Studies with *Cromolyn, Dapsone, Cyclosporin A and Pioglitazone* are still in progress [146–149].

6. Conclusion and future perspective

Currently, the predominant atmosphere in the field of neuroprotectant research is frustrating. In the past decades, over a thousand neuro-protective agents were proved to be safe and effective in animal trials but failed to show proper effect in human trials. Since 1996, when FDA approved rtPA, there has not been any other drug that could be suitable in the treatment of AIS.

The main differences between animal and human studies were discussed above that can be a possible explanation for ineffectiveness. Therapeutic benefit from neuroprotection can only be appraisable, before ischemic damage is complete (we can only save tissue, if there is something left to save). Most studies aim the penumbra, the potentially salvageable region after ischemic stroke. An ideal neuroprotectant would be effective in safely halting or slowing stroke progression and improve clinical outcome. Unfortunately, the extent of the penumbra is highly individual and depends not only on stroke onset time, but also on a few other factors, such as site of arterial occlusion, collateral circulation, blood pressure, pre-stroke condition of the affected brain region, etc.

Another practical difficulty in neuroprotectant studies is that in developed countries, the rtPA is a standard of care and can be administered in a 3–4.5 hours time window. Even endovascular therapy of AIS is spreading in stroke centres recently, with a wider therapeutic timeframe (even 6 hours or more from stroke onset in selected patients). This is exactly the same time range, when neuroprotectants could also be effective according to animal studies, and clinical experience as well. It leads to a conflict in application of a test drug because only a heterogeneous patient population remains to enrol to a study, who somehow could not participate in either or other re-canalisation therapy (too mild or too sever stroke, haemorrhagic stroke, medical or surgical history, blood tests, etc.).

The first pre-hospital trial, the FAST-MAG evaded this difficulty, when the neuroprotectant was administered before hospital arrival, reaching a very favourable onset to treatment time. However, these populations with stroke-like symptoms were really heterogeneous, with no preceding brain imaging, and thus the lack of proper patient selection. But, this study raised the concept of safely administering a neuroprotective drug complementary with an already approved re-canalisation therapy, because these drugs not necessarily display adverse effects in patients treated otherwise.

In connection with mechanism of action, there is also a concept that an administered neuroprotectant should aim not only a single target of the ischemic cascade, but more, or administering a 'stroke cocktail' to a patient with a selection of drugs is also an interesting idea.

Anyway, researchers with grim determination are still on the issue of developing neuroprotectant drugs, and hopefully, we will have positive results in the near future.

Author details

Attila Sas[1]*, László Horváth[1], Csaba Oláh[2,3] and Attila Valikovics[1]

*Address all correspondence to: sas.attila@gmail.com

1 Department of Stroke, Vascular- and General Neurology, and Toxicology, Borsod County University Teaching Hospital, Miskolc, Hungary

2 Department of Neurosurgery, Borsod County University Teaching Hospital, Miskolc, Hungary

3 Department of Interventional Radiology, Borsod County University Teaching Hospital, Miskolc, Hungary

References

[1] Easton JD, Saver JL, Albers GW, Alberts MJ, Chaturvedi S, Feldmann E, Hatsukami TS, Higashida RT, Johnston SC, Kidwell CS, Lutsep HL, Miller E, Sacco RL. Definition and evaluation of transient ischemic attack: A scientific statement for healthcare professionals from the American Heart Association/American Stroke Association Stroke Council; Council on Cardiovascular Surgery and Anesthesia; Council on Cardiovascular Radiology and Intervention; Council on Cardiovascular Nursing; and the Interdisciplinary Council on Peripheral Vascular Disease. Stroke. 2009;**40**:2276-2293

[2] Lozano R, Naghavi M, Foreman K, et al. Global and regional mortality from 235 causes of death for 20 age groups in 1990 and 2010: A systematic analysis for the Global Burden of Disease Study 2010. Lancet. 2012;**380**:2095-2128

[3] Feigin VL, Lawes CM, Bennett DA, Barker-Collo SL, Parag V. Worldwide stroke incidence and early case fatality reported in 56 population-based studies: A systematic review. Lancet Neurology. 2009;**8**:355-369

[4] Feigin VL, Forouzanfar MH, Krishnamurthi R, Mensah GA, Connor M, Bennett DA, Moran AE, Sacco RL, Anderson L, Truelsen T, O'Donnell M, Venketasubramanian N, Barker-Collo S, Lawes CMM, Wang W, Shinohara Y, Witt E, Ezzati M, Naghavi M,

Murray C. Global and regional burden of stroke during 1990-2010: Findings from the Global Burden of Disease Study 2010. Lancet. 2014;**383**(9913):245-254

[5] Samsa GP, Matchar DB, Goldstein L, Bonito A, Duncan PW, Lipscomb J, Enarson C, Witter D, Venus P, Paul JE, Weinberger M. Utilities for major stroke: Results from a survey of preferences among persons at increased risk for stroke. American Heart Journal. 1998;**136**(pt 1):703-713

[6] Sacco RL, Kasner SE, Broderick JP, Caplan LR, Connors JJ, Culebras A, Elkind MS, George MG, Hamdan AD, Higashida RT, Hoh BL, Janis LS, Kase CS, Kleindorfer DO, Lee JM, Moseley ME, Peterson ED, Turan TN, Valderrama AL, Vinters HV; American Heart Association Stroke Council, Council on Cardiovascular Surgery and Anesthesia; Council on Cardiovascular Radiology and Intervention; Council on Cardiovascular and Stroke Nursing; Council on Epidemiology and Prevention; Council on Peripheral Vascular Disease; Council on Nutrition, Physical Activity and Metabolism. Stroke. 2013;**44**:2064-2089

[7] O'Donnell MJ, Xavier D, Liu L, Zhang H, Chin SL, Rao-Melacini P, Rangarajan S, Islam S, Pais P, McQueen MJ, Mondo C, Damasceno A, Lopez-Jaramillo P, Hankey GJ, Dans AL, Yusoff K, Truelsen T, Diener HC, Sacco RL, Ryglewicz D, Czlonkowska A, Weimar C, Wang X, Yusuf S, INTERSTROKE Investigators. Risk factors for ischaemic and intracerebral haemorrhagic stroke in 22 countries (the INTERSTROKE study): A case-control study. Lancet. 2010;**376**:112-123

[8] Meschia JF, Bushnell C, Boden-Albala B, Braun LT, Bravata DM, Chaturvedi S, Creager MA, Eckel RH, Elkind MS, Fornage M, Goldstein LB, Greenberg SM,Horvath SE, Iadecola C, Jauch EC, Moore WS, Wilson JA; American Heart Association Stroke Council; Council on Cardiovascular and Stroke Nursing;Council on Clinical Cardiology; Council on Functional Genomics and Translational Biology; Council on Hypertension. Stroke. 2014;**45**(12):3754-3832

[9] Zivin JA. Acute stroke therapy with tissue plasminogen activator (tPA) since it was approved by the U.S. Food and Drug Administration (FDA). Annals of Neurology. 2009;**66**(1):6-10. DOI: 10.1002/ana.21750

[10] Kernan WN, Ovbiagele B, Black HR, Bravata DM, Chimowitz MI, Ezekowitz MD, Fang MC, Fisher M, Furie KL, Heck DV, Johnston SC, Kasner SE, Kittner SJ,Mitchell PH, Rich MW, Richardson D, Schwamm LH, Wilson JA; American Heart Association Stroke Council, Council on Cardiovascular and Stroke Nursing, Council on Clinical Cardiology, and Council on Peripheral Vascular Disease. Stroke. 2014;**45**(7):2160-2236

[11] von Gadow N, Nikoubashman O, Freiherr J, Block F, Reich A, Fesl G, Wiesmann M. Endovascular stroke treatment now and then—procedural and clinical effectiveness and safety of different mechanical thrombectomy techniques over time. Quantitative Imaging in Medicine and Surgery. 2017;**7**(1):1-7

[12] Moskowitz MA, Lo EH, Iadecola C. The science of stroke: Mechanisms in search of treatments. Neuron. 2010;**67**:181-198. [PubMed: 20670828]

[13] Lipton P. Ischemic cell death in brain neurons. Physiological Reviews. 1999;**79**:1431-1568. [PubMed: 10508238]

[14] Payabvash S, Souza LC, Wang Y, Schaefer PW, Furie KL, Halpern EF, et al. Regional ischemic vulnerability of the brain to hypoperfusion: The need for location specific computed tomography perfusion thresholds in acute stroke patients. Stroke. 2011;**42**:1255-1260

[15] Hertz L. Bioenergetics of cerebral ischemia: A cellular perspective. Neuropharmacology. 2008;**55**:289-309

[16] Rossi DJ, Brady JD, Mohr C. Astrocyte metabolism and signaling during brain ischemia. Nature Neuroscience. 2007;**10**:1377-1386

[17] Kaplan JH. Biochemistry of Na,K-ATPase. Annual Review of Biochemistry. 2002;**71**:511-535

[18] Kahlert S, Zündorf G, Reiser G. Glutamate-mediated influx of extracellular Ca^{2+} is coupled with reactive oxygen species generation in cultured hippocampal neurons but not in astrocytes. Journal of Neuroscience Research. 2005;**79**:262-271

[19] Sherwood TW, Lee KG, Gormley MG, Askwith CC. Heteromeric acid-sensing ion channels (ASICs) composed of ASIC2b and ASIC1a display novel channel properties and contribute to acidosis-induced neuronal death. Journal of Neuroscience Research. 2011;**31**:9723-9734

[20] Xiang Z, Yuan M, Hassen GW, Gampel M, Bergold PJ. Lactate induced excitotoxicity in hippocampal slice cultures. Experimental Neurology. 2004;**186**:70-77

[21] Xiong ZG, Zhu XM, Chu XP, Minami M, Hey J, Wei WL, et al. Neuroprotection in ischemia: Blocking calcium-permeable acid-sensing ion channels. Cell. 2004;**118**:687-698

[22] Abbas AK. Basic Immunology Updated Edition: Functions and Disorders of the Immune System. Antigen recognition in the adaptive immune system. Saunders; 2010;204-250

[23] Carden DL, Granger DN. Pathophysiology of ischaemia-reperfusion injury. Journal of Pathology. 2000;**190**:255-266

[24] Peerschke EI, Yin W, Ghebrehiwet B. Complement activation on platelets: Implications for vascular inflammation and thrombosis. Molecular Immunology. 2010;**47**:2170-2175

[25] Iadecola C, Zhang F, Xu X. Inhibition of inducible nitric oxide synthase ameliorates cerebral ischemic damage. American Journal of Physiology. 1995;**268**:R286–R292. [PubMed: 7530927]

[26] Kim JY, Kawabori M, Yenari MA. Innate inflammatory responses in stroke: Mechanisms and potential therapeutic targets. Current Medicinal Chemistry. 2014;**21**:2076-2097

[27] Hall CN, Reynell C, Gesslein B, Hamilton NB, Mishra A, Sutherland BA, et al. Capillary pericytes regulate cerebral blood flow in health and disease. Nature. 2014;**508**:55-60

[28] Caso JR, et al. Toll-like receptor 4 is involved in brain damage and inflammation after experimental stroke. Circulation. 2007;**115**:1599-1608

[29] Sansing LH, et al. Toll-like receptor 4 contributes to poor outcome after intracerebral hemorrhage. Annals of Neurology. 2011;**70**:646-656

[30] Schroeter M, Jander S, Witte OW, Stoll G. Local immune responses in the rat cerebral cortex after middle cerebral artery occlusion. Journal of Neuroimmunology. 1994;**55**: 195-203

[31] Savage CD, Lopez-Castejon G, Denes A, Brough D. NLRP3-Inflammasome activating DAMPs stimulate an inflammatory response in glia in the absence of priming which contributes to brain inflammation after injury. Frontiers in Immunology. 2012;**3**:288

[32] Fann DY, Lee SY, Manzanero S, Chunduri P, Sobey CG, Arumugam TV. Pathogenesis of acute stroke and the role of inflammasomes. Ageing Research Reviews. 2013;**12**: 941-966

[33] Mocco J, et al. Alterations in plasma complement levels after human ischemic stroke. Neurosurgery. 2006;**59**:28-33

[34] Lindsberg PJ, et al. Complement activation in the central nervous system following blood-brain barrier damage in man. Annals of Neurology. 1996;**40**:587-596

[35] Cervera A, et al. Genetically-defined deficiency of mannose-binding lectin is associated with protection after experimental stroke in mice and outcome in human stroke. PLoS One. 2010;**5**:e8433

[36] Geissmann F, et al. Development of monocytes, macrophages, and dendritic cells. Science. 2010;**327**:656-661

[37] Garcia JH, et al. Influx of leukocytes and platelets in an evolving brain infarct (Wistar rat). The American Journal of Pathology. 1994;**144**:188-199

[38] Harms H, et al. Preventive antibacterial therapy in acute ischemic stroke: A randomized controlled trial. PLoS ONE. 2008;**3**:e2158

[39] Klehmet J, et al. Stroke-induced immunodepression and post-stroke infections: Lessons from the Preventive Antibacterial Therapy in Stroke trial. Neuroscience. 2009;**158**: 1184-1193

[40] Allan SM, Rothwell NJ. Cytokines and acute neurodegeneration. Nature Reviews Neuro science. 2001;**2**:734-744

[41] Burnstock G. Purinergic signalling and disorders of the central nervous system. Nature Reviews Drug Discovery. 2008;**7**:575-590

[42] Liesz A, et al. Regulatory T cells are key cerebroprotective immunomodulators in acute experimental stroke. Journal of Natural Medicines. 2009;**15**:192-199

[43] Liesz A, et al. FTY720 reduces post-ischemic brain lymphocyte influx but does not improve outcome in permanent murine cerebral ischemia. PLoS One. 2011;**6**:e21312

[44] Konoeda F, et al. Therapeutic effect of IL 12/23 and their signaling pathway blockade on brain ischemia model. Biochemical and Biophysical Research Communications. 2010; **402**:500-506

[45] Planas AM, et al. Brain-derived antigens in lymphoid tissue of patients with acute stroke. Journal of Immunology. 2012;**188**:2156-2163

[46] Moalem G, et al. Autoimmune T cells protect neurons from secondary degeneration after central nervous system axotomy. Journal of Natural Medicines. 1999;**5**:49-55

[47] Frenkel D, et al. Nasal vaccination with myelin oligodendrocyte glycoprotein reduces stroke size by inducing IL 10 producing CD4+ T cells. Journal of Immunology. 2003;**171**: 6549-6555

[48] Hallenbeck J. How inflammation modulates central nervous system vessel activation and provides targets for intervention—a personal perspective. Annals of the New York Academy of Sciences. 2010;**1207**:1-7

[49] Gee JM, et al. Long term immunologic consequences of experimental stroke and mucosal tolerance. Experimental & Translational Stroke Medicine. 2009;**1**:3

[50] Sakaguchi S, Yamaguchi T, Nomura T, Ono M. Regulatory T cells and immune tolerance. Cell. 2008;**133**:775-787

[51] Ooboshi H, et al. Postischemic gene transfer of interleukin 10 protects against both focal and global brain ischemia. Circulation. 2005;**2**:913-919

[52] Ren X, et al. Regulatory B cells limit CNS inflammation and neurologic deficits in murine experimental stroke. Journal of Neuroscience. 2011;**31**:8556-8563

[53] Li S, Overman JJ, Katsman D, Kozlov SV, Donnelly CJ, Twiss JL, et al. An age-related sprouting transcriptome provides molecular control of axonal sprouting after stroke. Nature Neuroscience. 2010;**13**:1496-1504

[54] Hayakawa K, Nakano T, Irie K, Higuchi S, Fujioka M, Orito K, et al. Inhibition of reactive astrocytes with fluorocitrate retards neurovascular remodeling and recovery after focal cerebral ischemia in mice. Journal of Cerebral Blood Flow & Metabolism. 2010;**30**:871-882

[55] Hao Q, Chen Y, Zhu Y, Fan Y, Palmer D, Su H, et al. Neutrophil depletion decreases VEGF-induced focal angiogenesis in the mature mouse brain. Journal of Cerebral Blood Flow & Metabolism. 2007;**27**:1853-1860

[56] Prass K, et al. Stroke-induced immunodeficiency promotes spontaneous bacterial infections and is mediated by sympathetic activation reversal by poststroke T helper cell type 1-like immunostimulation. Journal of Experimental Medicine. 2003;**198**:725-736

[57] Meisel C, Schwab JM, Prass K, Meisel A, Dirnagl U. Central nervous system injury-induced immune deficiency syndrome. Nature Reviews Neuroscience. 2005;**6**:775-786

[58] Westendorp WF, Nederkoorn PJ, Vermeij JD, Dijkgraaf MG, van de Beek D. Post-stroke infection: A systematic review and meta-analysis. BMC Neurology. 2011;**11**:110

[59] Finlayson O, et al. Risk factors, inpatient care, and outcomes of pneumonia after ischemic stroke. Neurology. 2011;**77**:1338-1345

[60] Katzan IL, Cebul RD, Husak SH, Dawson NV, Baker DW. The effect of pneumonia on mortality among patients hospitalized for acute stroke. Neurology. 2003;60:620-625

[61] Martino R, et al. Dysphagia after stroke: Incidence, diagnosis, and pulmonary complications. Stroke. 2005;**36**:2756-2763

[62] Sellars C, et al. Risk factors for chest infection in acute stroke: A prospective cohort study. Stroke. 2007;**38**:2284-2291

[63] Stott DJ, Falconer A, Miller H, Tilston JC, Langhorne P. Urinary tract infection after stroke. QJM. 2009;**102**:243-249

[64] Chamorro A, et al. Catecholamines, infection, and death in acute ischemic stroke. Journal of the Neurological Sciences. 2007;**252**:29-35

[65] Chamorro A, et al. Interleukin 10, monocytes and increased risk of early infection in ischemic stroke. Journal of Neurology, Neurosurgery, and Psychiatry. 2006;**77**:1279-1281

[66] Woiciechowsky C, Schöning B, Lanksch WR, Volk HD, Döcke WD. Mechanisms of brain-mediated systemic anti-inflammatory syndrome causing immunodepression. Journal of Molecular Medicine. 1999;**77**:769-780

[67] Listed NA. The bitterest pill. Nature. 2006;**444**:532-533

[68] O'Collins VE, Macleod MR, Donnan GA, Horky LL, van der Worp BH, Howells DW. 1026 experimental treatments in acute stroke. Annals of Neurology. 2006;**59**:467-477

[69] Sacchetti ML. Is it time to definitely abandon neuroprotection in acuteischemic stroke? Stroke. 2008;**39**:1659-1660

[70] Zivin JA, Grotta JC. Animal stroke models: They are relevant to human disease. Stroke. 1990;**21**:981-983

[71] Gorelick PB. Neuroprotection in acute ischemic stroke: A tale of for whom the bell tolls. Lancet. 2000;**355**;1925-1926

[72] Morgenstern LB. What have we learned from clinical neuroprotective trials? Neurology. 2001;**57**:345-347

[73] Gladstone DJ, Black SE, Hakim AM. Toward wisdom from failure lesions from neuroprotective stroke trials and new therapeutic direction. Stroke. 2002;**33**:2123-2136

[74] Cheng YD, Al-Khoury L, Zivin JA. Neuroprotection for ischemic stroke: Two decades ofsuccess and failure. NeuroRx. 2004;**1**:36-45

[75] Albers GW, Atkinson RP, Kelley RE, Rosenbaum DM. Safety, tolerability, and pharmacokinetics of the N-methyl-D-aspartate antagonist dextrorphan in patients with acute stroke. Dextrorphan Study Group. Stroke. 1995;**26**(2):254-258

[76] Miyabe M, Kirsch JR, Nishikawa T, Koehler RC, Traystman RJ. Comparative analysis of brain protection by N-methyl-D-aspartate receptor antagonists after transient focal ischemia in cats. Critical Care Medicine. 1997;**25**:1037-1043

[77] Grotta J, Clark W, Coull B, Pettigrew LC, Mackay B, Goldstein LB, Meissner I, MurphyD, LaRue L. Safety and tolerability of the glutamate antagonist CGS 19755 (Selfotel) in patients with acute ischemic stroke: Results of a phase IIa randomized trial. Stroke. 1995;**26**:602-605

[78] Davis SM, Lees KR, Albers GW, Diener HC, Markabi S, Karlsson G, Norris J. Selfotel in acute ischemic stroke: Possible neurotoxic effects of an NMDA antagonist. Stroke. 2000;**31**:347-354

[79] Davis SM, Albers GW, Diener HC, Lees KR, Norris J. Termination of acute stroke studies involving selfotel treatment. ASSIST Steering Committed. Lancet. 1997;**349**(9044):32

[80] Lees KR. Cerestat and other NMDA antagonists in ischemic stroke. Neurology. 1997. **49**(5 Suppl 4):S66-S69

[81] Albers GW, Clark WM, Atkinson RP. Dose escalation study of the NMDA glycine-site antagonist ACEA 1021 in acute ischemic stroke. Stroke. 1999;**30**:508-513

[82] Sacco RL, DeRosa JT, Haley Jr EC, Levin B, Ordronneau P, Phillips SJ, et al. Glycine antagonist in neuroprotection for patients with acute stroke: GAIN Americas: A randomized controlled trial. Journal of the American Medical Association. 2001;**285**(13):1719-1728

[83] Cook DJ, Teves L, Tymianski M. Treatment of stroke with a PSD-95 inhibitor in the gyrencephalic primate brain. Nature. 2012;**483**:213-217

[84] Hill MD, Martin RH, Mikulis D, Wong JH, Silver FL, Terbrugge KG, et al., ENACT Trial Investigators. Safety and efficacy of NA-1 in patients with iatrogenic stroke after endovascular aneurysm repair (ENACT): Aphase 2, randomised, double-blind, placebo-controlled trial. The Lancet Neurology. 2012;**11**:942-950

[85] Rajanikant K, Zemek D, Senut MC, et al. Carnosine is neuroprotective against permanent focal cerebral ischemia in mice. Stroke. 2007;**38**;3023-3031

[86] Min J, Senut MC, Rajanikant K, et al. Differential neuroprotective effects of carnosine, anserine, and N-acetyl carnosineagainst permanent focal ischemia. Journal of Neuroscience Research. 2008;**86**:2984-2991

[87] Min J, Yu SW, Baek SH, et al. Neuroprotective effect of cyanidin-3-Oglucosideanthocyanin in mice with focalcerebral ischemia. Neuroscience Letters. 2011;**500**:157-161

[88] Yamaguchi T, Sano K, Takakura K, et al. Ebselen in acute ischemic stroke: A placebocontrolled, double-blind clinical trial. EbselenStudy Group. Stroke. 1998;**29**:12-17

[89] Ebselen Trial—Phase III. 2009. Available from: http://www.strokecenter.org/trials/clinicalstudies/298

[90] Edaravone Acute Infarction Study Group. Effect of a novel free radical scavenger, edaravone (MCI-186), on acute brain infarction. Randomized, placebo-controlled, double-blind study at multicenters. Cerebrovascular Diseases. 2003;**15**:222-229

[91] Nakase T, Yoshioka S, Suzuki A. Free radical scavenger, edaravone, reduces the lesion size of lacunar infarction in human brain ischemic stroke. BMC Neurology. 2011;**11**:1-7 (p. 39)

[92] Marshall JWB, Duffin KJ, Green AR, Ridley RM. NXY-059, a free radical-trapping agent, substantially lessens the functional disability resulting from cerebral ischemia in aprimate species. Stroke. 2001;**32**:190-198

[93] Lees KR, Zivin JA, Ashwood T, et al., Stroke–Acute Ischemic NXY Treatment (SAINT I) Trial Investigators. NXY-059 for acute ischemic stroke. New England Journal of Medicine. 2006;**354**:588-600

[94] Shuaib A, Lees K, Lyde P, et al., For the SAINT II Trial Investigators. NXY-059 for the treatment of acute ischemic stroke. New England Journal of Medicine. 2007;**357**:562-571

[95] Diener HC, Lees KR, Lyden P, et al., SAINT I and II Investigators. NXY-059 for the treatment of acute stroke: Pooled analysis of the SAINT I and II Trials. Stroke. 2008; **39**(6):1751-1758

[96] Adibhatla RM, Hatcher JF. Citicoline mechanisms and clinical efficacy in cerebral ischemia. Journal of Neuroscience Research. 2002;**70**(2):133-139

[97] Dávalos A, Alvarez-Sabín J, Castillo J, et al., International Citicoline Trial on Acute Stroke(ICTUS) Trial Investigators. Citicoline in the treatment of acute ischaemic stroke: An international, randomised, multicentre, placebo-controlled study (ICTUS trial). Lancet. 2012;**380**(9839):349-357

[98] Mitta M, Goel D, Bansal KK, Puri P. Edaravone-Citicoline comparative study in acute ischemic stroke (ECCS-AIS). The Journal of the Association of Physicians of India. 2012;**60**:36-38

[99] Heiss WD, Brainin M, Bornstein NM, Tuomilehto J, Hong Z, For the Cerebrolysin Acute Stroke Treatment in Asia (CASTA) Investigators. Cerebrolysin in patients with acute ischemic stroke in Asia: Results of a double-blind, placebo-controlled randomized trial. Stroke. 2012;**43**:630-636

[100] Sena E, Wheble P, Sandercock P, Macleod M. Systematic review and meta-analysis of the efficacy of tirilazad in experimental stroke. Stroke. 2007;**38**:388-394

[101] van der Worp HB, Kappelle LJ, Algra A, Bar PR, Orgogozo JM, Ringelstein EB, Bath PM, van Gijn J, TESS Investigators, TESS II Investigators. The effect of tirilazad mesylate on infarct volume of patients with acute ischemic stroke. Neurology. 2002;**58**:133-135

[102] Aisenbrey GA, Corwin E, Catanzarite V. Effect of magnesium sulfate on the vascularactions of norepinephrine and angiotensin II. American Journal of Perinatology. 1992;**9**:477-480

[103] Kemp PA, Gardiner SM, Bennett T, et al. Magnesium sulphate reverses the carotidvasoconstriction caused by endothelin-I, angiotensin II and neuropeptide-Y, but notthat caused by *N*(G)-nitro-l-argininemethylester, in conscious rats. Clinical Science. 1993;**85**:175-181

[104] Altura BT, Memon ZI, Zhang A, et al. Low levels of serum ionized magnesium are foundin patients early after stroke which result in rapid elevation in cytosolic free calcium and spasm in cerebral vascular muscle cells. Neuroscience Letters. 1997;**230**:37-40

[105] Saver JL, Kidwell C, Eckstein M, Starkman S. Prehospital neuroprotective therapy for acute stroke: Results of the Field Administration of Stroke Therapy-Magnesium (FAST-MAG) pilot trial. Stroke. 2004;**35**:e106-e108

[106] Clinical Trials database. Available from: www.clinicaltrials.gov

[107] Sydserff SG, Cross AJ, Murray TK, Jones JA, Green AR. Clomethiazole is neuroprotective in models of global and focal cerebral ischemia when infused at doses producing clinically relevant plasma concentrations. Brain Reserach. 2000;**862**:59-62

[108] Lyden P, Shuaib A, Ng K, Levin K, Atkinson RP, Rajput A, Wechsler L, Ashwood T, Claesson L, Odergren T, Salazar-Grueso E, CLASSI/H/T Investigators. Clomethiazole acutestroke study in ischemic stroke (CLASS-I): Final results. Stroke. 2002;**33**:122-128

[109] Turski L, Huth A, Sheardown M, McDonald F, Neuhaus R, Schneider HH, Dirnagl U, Wiegand F, Jacobsen P, Ottow E. ZK200775: A phosphonate quinoxalinedione AMPA antagonist for neuroprotection in stroke and trauma. Proceedings of the National Academy of Sciences of the United States of America. 1998;**95**:10960-10965

[110] Walters MR, Kaste M, Lees KR, Diener HC, Hommel M, de Keyser J, Steiner H, Versavel M. The AMPA antagonist ZK 200775 in patients with acute ischaemic stroke: A double-blind, multicentre, placebo-controlled safety and tolerability study. Cerebrovascular Diseases. 2005;**20**:304-309

[111] Furukawa T, Hoshino S, Kobayashi S, Asakura T, Takahashi M, Atsumi T, Teramoto A. The glutamate AMPA receptor antagonist, YM872, attenuates cortical tissue loss, regionalcerebral edema, and neurological motor deficits after experimental brain injury in rats. Journal of Neurotrauma. 2003;**20**:269-278

[112] A Study to Evaluate the Effects of YM872 on Stroke Lesion Volume in Acute StrokePatients. 2002. Available from: http://clinicaltrials.gov/ct2/show/NCT00044070

[113] Erecinska M, Silver IA. Ions and energy in mammalian brain. Progress in Neurobiology. 1994;**43**:37-71

[114] Onteniente B, Rasika S, Benchoua NA, Guegan C. Molecular pathway in cerebral ischemia. Cues to novel therapeutic strategies. Molecular Neurobiology. 2003;**27**:33-72

[115] Fabricius M, Fuhr S, Buatia R, et al. Cortical spreading depression and peri-infarct depolarization in acute injured human cerebral cortex. Brain. 2006;**129**:778-790

[116] Rataud J, Debarnot E, Mary V, Pratt J, Stutzmann JM. Comparative study of voltagesensitive sodium channel blockers in focal ischaemia and electric convulsions in rodents. Neuroscience Letters. 1994;**172**:19-23

[117] Taft WC, Clifton GL, Blair RE, DeLorenzo RJ. Phenytoin protects againstischemia-produced neuron cell death. Brain Research. 1989;**483**:143-148

[118] Pratt J, Rataud J, Bardot F, et al. Neuroprotective actions of riluzole in rodentmodels of global and focal cerebral ischaemia. Neuroscience Letters. 1992;**140**:225-230

[119] Smith SE, Hodges H, Sowinski P, et al. Longterm beneficial effects of BW619C89 on neurological deficit, cognitive deficit and brain damage after middle cerebral artery occlusion in the rat. Neuroscience. 1997;**77**:1123-1135

[120] Muir KW, Holzafel L, Lees KR. Phase II clinical trial of sipatrigine (619C89) by continuous infusion in acute stroke. Cerebrovascular Diseases. 2000;**10**:431-436

[121] Grotta J. Lubeluzole treatment of acute ischemic stroke. The US and Canadian Lubeluzole Ischemic Stroke Study Group. Stroke. 1997;**28**(12):2338-2346

[122] Hantson L, Wessel T. Therapeutic benefits of lubeluzole in ischemic stroke. Stroke. 1998;**29**(1):75-75

[123] Horn J, Haan R, Vermeulen M. Very Early nimodipine use in stroke (VENUS): A randomized, double-blind placebo-controlled trial. Stroke. 2001;**32**:461-465

[124] Kobayashi T, Mori Y. Ca2+ channel antagonists and neuroprotection from cerebral ischemia. European Journal of Pharmacology. 1998;**363**:1-15

[125] Bozik ME, Smith JM, Douglass A, et al. POST: Double-blind placebo controlled, safety and efficacy trial of intravenous BMS-204352 in patients with acute stroke. Stroke. 2000;**31**:1-270

[126] Zoellner H, Hofler M, Beckmann R, et al. Serum albumin is a specific inhibitor of a poptosis in human endothelial cells. Journal of Cell Science. 1996;**109**:2571-2580

[127] Ginsberg MD, Hill MD, Palesch YY, et al. The ALIAS Pilot Trial: A dose-escalation and safety study of albumin therapy for acute ischemic stroke-I: Physiological responses and safety results. Stroke. 2006;**37**:2100-2106

[128] Ginsberg MD, Palesch YY, Martin RH, et al., ALIAS Investigators. The albumin in acute stroke (ALIAS) multicenter clinical trial: Safety analysis of part 1 and rationale and design ofpart 2. Stroke. 2011;**42**:119-127

[129] Stanimirovich D, Satoh K. Inflammatory mediators of cerebral endothelium: A role inischemic brain inflammation. Brain Pathology. 2000;**10**:113-126

[130] Zhang RL, Chopp M, Jiang N, et al. Antiintercellular adhesion molecule–1 antibodyreduces ischemic cell damage after transient but not permanent middle cerebral artery occlusion in the Wistar rat. Stroke. 1995;**26**:1438-1443

[131] Enlimomab Acute Stroke Trial Investigators. Use of anti-ICAM-a therapy in ischemic stroke: Results of the enlimomab acute stroke trial. Neurology. 2001;**57**:1428-1434

[132] Furuichi Y, Maeda M, Matsuoka N, et al. Therapeutic time window of tacrolimus(FK506) in a nonhuman primate stroke model: Comparison with tissue plasminogen activator. Experimental Neurology. 2007;**204**:138-146

[133] Salat D, Ribosa R, Garcia-Bonilla L, Montaner J. Perspective: Statin use before andafter acute ischemic stroke onset improves neurological outcome. Expert Review of Cardiovascular Therapy. 2009;7:1219-1230

[134] Elkind MS, Sacco RL, Macarthur RB, et al. High-dose lovastatin for acute ischemic stroke: Results of the Phase I dose escalationneuroprotection with statin therapy for acuterecovery trial (NeuSTART). Cerebrovascular Diseases. 2009;**28**:266-275

[135] Fagan SC, Waller JL, Nichols FT, Edwards DJ, Pettigrew LC, Clark WM. Minocycline to improve neurologic outcome in stroke (MINOS): A dose-finding study. Stroke. 2010;**41**(10):2283-2287

[136] Adams Jr HP, Effron MB, Torner J, et al. Emergency administration of abciximab for treatment of patients with acute ischemic stroke: Results of an international phase III trial: Abciximab in Emergency Treatment of Stroke Trial (AbESTT-II). Stroke. 2008;**39**(1):87-99

[137] Clark WM, Warach SJ, Pettigrew LC, Gammans RE, Sabounjian LA. A randomized dose-response trial of citicoline in acute ischemic stroke patients. Citicoline Stroke Study Group. Neurology. 1997;**49**(3):671-678

[138] Clark WM, Williams BJ, Selzer KA, Zweifler RM, Sabounjian LA, Gammans RE. A randomized efficacy trial of citicoline in patients with acute ischemic stroke. Stroke. 1999;**30**(12):2592-2597

[139] Dávalos A, Castillo J, Alvarez-Sabín J, et al. Oral citicoline in acute ischemic stroke: An individual patient data pooling analysis of clinical trials. Stroke. 2002;**33**(12):2850-2857

[140] Clark WM, Schim JD, Kasner SE, Victor S. Trafermin in acute ischemic stroke: Results of a phase II/III randomized efficacy study. Neurology. 2000;**54**:A88

[141] Honmou O, Houkin K, Matsunaga T, et al. Intravenous administration of auto serum-expanded autologous mesenchymal stem cells in stroke. Brain. 2011;**134**:1790-1807

[142] Cramer SC, Abila B, Scott NE, Simeoni M, Enney LA,. Safety, pharmacokinetics, and pharmacodynamics of escalating repeat doses of GSK249320 in patients with stroke. Stroke. 2013;**44**(5):1337-1342

[143] Schwab S. Cooling plus Best Medical Treatment versus Best Medical Treatment Alonefor Acute Ischaemic Stroke (EuroHYP- 1). 2013

[144] Macleod MR, Petersson J, Norrving B, Hacke W, Dirnagl U, Wagner M, Schwab S, European Hypothermia Stroke Research Workshop. Hypothermia for Stroke: Call to action 2010. International Journal of Stroke. 2010;**5**:489-492

[145] Amaro S, Canovas D, Castellanos M, Gallego J, Marti-Febregas J, Segura T, Chamorro A. The URICO-ICTUS study, a phase 3 study of combined treatment with uric acid and rtPAadministered intravenously in acute ischaemic stroke patients within the first 4.5 h of onset of symptoms. International Journal of Stroke. 2010;**5**:325-328

[146] Dapsone for Acute Ischemia Stroke Study (DAISY). 2010. Available from: http://clinicaltrials.gov/show/NCT01144650

[147] Treatment of Acute Stroke with Cromolyn (Single Dose). 2010. Available from: http://clinicaltrials.gov/ct2/show/NCT01175525

[148] Nighoghossian N. Neuroprotection Impactof Cyclosporin A in Cerebral Infarction (CsAStroke). 2012. Available from: http://clinicaltrials.gov/show/NCT01527240

[149] Neuroprotection of Pioglitazone in Acute Ischemic Stroke. Available from: https://clinicaltrials.gov/ct2/show/NCT02195791

Chapter 7

On Overcoming Barriers to Application of Neuroinflammation Research

Edward L. Tobinick, Tracey A. Ignatowski and Robert N. Spengler

Additional information is available at the end of the chapter

http://dx.doi.org/10.5772/intechopen.68940

Abstract

Throughout history, new ideas in medicine or science have met initial resistance by entrenched medical or scientific communities. Barriers to medical innovation fall into six main categories as listed here in order of historical chronology: (1) Theological, (2) Academic, (3) Scientific, (4) Financial, (5) Governmental, and (6) Commercial. Researchers in the field of neuroinflammation often encounter such obstacles that may include denialism. Despite these barriers, recognition of the therapeutic potential of targeting neuroinflammation for treatment of stroke, traumatic brain injury, Alzheimer's disease, spinal pain, and a variety of additional brain disorders has accelerated in the past 10 years. Consequently, a paradigm shift in scientific thinking regarding neuroinflammation as a therapeutic target is now underway.

Keywords: denialism, perispinal, etanercept, stroke, traumatic brain injury, Alzheimer's, sciatica, neuroinflammation, spasticity, cognitive dysfunction, TNF

1. Introduction

> *I remember at an early period of my own life showing to a man of high reputation as a teacher some matters which I happened to have observed. And I was very much struck and grieved to find that, while all the facts lay equally clear before him, those only which squared with his previous theories seemed to affect his organs of vision.* (Lister [1]).

There is growing scientific evidence of the central involvement of neuroinflammation in the pathogenesis of a diverse group of neurological disorders [2–31]. This is particularly important since basic research fuels applied science's innovations. Despite this evidence, translation of neuroinflammation research findings by basic scientists into therapeutic methods that are widely employed has been hindered by the traditional barriers that are put into place by entrenched medical and scientific communities [32–40]. Of these barriers, denialism, the refusal to accept or even examine verifiable facts that conflict with one's philosophy, is particularly onerous and may undermine public health [40, 41]. Recognition of the existence of these barriers and careful consideration of their nature promise to facilitate the treatment of neuroinflammatory disorders [22, 38, 42, 43].

2. Barriers to translation of medical innovation

> *A new scientific truth does not triumph by convincing its opponents and making them see the light, but rather because its opponents eventually die, and a new generation grows up that is familiar with it.* (Planck [33]).

Barriers to medical innovation fall into six main categories, in approximate order of chronology: (1) Theological, (2) Academic, (3) Scientific, (4) Financial, (5) Governmental, and (6) Commercial. Any one of these barriers by itself can present an insurmountable blockade to the translational practice of a new medical discovery. Within each of these categories, denialism often operates to obstruct the progress of a new scientific discovery.

Historically, *theological barriers* to the acceptance of new scientific concepts have been formidable [34]. Prominent historical examples include the resistance of the Church to the scientific ideas of Galileo and Darwin [32, 34, 35, 40]. While theological barriers have diminished, they remain to the present day, including theological barriers to stem-cell and contraception research and practice.

Academic barriers can also impede or prevent scientific progress [32, 34, 35, 38, 39]. Ever since scientists and physicians organized into special societies, these societies have wielded their political and economic power to influence the acceptance [or nonacceptance] of new scientific concepts relevant to their interests [32, 34, 35, 38–40].

Scientific barriers are complex and multifaceted [32, 34–37, 39]. Scientific communities organize around certain shared assumptions, termed "paradigms," that form the foundations of their scientific beliefs [35]. New scientific discoveries, at odds with existing scientific dogma, have historically been attacked and willfully ignored, often by the reigning scientific "authorities" of the time [32, 34–40].

Financial barriers have always created difficulties for scientists because hypothesis generation, scientific discovery, data confirmation, and publication of a new scientific concept necessitates the gathering of sufficient financial resources to support what is characteristically a lengthy and expensive endeavor [39, 44]. Particularly expensive is drug development, which typically requires hundreds of millions of dollars of investment to achieve a new FDA indication, with some recent Alzheimer clinical trials costing more than a billion dollars [44, 45].

Governmental barriers have become increasingly complex over time, particularly so in recent decades. These barriers are justified by ethical, humanitarian, and public interest considerations as illustrated, for example, by the Tuskegee experiment. Nevertheless, as exemplified by the considerations that led to the passage of the recent twenty-first century Cures Act, governmental regulations have the potential to slow the pace of medical progress and may be subject to misuse.

Viewed in totality, the difficulty in achieving translation of any radically new or different medical innovation, particularly one that breaks new scientific ground, is readily appreciated [32, 34, 35, 38–40, 46]. Awareness of these barriers may help facilitate the process of successfully surmounting them [32, 34, 35, 38–40, 46–48].

3. Galileo: denialism during the dawning of the scientific method

> *What do you say to the leading philosophers of the university faculty here who, with the lazy obstinacy of a glutted adder, despite invitations a thousand times repeated, refuse even to glance either at the planets or the moon, or even at the telescope itself? Truly the eyes of these men are closed to the light of truth.* (Galileo [40]).

Galileo is considered by many to be the father of the scientific method. Despite his many pioneering scientific discoveries, it is well known that his scientific work was actively resisted by the Church. The denialism regarding Galileo's observational astronomical discoveries, including his discovery of the four largest moons of Jupiter, was, however, not limited to the *theological barrier* promulgated by Cardinal Bellarmine and the Roman Catholic Church, the dominant religion of Galileo's Italy. Rather it notably included an *academic barrier*: denialism by the university academics of the time, who joined the Church in refusing to even look through the telescope that Galileo had invented [32].

Galileo's letter communicates the single reason he was imprisoned and his ideas obstructed: denialism, due to willful ignorance or "willful blindness" by the academics and theologians of his time to the natural scientific truths regarding astronomical bodies that he had discovered [32]. It is tragic that willful blindness to life-saving medical discoveries, epitomized by the example of Semmelweis, may persist for decades before such denialism is overcome and still operates today [1, 22, 32, 36–39, 43, 47, 49].

4. Denialism in the nineteenth century: Semmelweis

> *The innate resistance of science to revolutionary change means that when truly major change is called for, the scientific community often and wrongly opposes it at first.*
>
> *Dogmatism in science and medicine: how dominant theories monopolize research and stifle the search for truth.*(Bauer [39]).

New medical discoveries need to overcome all of the enumerated barriers to achieve widespread acceptance and translation [32, 34, 38, 39]. A well-known historical example is illustrative of the existence of many such barriers. In mid-nineteenth century Vienna, Ignaz Semmelweis, through astute observation and careful study, deduced and then provided compelling scientific evidence that handwashing by obstetricians prior to assisting in childbirth dramatically reduced maternal mortality [36, 37]. His ground-breaking discovery, however, failed to achieve acceptance during his lifetime, due to academic denialism [36, 37]. The entrenched obstetrical community of his time simply refused to recognize his life-saving findings for decades [36, 37].

> *[Semmelweis] made the intriguing observation that obstetrical mortality within the conveniences of a hospital setting, and in the hands of sophisticated physicians, was far greater than that in the hands of simple midwives....He postulated that doctors coming from the autopsy room to the maternity ward brought with them the cause of childbed fever. His crude antiseptic measures, years before Lister, were sufficient to bring the mortality rate down from 25% to around 1%.*
>
> *Semmelweis's thinking was greeted with skepticism, and, at times, derision. His colleagues resented the constraints he had placed on them and the implications that they were the agents of death [49].*

It is not difficult to see how Semmelweis's findings threatened their specialty [36, 37, 49]. Semmelweis faced denialism by the leading obstetrical specialists of his time, a barrier he was unable to overcome [32, 34–39]. Additionally, Semmelweis's discovery that handwashing prevented life-threatening maternal infection conflicted with the scientific dogma followed by the obstetricians and general medical community of his time [32, 34–39].

A different and opposite historical example demonstrates the value of medical specialty support for the dissemination of medical innovation. In 1884 Sigmund Freud and his colleague Carl Koller were studying the medicinal effects of cocaine in Vienna [50, 51]. Koller discovered that topical eyedrops containing cocaine could be fashioned into an aqueous solution that produced effective local anesthesia of the cornea [50, 51]. On September 11, 1884, he performed the first ophthalmologic surgery using cocaine as a local anesthetic on a patient [50]. Koller's preliminary report was presented by his friend, opthalmologist Joseph Brettauer, at the conference of the German Opthalmologic Society in Heidelberg on September 15, 1884 [50]. Koller's discovery was rapidly embraced by the world-wide opthalmology community [50]. Within months cocaine was being used to achieve painless eye surgery around the world [50].

5. Commercial barriers to application of scientific discoveries

> *When the work was presented, my results were disputed and disbelieved, not on the basis of science but because they simply could not be true.* (Marshall [47]).

Neither Semmelweis nor Koller faced *commercial barriers* to application of their medical discoveries. In the twenty-first century, commercial barriers may be those most significant in preventing translation of a new scientific discovery [39]. This is particularly true with respect to translation of new discoveries regarding drugs and biologics [39, 44]. Marshall faced years of skepticism and resistance from gastroenterologists prior to his 2005 Nobel Prize for the discovery of *Helicobacter pylori* as a cause of peptic ulcers, recognition that led to the commercialization of his discoveries by Procter and Gamble [47]. Regulatory approval of new indications for existing drugs or biologics requires voluminous specialized regulatory filings and, traditionally, the completion of multiple, large, randomized, controlled clinical trials [44]. These requirements routinely necessitate not only the expenditure of hundreds of millions of dollars but also the explicit cooperation of the drug's manufacturer [44, 45]. Without such cooperation, regulatory approval is not possible.

There is a widespread misconception that drug manufacturers readily provide financial support for the implementation of randomized clinical trials (RCTs) of their drugs for any new indication supported by the peer-reviewed medical literature [52]. In fact, many novel uses of drugs are discovered by clinicians, rather than by drug manufacturers [44, 52]. In reality, companies consider the competitive landscape, market size, cost and difficulty of manufacturing, anticipated regulatory hurdles, patent structure (indications, patent life, etc.) covering their drug and its competitors and their projected earnings in their calculus [44]. Additional difficulties involved in successful RCT design include selection of indication, suitable patient population and inclusion criteria, exclusion criteria, drug dosing (amount and dosing interval), drug formulation (vehicle, pH, viscosity), and delivery method (particularly critical for central nervous system indications) [44, 51]. Independent drug discovery start-ups and academic research centers are, in many ways, more suited to performing such research, but have difficulty independently financing such costly undertakings. Alternative funding sources, such as government research grants, are extraordinarily competitive, particularly for researchers unaffiliated with leading research universities.

6. Medical dogma as a barrier to neuroinflammation research

> *The Semmelweis case shows in striking fashion that too much respect for the dominant paradigm can damage the interests of patients.* (Gillies [36]).

Today, more than 150 years after Semmelweis and 30 years after Marshall's discovery, medical dogma still operates to interfere with medical progress [32, 34, 35, 38, 39, 47, 53]. The example of most relevance to neuroinflammation research is the dogma surrounding the use of antiamyloid therapeutics for Alzheimer's disease [53, 54]. The continuing clinical trial failure of these drugs suggests that the underlying hypothesis is, in some way, faulty [45, 53, 54]. It is well known that investments in developing and testing antiamyloid drugs [all of which have failed] have dominated Alzheimer research funding for more than two decades, effectively funneling billions of dollars of research money away from competing drugs, such as therapeutics directly targeting neuroinflammation [45, 53, 54]. The recent announcement from the new UK Dementia Research Institute acknowledges these accumulated failures and indicates a resulting shift in research direction [53]. As Bart De Strooper, the new head of the institute, recently said, "The evidence suggests that inflammation is another key factor in killing brain cells and we should be targeting that" [53].

7. Perispinal injection as a novel method for delivery of CNS drugs

> *So how should scientists respond to denialism? The first step is to recognize when it is present. Denialism changes the rules of the game. Conventional approaches to scientific progress such as hypothesis generation and testing, and argument and counterargument which seek to elicit the underlying truth no longer apply.* (McKee and Diethelm [41]).

Rapid neurological improvement after perispinal etanercept challenges the dogma that etanercept, and other large molecules, cannot reach the brain in therapeutically effective amounts after perispinal delivery[1] [51]. In fact, the ability of perispinal injection to deliver a physiologically effective dose of a drug to the spinal cord was first demonstrated by Corning in 1885 [51]. The difficulty of delivering large molecules to the central nervous system (CNS) after peripheral delivery has long presented an obstacle to neuroinflammation research and translation of that research into viable commercial products in humans [10, 22, 51]. The unique anatomy of the cerebrospinal venous system (CSVS) (**Figure 1**), the anatomic route by which perispinal etanercept is delivered to the CNS, has been confirmed by independent authorities [51, 55–59]. Increasing awareness of the potential of perispinal injection as a method for effective delivery of large molecules to the CNS promises to dramatically alter the therapeutic possibilities for brain disorders [9, 10, 18, 21, 22, 25, 28, 30, 31, 42, 43, 55, 57, 59, 60].

8. Overcoming denialism in the twenty-first century: perispinal etanercept

> *Confronted with any illness of whatever type or severity, a doctor has two ethical imperatives. The first is to ensure that a specific patient receives the best available current medical care. The second is to develop new treatments so that the patient and others with the same problem can be treated completely, easily, and economically. The second ethical imperative will, if it leads to a successful outcome, have an enormous effect on the health and well-being of humankind.* (Horrobin [46]).

Denialism remains a potent barrier to scientific progress, even in the twenty-first century, as evidenced by holocaust denialism, tobacco-cancer denialism, AIDS denialism, and other examples of incorrect beliefs promulgated in the face of undeniable facts. Perispinal etanercept, a novel off-label treatment for four neuroinflammatory indications (spinal neuropathic pain, including sciatica; Alzheimer's disease; and chronic neurological dysfunction after stroke or traumatic brain injury) has emerged as a new therapeutic modality with unique clinical effects documented in the peer-reviewed medical literature [7, 8, 10, 51, 62–68]. The scientific rationale for the use of perispinal etanercept for these indications is extensive and has been previously reviewed [10, 19, 51, 65, 66, 68]. As the National Academy of Medicine has recently stated, "*Complementing randomized clinical trials, the ability to collect data from actual clinical practice presents a great opportunity to gain new insights about the efficacy and safety of new drugs*... [69]." This is exactly what has been done with perispinal etanercept and demonstrates

[1] "Perispinal delivery" is used here to denote perispinal injection superficial to the ligamentum flavum, utilizing the vertebral venous plexuses as a route to penetrate the relevant physiological barriers (ligamentum flavum and meninges).

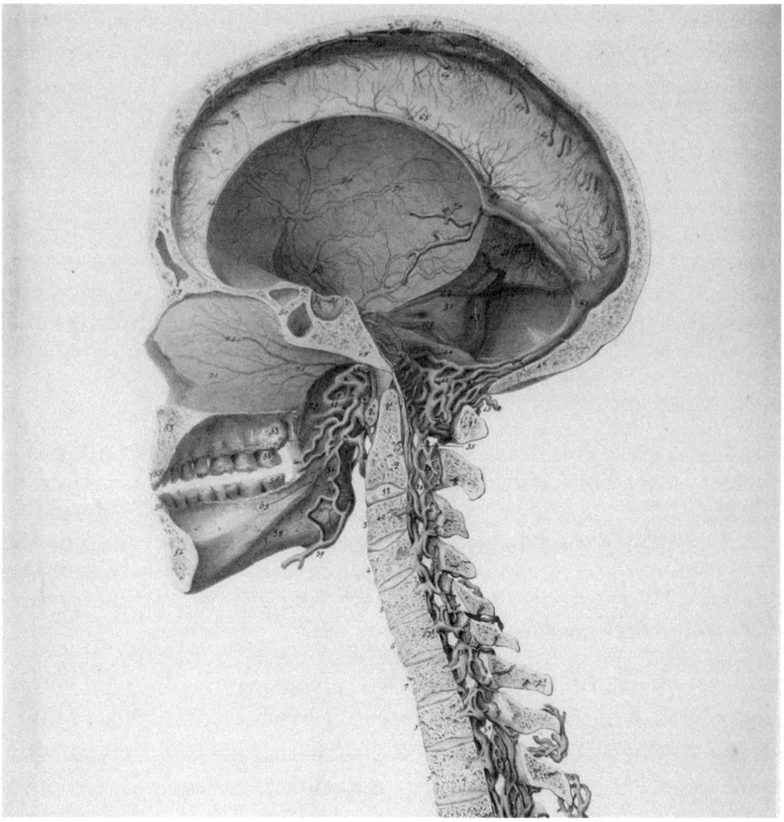

Figure 1. The cerebrospinal venous system, detail of Plate 5 from Breschet [61], Courtesy of the Sidney Tobinick Collection. ©2017 Edward Tobinick, used with permission.

the major role of clinicians in the discovery of new indications for existing drugs [7, 16, 51, 52, 62, 63, 67, 68].

Rapid neurological improvement is characteristic for each of the four off-label indications, often noticeable within minutes of the first dose [7, 8, 16, 51, 62, 64, 67, 68, 70, 71]. The spectrum of improvement as well as its rapidity are novel and may be attributed to the unique physiological effects of etanercept as well as the novel perispinal method of delivery enabled by the cerebrospinal venous system [8, 10, 16, 51, 55, 65, 68]. For example, in a series of 612 consecutive patients with chronic poststroke neurological dysfunction treated with perispinal etanercept, statistically significant improvements in motor impairment, spasticity, sensory impairment, cognition, psychological/behavioral function, aphasia, and pain, with evidence of a strong treatment effect even in the subgroup of patients treated more than 10 years after stroke, have been documented [16].

Significant neurological improvement of the degree documented after perispinal etanercept had not been previously noted with any therapeutic modality, but recently, the possibility of motor recovery years after stroke has been confirmed using modified bone marrow-derived mesenchymal stem cells [72]. This stem cell trial involved 18 patients with stable, chronic stroke treated with surgical transplantation of specialized allogeneic stem cells by needle injection into the peri-infarct brain after burr-hole craniostomy [72]. The clinical results in this trial were not attributed to the conversion of these specialized cells into neuronal cells [72–74]. Rather, as one scientist not involved with the trial suggested in his letter to the lead author,

> *....injecting SB623 cells into the chronic poststroke brain can be predicted to generate, over time, an increasingly anti-tumor necrosis factor state in this compartment. This would be consistent with clinical observations (http://www.strokebreakthrough.com/videos-by-category/) that introducing a widely used specific antitumor necrosis factor agent, etanercept, into this same compartment through Batson's plexus, followed by a short period of head-down positioning, has led to safe and rapid onset of poststroke improvements similar to those reported to evolve slowly after intracranial introduction of SB623 cells* [73].

The lead author of the stem cell study responded,

> *Immunomodulation related to protein and molecular factors secreted by the SB623 cells could be one of the mechanisms underlying the observed neurological recovery in our patients and could suggest that there is ongoing chronic inflammation >6 months after stroke that is suppressing intact neural circuits and rendering them nonfunctional. This concept has some support in the recent preclinical and clinical literature. In addition, it is conceivable that the transplanted SB623-secreted factors are enhancing native neurogenesis or synaptogenesis, potentially through blocking excess tumor necrosis factor effects after stroke, although this is unproven* [74].

Furthermore, the favorable effects of etanercept on spinal neuropathic pain, first documented clinically after perispinal injection [7, 10, 62, 65, 75], have been confirmed in four subsequent randomized, double-blind, placebo-controlled clinical trials [76–79]. These studies and others have led "to the emergence of TNF inhibitors as available strategies for clinical treatment of pain associated with intervertebral disc herniation" [60] and foreshadowed the reduction in central pain reported after stroke and traumatic brain injury (TBI) in patients treated with perispinal etanercept [16, 67, 68].

Additional scientific support for the perispinal etanercept stroke and TBI results has come from basic science studies of etanercept in stroke and TBI models, all of which demonstrated favorable results [80–86]. Recent independent scientific publications have also been supportive of these results [15, 18, 20–26, 28–31, 42, 59, 60, 79, 87–105].

Our current thinking regarding the rapid and sustained neurological improvement documented after perispinal etanercept for neuroinflammatory indications involves the following mechanisms, each of which involves amelioration of neuroinflammatory pathophysiology by etanercept (**Table 1**).

8.1. Immediate neutralization of excess TNF

Rapid neutralization of TNF by binding to excess circulating TNF is a known physiological effect of etanercept and the main scientific rationale behind its use for its approved indications [10]. Excess TNF has been implicated in the pathogenesis of Alzheimer's disease, stroke, TBI and neuropathic pain [10, 18, 21, 60, 65, 66, 68].

Physiological effect
1. Immediate neutralization of excess TNF
2. Modulation of neurotransmission at the individual synapse
3. Modulation of neuronal network function (synaptic scaling)
4. Reduction of microglial activation
5. Reduction in neuropathic pain
6. Activation of neurogenesis

Table 1. Mechanisms of amelioration of neuroinflammatory pathophysiology by etanercept.

8.2. Modulation of neurotransmission at the individual synapse

TNF's role as a gliotransmitter that modulates synaptic transmission and synaptic strength supports this as a physiological mechanism underlying the clinical effects of perispinal etanercept [8, 10, 15, 16, 65, 66, 68, 71, 106]. When applied exogenously to superfused brain tissue, TNF inhibits the stimulation (stimulations 1 and 2, S1 and S2, at 2 Hz, 120 shocks) evoked release of norepinephrine from noradrenergic axon terminals in the isolated median eminence [107]. Similarly, when TNF is applied to slices of the hippocampus, it inhibits stimulated (S1 at 1 HZ and S2 at 4 Hz) norepinephrine release in a concentration- and frequency-dependent manner [108–110]. In both studies, the addition of TNF was 15–16 minutes prior to stimulation, indicating that TNF does not require a long exposure time to develop modulatory effects. Interestingly, TNF inhibition of stimulated norepinephrine release under physiological conditions is altered in pathophysiological conditions. For example, the inhibition of stimulated norepinephrine release by TNF is supersensitized, or increased, during conditions whereby TNF expression is enhanced in the brain (chronic pain) [111, 112]. Thus, it is proposed that descending monoaminergic pain pathways providing endogenous analgesia are no longer engaged [23]. The rapid alleviation of chronic pain experienced by patients receiving perispinal etanercept may be explained by disinhibition of norepinephrine release and descending pain modulation.

8.3. Modulation of neuronal network function by mediation of synaptic scaling

The central role of TNF in modulating synaptic scaling and synaptic strength and thereby modulating neuronal network function may help explain the rapid and widespread neurological effects of perispinal etanercept, including its rapid improvement of cognition in Alzheimer's disease, poststroke cognitive dysfunction, and cognitive dysfunction after traumatic brain injury [8, 15, 16, 62, 67, 68, 71, 106].

8.4. Reduction of microglial activation

Etanercept has been shown to reduce microglial activation in multiple experimental models [81, 113, 114]; reviews: [10, 19]. Activated microglia release excess TNF, contributing to the neurotoxicity and perturbations in synaptic mechanisms seen in neuroinflammatory disorders [10, 19, 26, 63, 68, 81, 93, 114, 115]. Reduction of microglial activation may be a mechanism whereby perispinal etanercept reduces central homeostatic dysregulation of TNF levels induced by microglial activation after stroke or traumatic brain injury.

8.5. Reduction in neuropathic pain

Brain TNF is overexpressed during the development of neuropathic pain [4, 111, 116, 117]. Treatment using TNF inhibitors has been shown to reduce neuropathic pain in both basic science models and in the clinical setting [5, 10, 16, 19, 25, 60, 62, 68, 76–79, 99, 114]. Preclinical studies have shown that blockade of TNF synthesis in the brain is antinociceptive [99]. Also, clinical case studies report that targeting TNF centrally is analgesic [62, 71, 79]. This may be due to blockade of TNF that restores neurotransmission homeostasis along pain pathways.

8.6. Activation of neurogenesis

Although there is some conflicting data, a variety of experimental models suggest that TNF or other pro-inflammatory cytokines, if present in excess, may inhibit neurogenesis [118–122]. TNF and interleukin-1 are involved in the decrease of neurogenesis evidenced in pain and depression models [123–125]. Mice receiving sciatic nerve chronic constriction injury to induce neuropathic pain developed depressive-like behavior for 4 weeks following ligature placement that was associated with increased hippocampal TNF and impaired dentate gyrus neurogenesis dependent on TNF receptor-1 signaling [126]. There is data suggesting that inflammatory blockade may restore adult neurogenesis [122]. This, theoretically, might be a potential mechanism that could contribute to the increasing neurological improvement observed after perispinal etanercept treatment over the course of months in some patients [16, 63, 68, 120–122].

Perispinal etanercept has successfully traversed a variety of scientific, academic, and governmental barriers to achieve scientific acceptance and recognition [9, 11, 13, 15, 18, 20–26, 28–31, 42, 57, 59, 60, 79, 81, 82, 88–91, 93–98, 100–105, 114, 115, 123, 125, 127–133]. This was accomplished despite considerable misinformation published online by competing medical specialists, who refused the opportunity to observe, first-hand, the rapid neurological effects of perispinal etanercept, despite repeated invitations to do so [43, 48]. Such denialism is in the tradition of that faced by Galileo, Semmelweis, Lister and Marshall, but it has no place in science or medicine [1, 22, 32, 33, 35–39, 41–43, 47].

As Glaziou and colleagues have stated [134]:

> *Confident inferences about the effects of treatment are justified in several situations in which treatment effects are unlikely to be confused with the effects of biases. These include, in particular, ... interventions ... where there is a rapid response on a stable background [134].*

The rapid neurological improvement repeatedly observed in thousands of patients with chronic, intractable neurological dysfunction after treatment with perispinal etanercept, combined with strong, independent, basic science support, constitutes compelling evidence that mandates the recognition of these clinical effects and the initiation of the necessary actions, including the funding of randomized clinical trials, by the relevant medical specialties and governmental agencies, for the benefit of the public.

9. Overcoming barriers to the application of neuroinflammation research

I by no means expect to convince experienced naturalists whose minds are shocked with a multitude of facts all viewed, during a long course of years, from a point of view directly opposite to mine....But I look with confidence to the future, to young and rising naturalists, who will be able to look at both sides of the question with impartiality.

Charles Darwin [135], *The Origin of Species,* 1845.

The key to overcoming barriers to application of neuroinflammation research is education. It is essential that medical students and neuroscientists receive training in basic immunology, the role of cytokines in physiology and pathophysiology and the essential concepts underlying neuroinflammation. Because neuroinflammation is not concrete and visible under the microscope in the same way that pathology such as amyloid plaques are, improved methods, access and utilization of new and emerging methods for imaging neuroinflammation are also essential. Today, fortunately, the initial promise of neuroinflammation research is bearing fruit, and a paradigm shift in scientific thinking in this regard is well underway. Recognition of the necessity of neuroinflammation research for the successful development of new treatments for neurological disease must be a key goal of society. The allocation of sufficient research and educational funding to this end is essential.

Conflict disclosures

Edward Tobinick has multiple issued and pending US and foreign patents, assigned to TACT IP, LLC, that claim perispinal methods of use of etanercept and other drugs for treatment of neurological disorders, including but not limited to US patents 6419944, 6537549, 6982089, 7214658, 7629311, 8119127, 8236306, 8349323, 8900583; and Australian patents 758523 and 2011323616 B2. Dr. Tobinick is the CEO of TACT IP, LLC and founder of the Institute of Neurological Recovery, a medical practice that utilizes perispinal etanercept and trains physicians in its use as a therapeutic modality. Tracey Ignatowski and Robert Spengler have been unpaid expert witnesses for the INR. Tracey Ignatowski and Robert Spengler's professional activities include their work as co-directors of neuroscience at NanoAxis, LLC, a company formed to foster the commercial development of products and applications in the field of nanomedicine that include novel methods of inhibiting TNF. The article represents the authors' own work in which NanoAxis, LLC was not involved.

Author details

Edward L. Tobinick[1]*, Tracey A. Ignatowski[2] and Robert N. Spengler[3]

*Address all correspondence to: nrimed@gmail.com

1 Institute of Neurological Recovery, Boca Raton, FL, USA

2 Pathology and Anatomical Sciences, University at Buffalo-SUNY, Buffalo, NY, USA

3 Nanoaxis LLC, Buffalo, NY, USA

References

[1] Lister J. Edinburgh graduation address. Edinburgh Medical Journal. 1876;**xxii**:280-284

[2] Clark IA, Rockett KA, Cowden WB. Role of TNF in cerebral malaria. Lancet. 1991;**337**(8736):302-303

[3] Barone FC, Arvin B, White RF, et al. Tumor necrosis factor-alpha. A mediator of focal ischemic brain injury. Stroke. 1997;**28**(6):1233-1244

[4] Ignatowski TA, Covey WC, Knight PR, et al. Brain-derived TNF-α mediates neuropathic pain. Brain Research. 1999;**841**(1-2):70-77

[5] Sommer C, Schafers M, Marziniak M, et al. Etanercept reduces hyperalgesia in experimental painful neuropathy. Journal of the Peripheral Nervous System. 2001;**6**(2):67-72

[6] Tarkowski E, Andreasen N, Tarkowski A, et al. Intrathecal inflammation precedes development of Alzheimer's disease. Journal of Neurology, Neurosurgery, and Psychiatry. 2003;**74**(9):1200-1205

[7] Tobinick EL, Britschgi-Davoodifar S. Perispinal TNF-α inhibition for discogenic pain. Swiss Medical Weekly. 2003;**133**(11-12):170-177

[8] Tobinick E. Perispinal etanercept for treatment of Alzheimer's disease. Current Alzheimer Research. 2007;**4**(5):550-552

[9] Griffin WS. Perispinal etanercept: Potential as an Alzheimer therapeutic. Journal of Neuroinflammation. 2008;**5**:3

[10] Tobinick E. Perispinal etanercept: A new therapeutic paradigm in neurology. Expert Review of Neurotherapeutics. 2010;**10**(6):985-1002

[11] Esposito E, Cuzzocrea S. Anti-TNF therapy in the injured spinal cord. Trends in Pharmacological Sciences. 2011;**32**(2):107-115

[12] Folkersma H, Boellaard R, Yaqub M, et al. Widespread and prolonged increase in (R)-(11)C-PK11195 binding after traumatic brain injury. Journal of Nuclear Medicine. 2011;**52**(8):1235-1239

[13] Frankola KA, Greig NH, Luo W, et al. Targeting TNF-α to elucidate and ameliorate neuroinflammation in neurodegenerative diseases. Central Nervous System & Neurological Disorders – Drug Targets. 2011;**10**(3):391-403

[14] Ramlackhansingh AF, Brooks DJ, Greenwood RJ, et al. Inflammation after trauma: Microglial activation and traumatic brain injury. Annals of Neurology. 2011;**70**(3): 374-383

[15] Santello, M, Volterra A. TNF-α in synaptic function: Switching gears. Trends in Neuro sciences. 2012;**35**(10):638-647

[16] Tobinick E, Kim NM, Reyzin G, et al. Selective TNF inhibition for chronic stroke and traumatic brain injury: An observational study involving 629 consecutive patients treated with perispinal etanercept. CNS Drugs. 2012;**26**(12):1051-1070

[17] Johnson VE, Stewart JE, Begbie FD, et al. Inflammation and white matter degeneration persist for years after a single traumatic brain injury. Brain. 2013;**136**(Pt 1):28-42

[18] Cheng X, Shen Y, Li R. Targeting TNF: A therapeutic strategy for Alzheimer's disease. Drug Discovery Today. 2014;**19**(11):1822-1827

[19] Ignatowski TA, Spengler RN, Dhandapani KM, et al. Perispinal etanercept for post-stroke neurological and cognitive dysfunction: Scientific rationale and current evidence. CNS Drugs. 2014;**28**(8):679-697

[20] Olmos G, Llado J. Tumor necrosis factor alpha: A link between neuroinflammation and excitotoxicity. Mediators of Inflammation. 2014;**2014**:861231

[21] Tuttolomondo A, Pecoraro R, Pinto A. Studies of selective TNF inhibitors in the treatment of brain injury from stroke and trauma: A review of evidence to date. Drug Design, Development and Therapy. 2014;**8**:2221-2239

[22] Clark IA, Vissel B. A Neurologist's guide to TNF biology and to the principles behind the therapeutic removal of excess TNF in disease. Neural Plasticity. 2015;**2015**:358263

[23] Fasick V, Spengler RN, Samankan S, et al. The hippocampus and TNF: Common links between chronic pain and depression. Neuroscience & Biobehavioral Reviews. 2015;**53**: 139-159

[24] McCaulley ME, Grush KA. Alzheimer's disease: Exploring the role of inflammation and implications for treatment. International Journal of Alzheimer's Disease. 2015;**2015**:515248

[25] Ohtori S, Inoue G, Miyagi M, et al. Pathomechanisms of discogenic low back pain in humans and animal models. Spine Journal. 2015;**15**(6):1347-1355

[26] Rossi D. Astrocyte physiopathology: At the crossroads of intercellular networking, inflammation and cell death. Progress in Neurobiology. 2015;**130**:86-120

[27] Witcher KG, Eiferman DS, Godbout JP. Priming the inflammatory pump of the CNS after traumatic brain injury. Trends in Neurosciences. 2015;**38**(10):609-620

[28] Bergold PJ. Treatment of traumatic brain injury with anti-inflammatory drugs. Experimental Neurology. 2016;**275** (Pt 3):367-380

[29] Clark IA Vissel B. Excess cerebral TNF causing glutamate excitotoxicity rationalizes treatment of neurodegenerative diseases and neurogenic pain by anti-TNF agents. Journal of Neuroinflammation. 2016;**13**(1):236

[30] Hellewell S, Semple BD, Morganti-Kossmann MC. Therapies negating neuroinflammation after brain trauma. Brain Research. 2016;**1640**(Pt A):36-56

[31] Walters A, Phillips E, Zheng R, et al. Evidence for neuroinflammation in Alzheimer's disease. Progress in Neurology and Psychiatry. 2016;**20**(Sept./Oct.):25-31

[32] Stern BJ. Resistances to Medical Change, in Society and Medical Progress.London: The Scientific Book Club/Oxford University Press; 1941

[33] Planck M. Scientific Autobiography, and Other Papers. London: Williams & Norgate; 1950. 192 p

[34] Barber B. Resistance by scientists to scientific discovery. Science. 1961;**134**(3479):596-602

[35] Kuhn TS. The Structure of Scientific Revolutions. Vol. xv. Chicago: University of Chicago Press; 1962. p. 172.

[36] Gillies D. Hempelian and Kuhnian approaches in the philosophy of medicine: The Semmelweis case. Studies in History and Philosophy of Science. 2005;**36**(1):159-181

[37] Hauzman, E.E., Semmelweis and his German Contemporaries, in 40th International Congress on the History of Medicine, ISHM 2006. 2006: Budapest, Hungary

[38] Wolinsky H. Paths to acceptance. The advancement of scientific knowledge is an uphill struggle against 'accepted wisdom'. EMBO Reports. 2008;**9**(5):416-418

[39] Bauer HH. Dogmatism in Science and Medicine: How Dominant Theories Monopolize Research and Stifle the Search for Truth. Vol. vii. Jefferson, N.C.: McFarland & Co., Inc., Publishers; 2012. p. 293

[40] Galileo Galilei. Letter to Johannes Kepler, August 10, 1610

[41] McKee M, Diethelm P. How the growth of denialism undermines public health. British Medical Journal. 2010;**341**:c6950

[42] Clark I. New hope for survivors of stroke and traumatic brain injury. CNS Drugs. 2012;**26**(12):1071-1072

[43] Clark IA. An unsound AAN practice advisory on poststroke etanercept. Expert Review of Neurotherapeutics. 2017;**17**(3):215-217

[44] Tobinick EL. The value of drug repositioning in the current pharmaceutical market. Drug News Perspectives. 2009;**22**(2):119-125

[45] Sheridan C. J&J's billion dollar punt on anti-amyloid antibody. Nature Biotechnology. 2009;**27**(8):679-681

[46] Horrobin DF. Effective clinical innovation: An ethical imperative. Lancet. 2002;**359**(9320): 1857-1858

[47] Marshall BJ. Biographical. 2005. Available from: http://www.nobelprize.org/nobel_prizes/medicine/laureates/2005/marshall-bio.html.

[48] [O]n the Perispinal Use of Enbrel. 2016. Available from: http://novella-enbrel.blogspot.com

[49] Tavassoli M. Selected items from the history of pathology – Ignaz Philipp Semmelweis (1818-1865). American Journal of Pathology. 1980;**101**(1):114

[50] dos Reis Jr, A. Sigmund Freud (1856-1939) and Karl Koller (1857-1944) and the discovery of local anesthesia. Revista Brasileira de Anestesiologia. 2009;**59**(2):244-257

[51] Tobinick EL. Perispinal delivery of CNS drugs. CNS Drugs. 2016;**30** (6):469-480

[52] Demonaco HJ, Ali A, Hippel E. The major role of clinicians in the discovery of off-label drug therapies. Pharmacotherapy. 2006;**26**(3):323-332

[53] Leake J. Alzheimer's research chief orders shake-up after 20 years of failure. In: The Sunday Times, London. February 26, 2017: London.

[54] Mullane K, Williams M. Alzheimer's therapeutics: Continued clinical failures question the validity of the amyloid hypothesis-but what lies beyond? Biochemical Pharmacology. 2013;**85**(3):289-305

[55] Tobinick E. The cerebrospinal venous system: Anatomy, physiology, and clinical implications. Medscape General Medicine. 2006;**8**(1):53

[56] Pearce JM. The craniospinal venous system. European Neurology. 2006;**56**(2):136-138

[57] Nathoo N, Caris EC, Wiener JA, et al. History of the vertebral venous plexus and the significant contributions of Breschet and Batson. Neurosurgery. 2011;**69**(5):1007-1014; discussion 1014

[58] Stringer MD, Restieaux M, Fisher AL, et al. The vertebral venous plexuses: The internal veins are muscular and external veins have valves. Clinical Anatomy. 2012;**25**(5):609-618

[59] Griessenauer CJ, Raborn J, Foreman P, et al. Venous drainage of the spine and spinal cord: A comprehensive review of its history, embryology, anatomy, physiology, and pathology. Clinical Anatomy. 2015;**28**(1):75-87

[60] Winkelstein BA, Allen KD, Setton LA. Chapter 19: Intervertebral disc herniation: Pathophysiology and emerging therapies. In: Shapiro IM, Risbud MV, editors. The Intervertebral Disc. Wien, Austria: Springer-Verlag; 2014

[61] Breschet G. Recherches anatomiques physiologiques et pathologiques sur le systáeme veineux. Paris: Rouen fráeres; 1829

[62] Tobinick E, Davoodifar S. Efficacy of etanercept delivered by perispinal administration for chronic back and/or neck disc-related pain: A study of clinical observations in 143 patients. Current Medical Research and Opinion. 2004;**20**(7):1075-1085

[63] Tobinick E, Gross H, Weinberger A, et al. TNF-α modulation for treatment of Alzheimer's disease: A 6-month pilot study. Medscape General Medicine. 2006;**8**(2):25

[64] Tobinick EL, Gross H. Rapid improvement in verbal fluency and aphasia following perispinal etanercept in Alzheimer's disease. BMC Neurology. 2008;**8**:27

[65] Tobinick E. Perispinal etanercept for neuroinflammatory disorders. Drug Discovery Today. 2009;**14**(3-4):168-177

[66] Tobinick E. Tumour necrosis factor modulation for treatment of Alzheimer's disease: rationale and current evidence. CNS Drugs. 2009;**23**(9):713-725

[67] Tobinick E. Rapid improvement of chronic stroke deficits after perispinal etanercept: three consecutive cases. CNS Drugs. 2011;**25**(2):145-155

[68] Tobinick E, Rodriguez-Romanacce H, Kinssies R, et al. Chapter 7 – Perispinal etanercept for traumatic brain injury. In: Heidenreich KA, editor. New Therapeutics for Traumatic Brain Injury. New York: Academic Press/Elsevier; 2017. Available from: http://dx.doi.org/10.1016/B978-0-12-802686-1.00007-9

[69] Dzau VJ, McClellan MB, McGinnis JM, et al. Vital directions for health and health care: Priorities from a national academy of medicine initiative. London, UK. JAMA, 2017; **317**(14):p.1461-1470

[70] Tobinick EL, Gross H. Rapid cognitive improvement in Alzheimer's disease following perispinal etanercept administration. Journal of Neuroinflammation. 2008;**5**:2

[71] Tobinick E, Rodriguez-Romanacce H, Levine A, et al. Immediate neurological recovery following perispinal etanercept years after brain injury. Clinical Drug Investigation. 2014;**34**(5):361-366

[72] Steinberg GK, Kondziolka D, Wechsler LR, et al. Clinical outcomes of transplanted modified bone Marrow-Derived mesenchymal stem cells in stroke: A Phase 1/2a study. Stroke. 2016;**47**(7):1817-1824

[73] Clark IA. Letter to Clark regarding article, "clinical outcomes of transplanted modified bone Marrow-Derived mesenchymal stem cells in stroke: A phase 1/2a study". Stroke. 2016;**47**(12):e268

[74] Steinberg GK, Kondziolka D, Bates D, et al. Response by Steinberg et al to letter regarding article, "clinical outcomes of transplanted modified bone Marrow-Derived mesenchymal stem cells in stroke: A Phase 1/2A study". Stroke. 2016;**47**(12):e269

[75] Tobinick EL. Targeted etanercept for discogenic neck pain: Uncontrolled, open-label results in two adults. Clinical Therapeutics. 2003;**25**(4):1211-1218

[76] Cohen SP, Bogduk N, Dragovich A, et al. Randomized, double-blind, placebo-controlled, dose-response, and preclinical safety study of transforaminal epidural etanercept for the treatment of sciatica. Anesthesiology. 2009;**110**(5):1116-1126

[77] Freeman BJ, Ludbrook GL, Hall S, et al. Randomized, Double-blind, Placebo-Controlled, trial of transforaminal epidural etanercept for the treatment of symptomatic lumbar disc herniation. Spine (Phila Pa 1976). 2013;**38**(23):1986-1994

[78] Ohtori S, Miyagi M, Eguchi Y, et al. Epidural administration of spinal nerves with the tumor necrosis factor-alpha inhibitor, etanercept, compared with dexamethasone for treatment of sciatica in patients with lumbar spinal stenosis: A prospective randomized study. Spine (Phila Pa 1976). 2012;**37**(6):439-444

[79] Sainoh T, Orita S, Miyagi M, et al. Single intradiscal administration of the tumor necrosis Factor-Alpha inhibitor, etanercept, for patients with discogenic low back pain. Pain Medicine. 2016;**17**:40-45

[80] Arango-Davila CA, Vera A, Londono AC, et al. Soluble or soluble/membrane TNF-α inhibitors protect the brain from focal ischemic injury in rats. International Journal of Neuroscience. 2015;**125**(12):936-940

[81] Chio CC, Lin JW, Chang MW, et al. Therapeutic evaluation of etanercept in a model of traumatic brain injury. Journal of Neurochemistry. 2010;**115**(4):921-929

[82] Clausen B, Degn M, Martin N, et al. Systemically administered anti-TNF therapy ameliorates functional outcomes after focal cerebral ischemia. Journal of Neuroinflammation. 2014;**11**(1):203

[83] Iwata N, Takayama H, Xuan M, et al. Effects of etanercept against transient cerebral ischemia in diabetic rats. BioMed Research International. 2015;**2015**:189292

[84] Wu MH, Huang CC, Chio CC, et al. Inhibition of peripheral TNF-α and downregulation of microglial activation by Alpha-Lipoic acid and etanercept protect rat brain against ischemic stroke. Molecular Neurobiology. 2016;**53**(7):4961-4971

[85] Yagi K, Lidington D, Wan H, et al. Therapeutically targeting tumor necrosis Factor-alpha/Sphingosine-1-Phosphate signaling corrects myogenic reactivity in subarachnoid hemorrhage. Stroke. 2015;**46**(8):2260-2270

[86] Zhang BF, Song JN, Ma XD, et al. Etanercept alleviates early brain injury following experimental subarachnoid hemorrhage and the possible role of tumor necrosis Factor-alpha and c-Jun N-Terminal kinase pathway. Neurochemical Research. 2015;**40**(3):591-599

[87] Hess A, Axmann R, Rech J, et al. Blockade of TNF-α rapidly inhibits pain responses in the central nervous system. Proceedings of the National Academy of Sciences of the United States. 2011;**108**(9):3731-3736

[88] Kim CT. Stroke rehabilitation. In: Kim CT, editor. Rehabilitation Medicine. Rijeka, Croatia, InTech; 2012. ISBN 978-953-51-0683-8, DOI: 10.5772/38499

[89] Maccioni RB, Farias G, Rojo LE, et al. Chapter 6: In search of therapeutic solutions for Alzheimer's Disease. In: Mantamadiotis T, editor. When Things Go Wrong – Diseases and Disorders of the Human Brain. Rijeka, Croatia, InTech; 2012

[90] Maudsley S, Chadwick W. Progressive and unconventional pharmacotherapeutic approaches to Alzheimer's disease therapy. Current Alzheimer Research. 2012;**9**(1):1-4

[91] Williams M, Coyle JT. Chapter 7 – Historical perspectives on the discovery and development of drugs to treat neurological disorders. In: Barrett JE, Coyle JT, Williams M, editors. Translational Neuroscience: Applications in Psychiatry, Neurology, and Neurodevelopmental Disorders. New York, NY: Cambridge University Press; 2012. pp. 129-148

[92] Blaylock RL. Immunology primer for neurosurgeons and neurologists part 2: Innate brain immunity. Surgical Neurology International. 2013;**4**:118

[93] Brambilla L, Martorana F, Rossi D. Astrocyte signaling and neurodegeneration: New insights into CNS disorders. Prion. 2013;**7**(1):28-36

[94] Petzold A, Girbes A. Pain management in neurocritical care. Neurocrit Care. 2013;**19**(2): 232-256

[95] Faingold CL. Chapter 7: Network control mechanisms: Cellular inputs, neuroactive substances, and synaptic changes. In: Faingold CL, Blumenfeld H, editors. Neuronal Networks in Brain Function, CNS Disorders, and Therapeutics. Elsevier; 2014

[96] Sedger LM, McDermott MF. TNF and TNF-receptors: From mediators of cell death and inflammation to therapeutic giants – past, present and future. Cytokine Growth Factor Review. 2014;**25**(4):453-472

[97] Siniscalchi A, Gallelli L, Malferrari G, et al. Cerebral stroke injury: The role of cytokines and brain inflammation. Journal of Basic and Clinical Physiology and Pharmacology. 2014;**25**(2):131-137

[98] Clark IA, Vissel B. Amyloid beta: One of three danger-associated molecules that are secondary inducers of the proinflammatory cytokines that mediate Alzheimer's disease. British Journal of Pharmacology. 2015;**172**(15):3714-3727

[99] Gerard E, Spengler RN, Bonoiu AC, et al. Chronic constriction injury-induced nociception is relieved by nanomedicine-mediated decrease of rat hippocampal tumor necrosis factor. Pain. 2015;**156**(7):1320-1333

[100] Tai LM, Ghura S, Koster KP, et al. APOE-modulated Abeta-induced neuroinflammation in Alzheimer's disease: Current landscape, novel data and future perspective. Journal of Neurochemical. 2015;**133**(4):465-488

[101] Varley J, Brooks DJ, Edison P. Imaging neuroinflammation in Alzheimer's disease and other dementias: Recent advances and future directions. Alzheimers Dement. 2015;**11**(9):1110-1120

[102] Hsuan YC, Lin CH, Chang CP, et al. Mesenchymal stem cell-based treatments for stroke, neural trauma, and heat stroke. Brain and Behavior. 2016;**6**(10):e00526

[103] Jang SS, Chung HJ. Emerging link between alzheimer's disease and homeostatic synaptic plasticity. Neural Plasticity. 2016;**2016**:7969272

[104] Su F, Bai F, Zhang Z. Inflammatory cytokines and alzheimer's disease: A review from the perspective of genetic polymorphisms. Neuroscience Bulletin. 2016;**32**(5):469-480

[105] Yadav S, Gandham SK, Panicucci R, et al. Intranasal brain delivery of cationic nanoemulsion-encapsulated TNF-α siRNA in prevention of experimental neuroinflammation. Nanomedicine. 2016;**12**(4):987-1002

[106] Tobinick E. Deciphering the physiology underlying the rapid clinical effects of perispinal etanercept in Alzheimer's disease. Current Alzheimer Research. 2012;**9**(1):99-109

[107] Elenkov IJ, Kovacs K, Duda E, et al. Presynaptic inhibitory effect of TNF-α on the release of noradrenaline in isolated median eminence. Journal of Neuroimmunology. 1992;**41**(1):117-120

[108] Ignatowski TA, Chou RC, Spengler RN. Changes in noradrenergic sensitivity to tumor necrosis factor-alpha in brains of rats administered clonidine. Journal of Neuroimmunology. 1996;**70**(1):55-63

[109] Ignatowski TA, Noble BK, Wright JR, et al. Neuronal-associated tumor necrosis factor (TNF-α): its role in noradrenergic functioning and modification of its expression following antidepressant drug administration. Journal of Neuroimmunology. 1997; **79**(1):84-90

[110] Ignatowski TA, Spengler RN. Tumor necrosis factor-alpha: Presynaptic sensitivity is modified after antidepressant drug administration. Brain Research. 1994;**665**(2):293-299

[111] Covey WC, Ignatowski TA, Knight PR, et al. Brain-derived TNF-α: Involvement in neuroplastic changes implicated in the conscious perception of persistent pain. Brain Research. 2000;**859**(1):113-122

[112] Ignatowski TA, Sud R, Reynolds JL, et al. The dissipation of neuropathic pain paradoxically involves the presence of tumor necrosis factor-alpha (TNF). Neuropharmacology. 2005;**48**(3):448-460

[113] Marchand F, Tsantoulas C, Singh D, et al. Effects of Etanercept and Minocycline in a rat model of spinal cord injury. European Journal of Pain. 2009;**13**(7):673-681

[114] Shen CH, Tsai RY, Shih MS, et al. Etanercept restores the antinociceptive effect of morphine and suppresses spinal neuroinflammation in morphine-tolerant rats. Anesthesia & Analgesia. 2011;**112**(2):454-459

[115] Rossi D, Martorana F, Brambilla L. Implications of gliotransmission for the pharmacotherapy of CNS disorders. CNS Drugs. 2011;**25**(8):641-658

[116] Covey WC, Ignatowski TA, Renauld AE, et al. Expression of neuron-associated tumor necrosis factor alpha in the brain is increased during persistent pain. Regional Anesthesia and Pain Medicine. 2002;**27**(4):357-366

[117] Sud R, Ignatowski TA, Lo CP, et al. Uncovering molecular elements of brain-body communication during development and treatment of neuropathic pain. Brain, Behavior, and Immunity. 2007;**21**(1):112-124

[118] Cacci E, Claasen JH, Kokaia Z. Microglia-derived tumor necrosis factor-alpha exaggerates death of newborn hippocampal progenitor cells in vitro. The Journal of Neuroscience. 2005;**80**(6):789-797

[119] Ekdahl CT, Kokaia Z, Lindvall O. Brain inflammation and adult neurogenesis: The dual role of microglia. Neuroscience. 2009;**158**(3):1021-1029

[120] Iosif RE, Ahlenius H, Ekdahl CT, et al. Suppression of stroke-induced progenitor proliferation in adult subventricular zone by tumor necrosis factor receptor 1. The Journal of Neuroscience. 2008;**28**(9):1574-1587

[121] Iosif RE, Ekdahl CT, Ahlenius H, et al. Tumor necrosis factor receptor 1 is a negative regulator of progenitor proliferation in adult hippocampal neurogenesis. The Journal of Neuroscience. 2006;**26**(38):9703-9712

[122] Monje ML, Toda H, Palmer TD. Inflammatory blockade restores adult hippocampal neurogenesis. Science. 2003;**302**(5651):1760-1765

[123] Clark IA, Alleva LM, Vissel B. The roles of TNF in brain dysfunction and disease. Pharmacology & Therapeutics. 2010;**128**(3):519-548

[124] del Rey A, Yau HJ, Randolf A, et al. Chronic neuropathic pain-like behavior correlates with IL-1β expression and disrupts cytokine interactions in the hippocampus. Pain. 2011;**152**(12):2827-2835

[125] Ren WJ, Liu Y, Zhou LJ, et al. Peripheral nerve injury leads to working memory deficits and dysfunction of the hippocampus by upregulation of TNF-α in rodents. Neuropsychopharmacology. 2011;**36**(5):979-992

[126] Dellarole A, Morton P, Brambilla R, et al. Neuropathic pain-induced depressive-like behavior and hippocampal neurogenesis and plasticity are dependent on TNFR1 signaling. Brain, Behavior, and Immunity. 2014;**41**:65-81

[127] Auffray C. Evaluations for Tobinick, EL and Gross H J of Neuroinflammation. Faculty of 1000 Biology. 2008;**5**(1):2

[128] Kato K, Kikuchi S, Shubayev VI, et al. Distribution and tumor necrosis factor-alpha isoform binding specificity of locally administered etanercept into injured and uninjured rat sciatic nerve. Neuroscience. 2009;**160**(2):492-500

[129] Cavanagh C, Colby-Milley J, Farso M, et al. Early molecular and synaptic dysfunctions in the prodromal stages of Alzheimer's disease: Focus on TNF-α and IL-1β. Future Neurology. 2011;**6**(6):757-769

[130] Gabbita SP, Srivastava MK, Eslami P, et al. Early intervention with a small molecule inhibitor for tumor necrosis factor-alpha prevents cognitive deficits in a triple transgenic mouse model of Alzheimer's disease. Journal of Neuroinflammation. 2012;**9**:99

[131] Kaufman EL, Carl A. Biochemistry of back pain. The Open Spine Journal. 2013;**5**:12-18

[132] Muccigrosso MM, Ford J, Benner B, et al. Cognitive deficits develop 1 month after diffuse brain injury and are exaggerated by Microglia-Associated reactivity to peripheral immune challenge. Brain, Behavior, and Immunity. 2016;**54**:95-109

[133] Menzel L, Kleber L, Friedrich C, et al. Progranulin protects against exaggerated axonal injury and astrogliosis following traumatic brain injury. Glia. 2017;**65**(2):278-292

[134] Glasziou P, Chalmers I, Rawlins M, et al. When are randomised trials unnecessary? Picking signal from noise. Bitish Medical Journal. 2007;**334**(7589):349-351

[135] Darwin, C., J.F. Duthie, and W. Hopkins, On the origin of species by means of natural selection: or, The preservation of favoured races in the struggle for life. 1859, London: John Murray, Albemarle Street.

Chapter 8

The Role of NO/cGMP Signaling on Neuroinflammation: A New Therapeutic Opportunity

Christina A. Peixoto, Ana K.S. Nunes and Catarina Rapôso

Additional information is available at the end of the chapter

http://dx.doi.org/10.5772/intechopen.68990

Abstract

The nitric oxide/cyclic guanosine monophosphate (NO/cGMP) signaling appears to play a key role in inhibiting neuroinflammation and preventing the activation of a proapoptotic pathway, thereby promoting neural cell survival. In addition, evidence indicates that cGMP/protein kinase G (PKG) pathway is involved in the modulation of glial cell activity. Phosphodiesterase 5 (PDE5), which hydrolyzes cGMP in the inactive form, 5'GMP, is present throughout the body and brain and has emerged as a potential therapeutic target for diseases related to neuroinflammatory and neurodegenerative processes, since their inhibition leads to accumulation of cGMP. The objective of this chapter is to review current knowledge of NO/cGMP signaling pathways on neuroinflammation and the potential therapeutic use of PDE5 inhibitors (PDE5-Is) in neurological diseases. The extensive, while recent, literature on the effects of PDE-Is on Alzheimer's disease (AD), multiple sclerosis (MS), Parkinson's disease (PD), Huntington's disease (HD), and stroke has been reviewed.

Keywords: PDE5 inhibitors, neurological diseases, glial cells, cGMP signaling, neuroinflammation, neurodegeneration

1. Introduction

A growing number of studies have explored the interaction between the nervous and immune systems during the development of neurological disorders. The central nervous system (CNS) is an environment considered "immunologically privileged," as many antibodies and peripheral immune cells are blocked by the blood-brain barrier (BBB), a highly specialized brain endothelial structure composed of pericytes, astrocytes, and microglia, which does not allow the passage of peripheral immune cells and whose resident cells express little major histocompatibility complexes I and II (MHC-I and MHC-II) receptors, as well as low levels of proinflammatory cytokines. However, in damage situation, glial cells show increased expression of MHC, Toll-like receptors (TLRs), and proinflammatory cytokines (such as TNF-α, IFN-γ, IL-1β, and IL-6). Innate immune response mediated by glial cells seems to be crucial for the progression of many neurodegenerative diseases including Alzheimer's disease (AD), multiple sclerosis (MS), and Parkinson's disease (PD). Thus, neuroimmunology emerged as an intersection between the nervous system disease mechanism and therapeutic targets.

The nitric oxide/cyclic guanosine monophosphate (NO/cGMP) signaling appears to play an essential role in inhibiting neuroinflammation and in preventing the activation of a proapoptotic pathway, thus promoting neural cell survival. Phosphodiesterase type 5 inhibitors (PDE5-Is) have recently emerged as a potential therapeutic strategy to modulate neuroinflammation. Mechanistically, PDE5-Is exert anti-inflammatory and neuroprotection effects by inhibiting PDE5 with subsequent accumulation of cGMP and activation of protein kinase G (PKG). The objective of this chapter is to review present knowledge of the NO/cGMP signaling pathways on neuroinflammation and the potential therapeutic use of PDE5-Is on neurodiseases.

2. The role of NO/cGMP signaling on inflammation

Cyclic nucleotides, cyclic adenosine monophosphate (cAMP), and cyclic guanosine monophosphate (cGMP) exert many physiological roles such as the regulation of ion channels, relaxation of smooth muscle, immunomodulation, inflammation, cell proliferation and apoptosis, insulin secretion and glycogen synthesis/glycogenolysis, lipogenesis and lipolysis steroidogenesis, phototransduction as well as neuronal survival, and consolidation of memory. Both cAMP and cGMP can alter cell function by activating or inactivating proteins by phosphorylation. The most important regulation of cyclic nucleotides is achieved in negative feedback by activating phosphodiesterases (PDEs), which hydrolyses the cAMP and cGMP in their inactive forms, 5'AMP and 5'GMP, respectively [1–3].

Synthesis of intracellular cAMP from adenosine 5'-triphosphate (ATP) by membrane-bound adenylyl cyclase (AC) is mainly regulated by G proteins. The response to activation of G-protein-coupled receptors (GPCRs) transduces a variety of extracellular signals and then to intracellular signals, regulating cellular responses [4]. The key transducer of cAMP signals is the cAMP-dependent protein kinase A (PKA). Upon binding of cAMP to the regulatory PKA subunits, it dissociates into two free regulatory and two catalytic subunits. The liberated active catalytic PKA subunits can phosphorylate serine and threonine residues on substrate proteins, including the transcription factor cAMP-response element-binding protein (CREB). There are some alternative PKA-independent cAMP actions, such as the immunomodulatory effects in monocytes and macrophages of guanine exchange proteins directly activated by cAMP (EPAC-1 and EPAC-2) [5, 6].

Synthesis of cGMP is mediated by membrane-bound/particulate (pGC) and cytosolic/soluble (sGC) guanylate cyclases, which convert guanosine 5'-triphosphate (GTP) into cGMP. sGC is activated by NO released by the endothelium and neurons, whereas pGCs (GC-A, GC-B, and GC-C) are activated by binding of specific peptides. GC-A present in the kidney is responsible for controlling natriuresis and blood pressure through stimulation by atrial natriuretic peptide (ANP) and brain-type natriuretic peptide (BNP), which are released from the heart. In the small intestine, GC-C stimulates secretion of fluids through activation by intestinal peptide, guanylin [7]. The physiological effects of cGMP activities are determined by three types of intracellular targets: cGMP-dependent kinases (PKG), cyclic nucleotide-gated channels, and cGMP-binding PDEs [8]. In some cell types, it modulates the concentration of cAMP by activating PDE2 or inhibiting PDE3 activity [9, 10].

cGMP plays an important role as a mediator of the action of NO. NO is highly reactive and unstable free radical, which regulates a variety of cellular functions by diffusion from its originating cell to surrounding cells [11]. The NO can be synthesized by three NO synthase (NOS) isoforms, namely, neuronal synthase (nNOS or NOS-I), inducible form (iNOS or NOS-II), and the endothelial form (eNOS or NOS-III). The constitutive isoforms, eNOS and nNOS, are anchored on the internal surface of the cell membranes, and their activities by the endothelial cells and neurons are responsible for maintenance of physiological homeostasis such as blood pressure and blood flow, platelet aggregation, leukocyte adhesion to the endothelium, and neuronal signaling. eNOS and nNOS produce NO under physiological conditions and are primarily regulated by intracellular Ca^{2+}/calmodulin levels. The inducible isoform iNOS is Ca^{2+} independent and represents a newly synthesized enzyme, which is expressed in response to specific stimuli, such as endotoxin and cytokines. iNOS is present in macrophages, hepatocytes, smooth muscle, endothelium, and glial cells and produces NO after immunological stimulation [i.e., IFN-γ, TNF-α, lipopolysaccharide (LPS)]. Whereas eNOS and nNOS produce NO for a short period of time (seconds or minutes), iNOS produces NO for long period of time (hours to days) and typically synthesizes 100–1000 times more than constitutive NOS [12, 13]. At high levels, NO produced by iNOS exerts cytotoxic and pro-inflammatory effects; however, the low nanomolar concentrations of NO produced by the eNOS isoform exhibit anti-inflammatory effects via the cGMP signaling and perhaps other mechanisms [14, 15]. The NO pathway can inhibit vascular nuclear factor-kappaB (NF-κB), a key transcriptional mediator of inflammation, by increasing the expression of cytoplasmic and nuclear levels of its inhibitor, the IκB-α [16], or by directly inhibiting the NF-κB binding [17]. Moreover, eNOS regulates NF-κB expression in a negative feedback mechanism, limiting local inflammation [18].

Studies developed on knockout mice for NOS isoforms indicate that NO derived from eNOS and nNOS is critical in the regulation of leukocyte-endothelial cell interactions in postcapillary venules [19, 20]. NO produced by the vascular endothelium exerts a cytoprotective and antithrombotic role by preventing the activation and adherence of leukocytes and platelets. The anti-inflammatory effects of NO are mediated predominantly via the activation of sGC and subsequent formation of cGMP. The production of cGMP causes specific downregulation of the expression of P-selectin on endothelial cells and platelets to prevent leukocyte rolling, adhesion, and migration [21].

The NF-κB is the generic name of a family of transcription factors that functions as dimers and regulates gene expression of a plethora of inflammatory and immune mediators, including cyclooxygenase-2 (COX-2) and iNOS, both considered important mediators in the recruitment of inflammatory cells [22–24]. The NF-κB proteins are sequestered in the cytoplasm through physical interaction with IκB family proteins. Proinflammatory cytokines (IL-1, TNF-α), B- and T-cell activators, pathogen-associated molecular patterns (PAMPs), and oxidative stress activate IκB kinase (IKK), a cytoplasmic kinase complex, that phosphorylates the IκB molecules, leading to their subsequent degradation through the ubiquitin–proteasome pathway. NF-κB dimers then translocate to the nucleus where they can bind to κB consensus sequences and activates the transcription of various genes [4]

Cyclic AMP/PKA modulates the NF-κB function through several events; some of them include CREB-mediated transcription of the IκB gene, thus elevating the expression of resynthesized IκB, inhibiting IκB degradation via blocking of IKK activity, and enhancing IκB levels by interfering with Iκ ubiquitination and/or subsequent proteasomal degradation [25–28].

Intracellular levels of cGMP also exert a role in modulating inflammatory response. Initially, some studies demonstrated that inhibition of endogenous NO production markedly increased monocyte chemoattractant protein-1 (MCP-1) mRNA levels in endothelial cells, whereas exogenous addition of NO dose dependently decreased MCP-1 mRNA expression and secretion [29]. This NO modulating effect of MCP-1 expression occurs via suppression of NF-κB by reducing the degradation of IκB [30, 31]. In sequence, a detailed study described the NO/cGMP role in regulating the inflammatory response. According to Aiwaza and cols [9], NO and C-type natriuretic peptide (CNP) inhibit NF-κB activity via cGMP-dependent activation of PKA, but not of PKG. In summary, the cGMP elevated levels by NO donor or natriuretic peptide inhibited PDE3 activity, which lead to the increase of cAMP and activation of PKA. PKA inhibited NF-κB transcription activity and, subsequently, the downstream MCP-1 and vascular cell adhesion molecule-1 (VCAM-1) gene expressions.

Moreover, there are other mechanisms by which NO/cGMP regulates the NF-κB activation and MCP-1 expression, such as activation of mitogen-activated protein kinase (MAPK) phosphatase-1 (MKP-1) and, ultimately, inhibition of p38 MAPK, suggesting a counter-regulatory action of p38 MAPK and NF-κB [32].

In addition to anti-inflammatory effects, NO can have both pro- and anti-tumorigenic activities depending on NOS uncoupling that can occur under some conditions, such as low [Arg] or elevated levels of endogenous NOS inhibitors. Uncoupled NOS produces oxidants like peroxynitrite and O_2, which initiates different downstream signaling that for tumor cells are pro-proliferative and antiapoptotic, e.g., NF-κB. However, when the primary product of NOS is NO, downstream signaling is dominated by anti-tumorigenic NO-dependent pathways (sGC/cGMP/PKG) [33]. The NO/cGMP/PKG pathway appears to play an essential role in promoting apoptosis, thus inhibiting tumor growth. Activating cGMP/PKG pathway by PDE5 inhibitors selectively inhibits colon tumor growth, as well as the knockdown of PDE5 in colon cancer cell (HT-29) by siRNA efficiently promotes apoptosis and delayed proliferation [34, 35]. Recently, it was also demonstrated that increased intracellular levels of cGMP induced by the inhibition of PDE5 significantly inhibit colonic tumorigenesis dependent on inflammation [36].

However, NO/cGMP/PKG actions appear to be highly cell type and context dependent. In some neural cells, the NO/cGMP/PKG pathway has an essential role as an antiapoptotic/prosurvival factor [37]. This neuroprotective mechanism may be especially important during brain ischemia, inflammation, or trauma. In retinal neuroglial progenitor cells, NO/cGMP/PKG antiapoptotic cascade is activated through Akt-induced CREB1 activation [38, 39]. CREB is a transcription factor involved with neurotransmitters, growth factors, and other signaling molecules with essential functions for memory and neuronal survival [40, 41]. In cerebellar granule neurons, there is evidence that NO plays an active role in sustaining the neuronal survival through NO/cGMP/PKG [42].

cGMP/PKG1 is also considered as a key effector in cardioprotection induced by PDE5 inhibitors against ischemic injury in the infarcted heart and cardiomyocytes. The potential mechanisms include its antiapoptotic effect as is evident by increased phosphorylation of Akt (pAkt) and glycogen synthase kinase 3β (pGSK3β), Bcl-2 expression, and prevention of caspase-3/caspase-7 activation [43–45]. Other studies provided the evidence that PDE5 inhibition prolonged survival of transplanted of bone marrow-derived mesenchymal stem cells in ischemic heart via cGMP/PKG signaling, contributing to regeneration of the ischemic heart [46].

3. The role of glial cells on neuroinflammation: the modulation by NO/cGMP

Several lines of evidence strongly suggest that neuroinflammation is a crucial process involved in the progression of neuronal degeneration, a common feature observed in several neurodegenerative disorders. Therefore, the involvement of the local innate immune response can be a very complex process, contributing to perpetuate the damage to the CNS [47].

In the inflammatory process, there is an increase in blood flow and vascular permeability, venular dilatation, and recruitment of cells to the inflammatory site. Reactive oxygen species (ROS) play an important role in the inflammatory process, including endothelial cell damage and increased microvascular permeability, chemotactic factor production, neutrophil recruitment, oxidation, and lipid peroxidation [48]. These inflammatory mediators play a regulatory role in the growth, differentiation, and activation of immune cells [49]. Glial cells (microglia, astrocytes, and oligodendrocytes) define brain homeostasis and are responsible for defense against neural tissue injury [50, 51].

3.1. Astrocytes

Astrocytes constitute a very heterogeneous population of cells, which regulate pH, extracellular levels of ions, neurotransmitters, and energy metabolism. They are involved in the formation and functioning of BBB [52] and also actively participate in neurotransmission [53]. In situations of CNS damage, the typical response is some degree of reactive gliosis [54], an astrocytic response involving positive gene regulation of cytoskeletal proteins (e.g., glial fibrillary acid protein, GFAP), hypertrophy, hyperplasia, and rearrangement of astrocytes, which may form glial scars [50].

In addition, astrocytes play an important role in central immunity. The innate immune response is precisely adjusted by identifying the type of threat that is present. Molecular structures associated with the threat are recognized by pattern recognition receptors (PRRs). PRRs recognize PAMPs, expressed by bacteria, fungi, and viruses, or damage-associated molecular patterns (DAMPs), expressed by cells and tissues under stress or injury. One of the major classes of PRRs in mammals is TLRs. The response is rapid both to the presence of pathogens and to other types of damage to the tissue, activating the immune system, which releases cytokines and chemokines, and modulating the BBB [50].

Astrocytes express TLRs [55]. The brain and spinal cord of multiple sclerosis patients showed increased TLR3 and TLR4 in astrocytes in regions of inflammation [56]. Most TLRs, after detecting their respective ligands, initiate a signal that is mediated by the myeloid differentiation gene 88 (Myd88) and result in the activation of nuclear transcription factor NF-κB. Translocation of NF-κB to the nucleus culminates in the secretion of proinflammatory molecules (IL-1β, IL-6, TNF-α, and IL-12). Activated astrocytes may also produce chemokines that recruit microglial cells, lymphocytes, and dendritic cells to the site of injury [57].

In the astrocytic response, in addition to increased TLR4 levels, leading to the expression of a variety of chemokines and cytokines [55, 58], other important processes occur, such as alteration of intracellular calcium signaling. Under conditions that lead to neuroinflammation in the CNS, as in exposure to LPS, Ca^{2+} signaling in the astrocyte network is over activated, triggering astrocyte activation. The inhibition of the communicating junctions (gap junctions), with changes in intercellular Ca^{2+} waves and Na^+/K^+-ATPase activity, results in disorganization of the actin filaments (stress fibers) [58, 59], and these effects are hallmarks of astrocyte reaction on neuroinflammation.

Evidence indicates that the cGMP/PKG pathway is involved in the regulation of astrocytic activity [60]. The NO, through the cGMP/PKG, decreased intracellular Ca^{2+} in astrocytes, reducing intercellular Ca^{2+} waves [61]. In addition, cGMP inhibited IFN-γ-induced MHC-II expression, as well as the expression of LPS-induced matrix metalloproteinase-9 (MMP-9) and TNF-α in cultured astrocytes [13, 60, 62]. According to these studies, MMP-9 expression is dependent on extracellular signal-regulated kinase (ERK) activation via NF-κB. This data supports the hypothesis that the NO/cGMP/PKG pathway plays a role in astrocytic cells that contributes to the resolution of neuroinflammation.

3.2. Microglia

Microglia constitute the cells that are part of the innate immune system and are therefore considered as the pathological sensors of the CNS damage. The phenotypic changes of the microglia after activation are functionally identical to those observed in macrophages [63, 64]. The physiological functions of microglia are important for the maintenance of homeostasis. In addition, they have been shown to be responsible for the secretion of neurotrophic factors, such as the brain-derived neurotrophic factor (BDNF) [65] and for removing aggregates of proteins [66]. However, when exposed to infections, lesions, or dysfunction of the nervous system, microglial cells become activated. In the absence of pathology, the microglia "at rest" are small cells with long and thin processes ("branched phenotype"). When activated, the microglia loses the long extensions typical of the inactive microglia and exhibits ameboid extensions ("ameboid phenotype") [67]. Protein Iba-1, expressed on the microglia surface, is used as a marker of its activated state [68]. This physiological transformation is associated with changes in the expression of surface receptors and the release of cytokines, which may contribute to the damage of synaptic plasticity and the neurodegenerative disease aggravation [69].

Activated microglial cells become a source of TNF-α, IL-1β, IL-1α, superoxide, NO, chemokines, and glutamate, which may promote neuronal death. TNF-α, secreted both by microglia and astrocytes, can directly promote neuronal death by binding to its corresponding receptors (TNFRs). Evidence indicates that TNF-α induces apoptosis of mature oligodendrocytes in inflammatory demyelinating diseases such as multiple sclerosis [61, 70] and plays a key role in neurodegeneration process observed in Parkinson's and Alzheimer's diseases [57].

An in vitro study using N9 microglial cells demonstrated that the treatment with the PDE5 inhibitor, sildenafil, suppressed NO, IL-1β, and TNF-α production induced by LPS, due to suppression of the MAPKs/NF-κB pathways through the inhibition of NADPH oxidase, mediated ROS generation [71]. These results indicate that cGMP accumulation as a result of PDE5 inhibition might participate in the inhibition of microglial activation.

3.3. Oligodendrocytes

Oligodendrocytes are myelinizing CNS cells that arise from oligodendrocyte progenitor cells (OPCs). OPCs differentiate in mature or myelinizing oligodendrocyte, fixing extensions in axons to generate the concentric membrane layers to produce myelin. The presence of oligodendrocytes is more common in the white matter of neuronal tissue, such as the corpus callosum and cerebellum, and less frequent in gray [72]. In both compartments, myelin is necessary for the saltatory conduction of action potentials along axons [73].

Oligodendrocyte dysfunction and myelin abnormalities are found in a wide variety of neurological diseases and may be involved in the pathophysiology of various diseases, including genetic leukodystrophies [74], schizophrenia and bipolar disorder [75, 76], brain injury [77], and endocrine and metabolic abnormalities [78, 79] and neurodegenerative conditions such as strokes [80, 81], Parkinson's disease [82], Alzheimer's disease [83–85], multiple sclerosis [86], and diabetic encephalopathy [87].

In an attempt to repair myelin damage, increased differentiation of OPCs into mature oligodendrocytes promotes remyelination [88]. In later stages of injury, however, OPCs also enter into apoptosis. Recent studies have shown that treatment with sildenafil increases the levels of the protein expressed by oligodendrocytes, myelin basic protein (MBP), and also restores myelin sheath morphology, indicating remyelination. In addition, sildenafil induces the differentiation of OPCs into mature oligodendrocytes, as demonstrated by the increase of glutathione S-transferase pi (GST-pi, a marker of mature oligodendrocytes), indicating that cGMP signaling can modulate OPC survival and myelin production [89].

Oligodendrocytes are not inert immune cells, but secrete a wide variety of inflammatory mediators, such as the proinflammatory cytokines IL-1-β and IL-6 and CCL-2 and IL-8 chemokines involved in the recruitment of immune cells during inflammation [90]. In experimental multiple sclerosis models, oligodendrocytes in apoptosis also express increased levels of COX-2 at the demyelination beginning, which seem to make these cells more susceptible to death by glutamate-mediated excitotoxicity [91].

4. Therapeutic applications of phosphodiesterase 5 inhibitors in central neurological diseases

Faced with rising costs for the development of new drugs, researchers are looking for ways to repurpose older ones. Taking medications that have been developed for one disorder—and even some that fail in initial trials—and "repositioning" them to tackle another are a growing strategy for researchers in industry and academia [92].

The administration of selective PDE5-Is increases the levels of cGMP [93, 94], with effects on multiple organs and systems. The PDE5-I, sildenafil, is a medication for angina pectoris developed in 1989 [92]. For many years, sildenafil (Viagra®, Pfizer) has been the most representative molecule of the class of drugs to treat erectile dysfunction (ED) [95]. Under the trade name Revatio® (Pfizer), it was also approved for pulmonary artery hypertension therapy in June 2005 [96] and, more recently, for the Raynaud's phenomenon [97]. Therefore, sildenafil is a classic success story of repositioning.

PDE5 is present throughout the body and brain [95, 98] and has emerged as a potential therapeutic target for diseases related to neuroinflammatory and neurodegenerative processes because of its reported relation with them (for review, see [99]). To date, only four PDE5-Is have been approved by the US Food and Drug Administration (FDA) and by the European Medicines Agency: sildenafil, vardenafil, tadalafil, and avanafil. Sildenafil is reported to clearly cross the BBB [100], whereas evidence for vardenafil is indirect [101] and, while it was first considered that tadalafil does not cross it [102], later was demonstrated that this drug is able to cross the barrier [103]. Several studies indicate that sildenafil and other PDE5-Is may offer novel strategies for the treatment of neurological pathologies [12, 102, 104]. The beneficial effects of PDE5-Is were initially attributed to its mechanism in smooth muscle (regulating blood flow) and improving synaptic plasticity and neurogenesis. However, recent studies point to an important effect of these drugs on neuroinflammation, which may be, at least in part, responsible for their protective effects on central neurological diseases.

Thus, five major mechanisms of PDE5-Is have been described in neurological disease models: (1) by modulating the CREB pathway, inducing the formation of new synaptic connections and neurogenesis, improving cognition and memory; (2) through the modulation of Akt/GSK3β and calpain/p25/CDK5 pathways, decreasing aggregate formation of proteins; (3) through apoptosis inhibition; (4) by inducting angiogenesis and improving blood flow; and (5) through the modulation of neuroinflammation. Targeting multiple elements in the network underlying complex diseases, such as neurological diseases, may produce benefits beyond those of representative monotherapies [105, 106]. Repositioning PDE5-Is as therapeutic approaches that can be used in combination with other drugs can therefore be useful. This section aims to name and classify representative preclinical and clinical studies of PDE5-Is in central neurological diseases (Alzheimer's disease, multiple sclerosis, Parkinson's disease, Huntington's disease (HD), and stroke) and to describe the main known mechanisms, with emphasis on neuroinflammation (following a search of the Medline®/PubMed® database, during the period between 2000 and 2016).

4.1. Alzheimer's disease

Alzheimer's disease (AD) has become the fourth leading lethal disease among the elderly after cancer, heart disease, and stroke. It is an age-related neurodegenerative disease characterized by the presence of senile plaques (consisting of β-amyloid filaments, Aβ), neurofibrillary tangles (composed of hyperphosphorylated tau deposits), and neuronal degeneration accompanied by significant loss of synapses [107, 108] (**Figure 1A**). While early studies focused on assessing the beneficial effects of PDE5-Is on AD through the formation of synapses, neurogenesis, and protein aggregation pathways, more recent studies have shown that the role of these drugs in neuroinflammation may be an important mechanism in AD.

4.1.1. PDE5-Is' beneficial effects in AD through CREB/BDNF/Arc pathway, Akt/GSK3b pathway, and calpain/p25/CDK5 pathway modulation

cGMP/PKG pathway contributes to phosphorylation of the transcription factor CREB; Prickaerts et al. [109] suggested that the cGMP/PKG/CREB pathway induces the synthesis of proteins essential for memory consolidation, probably through the formation of new synaptic connections [110]. Therefore, the chronic administration of PDE5-Is may lead to gene transcription through CREB activation, by raising cGMP levels (**Figure 2A**).

Puzzo et al., in 2009 [102], and Cuadrado-Tejedor et al., in 2011 [111], showed that sildenafil has beneficial effects on AD models, modulating the CREB pathway. Puzzo et al. [102] demonstrated that sildenafil (3 mg/kg, i.p., for 3 weeks) may be beneficial against cognitive loss in the APP/PS1 mouse model of amyloid deposition, producing an immediate and lasting improvement of synaptic function, CREB phosphorylation, and memory. This effect was associated with a reduction in Aβ levels. Cuadrado-Tejedor et al. [111] showed that sildenafil (15 mg/kg, i.p., for 5 days) restored cognitive deficits in aged rat model of AD (Tg2576-AD transgenic mice); however, whereas pCREB was not significantly induced in mice treated with sildenafil, the BDNF and Arc (CREB downstream target molecules) increased, confirming that the drug acts through this pathway (CREB/BDNF/Arc), inducing synaptic formation and improving memory.

Cuadrado-Tejedor and coworkers [111] showed, however, that sildenafil did not affect Aβ-burden while decreased tau phosphorylation. The formation and aggregation of Aβ and tau involve some pathways, which can be plausible therapeutic target for the treatment of AD. GSK3β, which is inhibited by Akt, and cyclin-dependent kinase 5 (CDK5), which is activated by p25, are the most relevant kinases involved in the pathogenic mechanisms of AD

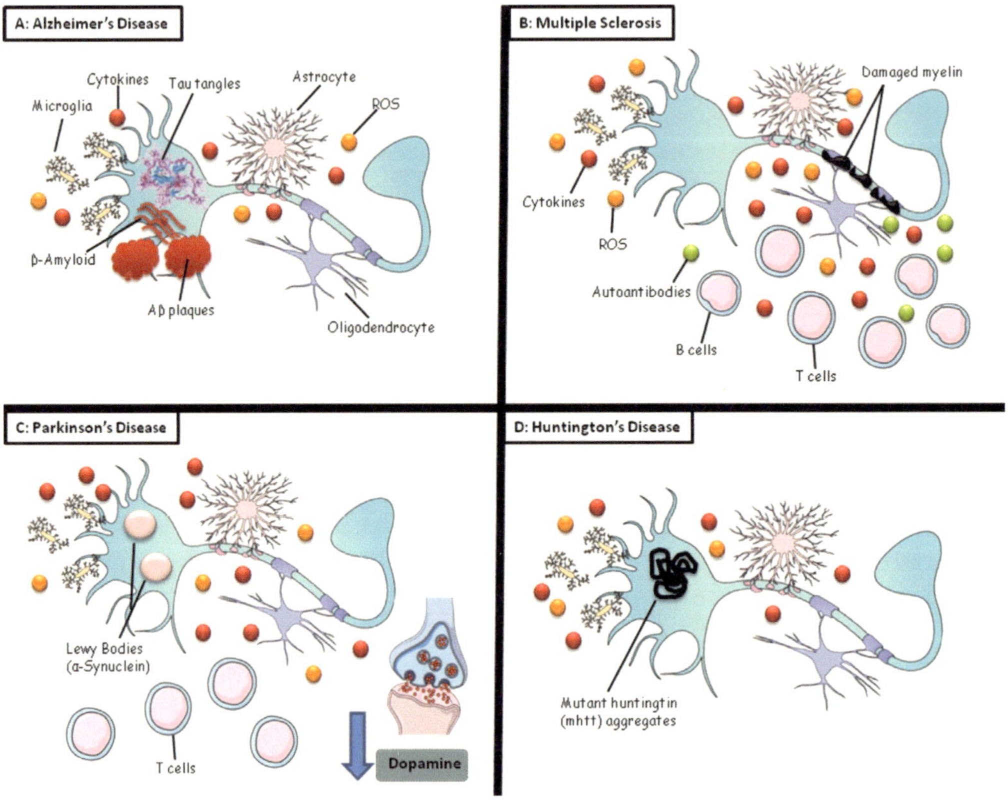

Figure 1. Hallmark pathologies of (A) Alzheimer's disease (AD), (B) multiple sclerosis (MS), (C) Parkinson's disease (PD), and (D) Huntington's disease (HD). (A) In AD, neurons contain intracellular neurofibrillary tangles composed of hyperphosphorylated tau protein and extracellular plaques of amyloid β (Aβ). The inflammatory reaction, with activation of microglia and astrocytes and the subsequent release of inflammatory cytokines and reactive oxygen species (ROS), plays a significant role in the pathological processing of AD. (B) MS is a chronic autoimmune/inflammatory disorder characterized by demyelination of axons, with associated acute and chronic inflammatory events involving the recruitment/activation of microglia/macrophages, astrocytes and B and T cells and release of proinflammatory cytokines, ROS, and autoantibodies. (C) In PD, neurons contain α-synuclein aggregates, forming Lewy bodies. Neuronal loss leads to lower production of dopamine. There is a persistent inflammatory response, T-cell infiltration, and glial cell activation in patients with PD and animal models, which play a crucial role in the degeneration of dopaminergic neurons. (D) In HD, mutant huntingtin protein (mhtt) containing an extended polyglutamine repeat, caused by at least 36 CAG repeats in the huntingtin gene, leads to intraneuronal aggregates. In all four diseases, the pathological events ultimately result in neuronal death. Over time, this either causes or contributes to neuroinflammation.

by phosphorylation at multiple sites of the microtubule-binding protein, tau [112, 113]. The activities of GSK3β and CDK5 were reduced by sildenafil, whereas the drug increased Akt and decreased p25. The decrease in kinase activity of GSK3β and CDK5 due to sildenafil may lead to a reduction in tau phosphorylation, possibly contributing to the reestablishment of cognitive function (**Figure 2B**). Then, according to Cuadrado-Tejedor et al. [111], sildenafil reversed the marked memory deficits of elderly Tg2576 animals by regulating the Akt/GSK3β/pTau and p25/CDK5/pTau pathways, not resulting from any decrease in the Aβ-load. However, the contrasts between Cuadrado-Tejedor et al. [111] and Puzzo et al. [102] may be

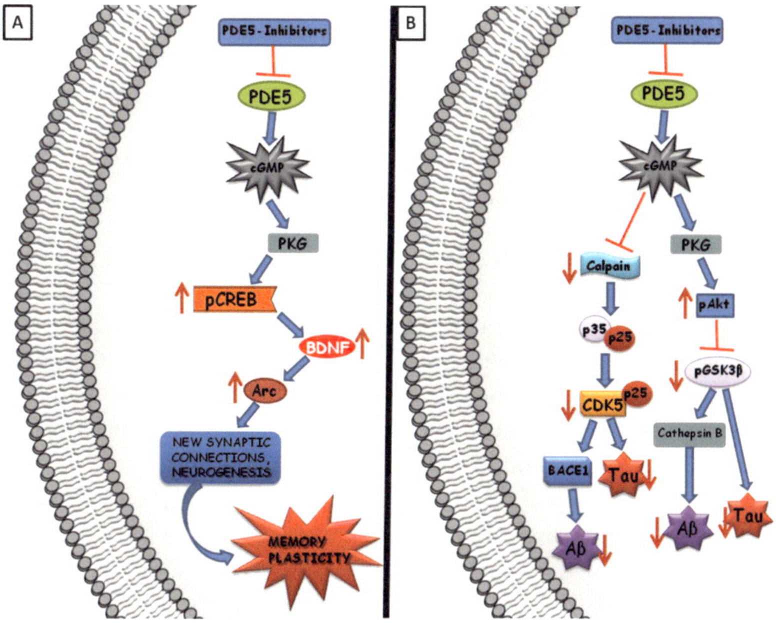

Figure 2. PDE5-I mechanisms in the CREB pathway and protein aggregation. (A) The PDE5 inhibitors (PDE5-Is) modulate the CREB pathway, increasing the expression of CREB and the downstream targets, BDNF, and Arc. The result is the induction of new synaptic connections and neurogenesis, leading to the restoration of pathological cognitive signs of neurological diseases, such as Alzheimer's disease and Huntington's disease. (B) PDE5-Is also modulate pathways involved in the protein aggregation. Calpain is an enzyme that cleavage p35 in its more stable isoform, p25. The formation of the p25/CDK5 complex is associated with tau hyperphosphorylation. In addition, p25/CDK5, via the downstream target BACE1, also leads to cleavage of amyloid precursor protein (APP), contributing to the formation of Aβ plaques. PDE5-Is induce a decrease in the activity of calpain, p25, and CDK5, with consequent decrease in protein aggregation. GSK3β is a kinase involved in the hyperphosphorylation of Tau. In addition, through the downstream target, cathepsin B, GSK3β leads to the formation of Aβ plaques. pAkt is a GSK3β inhibitor, modulating the pathway. PDE-Is increase Akt phosphorylation and decrease GSK3β activity and cathepsin B expression, which can contribute to control the protein aggregation. —┤ Inhibition ⟶ ; activation; ↑ increased expression/activity; ↓ decreased expression/activity.

due to differences between dose, duration of treatment, and animal models. In addition, both Akt/GSK3β and p25/CDK5 signaling are also involved in the regulation of Aβ [114], and it is possible that if the treatment was longer, this effect would be detected.

Following the same line of investigation, Orejana et al. [114] treated senescence-accelerated mouse-prone 8 (SAMP8, used as a model of aging, which displays many established pathological features of AD) with sildenafil (7.5 mg/kg, i.p., for 4 weeks) and showed that the mechanism of protection is through Aβ decrease, by pAkt/GSK3β /cathepsin B pathway and calpain/p25/CDK5/BACE1 pathway inhibition. pAkt inhibits GSK3β, which is an important activator of cathepsin B [115]. Calpain is an enzyme that cleavages p35 in p25, and p25/CDK5 regulates BACE1 (protein cleaving enzyme 1) expression levels. BACE1 and cathepsin B (both β-secretases) cleavage amyloid precursor protein (APP), contributing to the formation of Aβ. Sildenafil decreased the activity of calpain, p25, and CDK5 and markedly increased Akt phosphorylation and decreased GSK3β activity. Consequently, sildenafil decreased the expression of BACE1 and cathepsin B, leading to a reduction in APP and Aβ levels (**Figure 2B**). These findings demonstrate that sildenafil modulates calpain/p25/CDK5/BACE1 and pAkt/GSK3β/cathepsin B pathways, and these mechanisms are probably responsible for beneficial effects of this class of drugs in AD models.

4.1.2. PDE5-Is beneficial effects in AD through the control of neuroinflammation

Although the first PDE5-I studies in AD models have been focused on synapse formation, neurogenesis, and memory improvement, investigating primarily CREB, tau phosphorylation, and Aβ formation pathways, more recent studies also point to an important anti-inflammatory mechanism of this class of drugs in AD. The work by Orejana et al. [114] was perhaps one of the first studies to suggest and demonstrate that sildenafil modulates inflammatory cells in AD model. They showed that sildenafil decreased the GFAP, a marker of astrogliosis. However, Orejana et al. [114] could not differentiate whether the reduction in GFAP levels resulted from less accumulation of Aβ or if it was a direct modulation of inflammatory events by sildenafil. A recent study using sildenafil in cultured astrocytes confirmed that sildenafil has a direct mechanism on neuroinflammation [116].

Until 2013, it was unknown whether PDE5-Is reversed Aβ-induced neuroinflammation in APP/PS1 transgenic mice. Zhang et al. [117] showed that APP/PS1 mice presented impaired cognitive ability, neuroinflammatory response in the hippocampus, and downregulated cGMP; sildenafil reversed memory deficits and cGMP/PKG/pCREB signaling dysfunction and reduced Aβ levels in this model. In addition, sildenafil decreased the proinflammatory cytokines IL-1β, IL-6, and TNF-α. The inhibition of hippocampal PKG immediately prior to the injection of sildenafil significantly blocked these effects, further indicating the participation of PKG in the anti-inflammatory effects produced by sildenafil (**Figure 3A, B**).

An ongoing neuroinflammatory process has been considered a marker of AD [117]. The deposition of Aβ peptides and the activation of glial cells surrounding senile plaques in brain areas involved in cognitive functions are assumed to participate in the onset of a pathological cascade resulting in synaptic dysfunction, synaptic loss, and neuronal death [118, 119]. The inflammatory reaction, with activation of microglia and astroglia, and the subsequent release of inflammatory cytokines (IL-1β, TNF-α, and COX-2 and so on) play a significant role in the pathological processing of AD [108] (**Figure 1A**). Proinflammatory cytokines, such as TNF-α and IL-1β, may contribute to brain dysfunction and neurodegeneration, impair synaptic plasticity, and induce memory impairment, while the anti-inflammatory cytokine IL-4 has the opposite effect [120, 121]. NF-κB is well known as a key regulator that induces the expression of many proinflammatory cytokines and inducible effector enzymes linked to the inflammatory process. The degradation of IκB-α (NF-κB inhibitory protein) and NF-κB phosphorylation were enhanced after the Aβ injection [108].

Additionally to classical PDE5-Is, other drugs have been demonstrated to act on AD by inhibiting PDE5 and modulating neuroinflammation. It has recently been showed by Li et al. [108] that sodium hydrosulfide (NaHS), a hydrogen sulfide donor, decreased PDE5 levels, attenuated neuronal death, and suppressed apoptosis by inhibiting the activation of pro-caspase-3 in

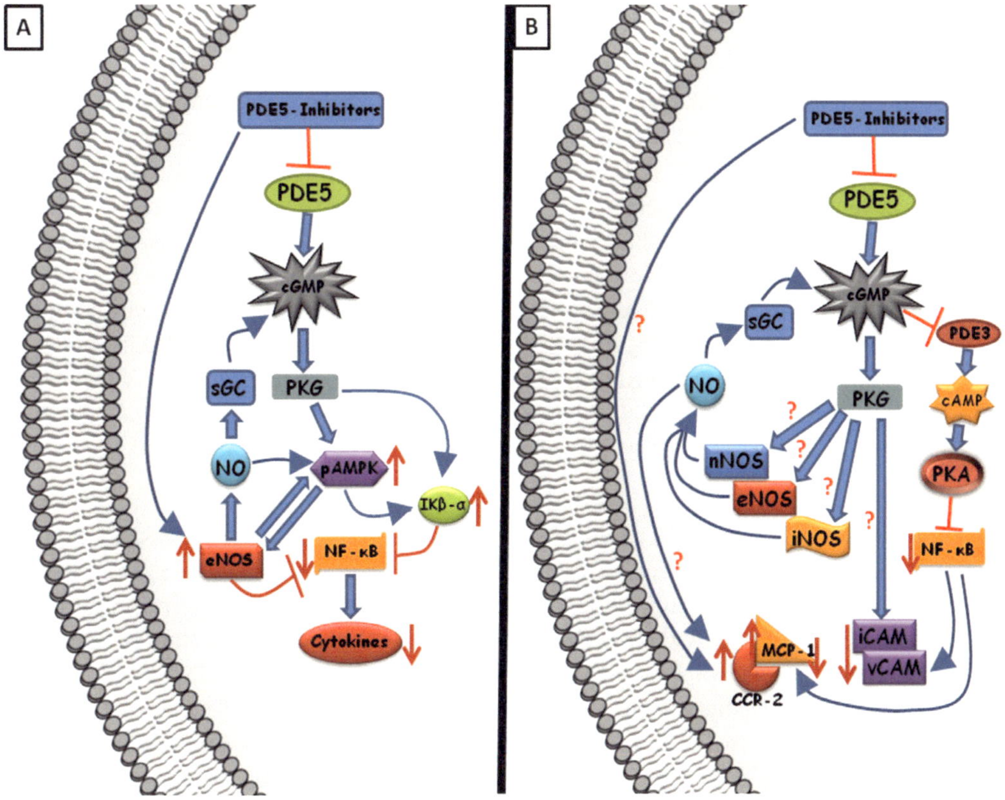

Figure 3. PDE5 inhibitors modulate neuroinflammation. (A) AMPK exerts its anti-inflammatory activity through multiple signaling pathways. The phospho-AMPK (pAMPK) suppresses NF-κB, by increasing its inhibitory protein, IKβ-α. Consequently, the production of cytokines is decreased. In addition, AMPK phosphorylates and activates eNOS, inducing NO production; eNOS increases AMPK, in a positive feedback, and NO can act as an endogenous activator of AMPK, suggesting a reciprocal relationship between AMPK and eNOS. eNOS also inhibits NF-κB, decreasing the inflammatory response. PDE5-Is increase pAMPK and eNOS expression, increase IKβ-α, and decrease NF-κB. NO activates sGC, inducing cGMP production, which can amplify the effect of PDE5-Is. (B) Some possible mechanisms of PDE5-Is in the control of neuroinflammation have been demonstrated while not fully understood. PDE5-Is increase levels of the chemokine MCP-1 and its receptor, CCR-2, which are typically overregulated in multiple sclerosis models. It is possible that this effect is indirect, through NO, since this gas was shown to increase MCP-1/CCR-2, but it has not been confirmed so far. In addition, PDE5-Is were shown to increase the three isoforms of nitric oxide synthase (nNOS, iNOS, and eNOS), along with increased levels of NO. However, the mechanism of NOS participation on the effects of PDE5-Is is unclear. ICAM-1 and VCAM-1 were decreased by PDE5-Is, which may be important for the control of leukocyte infiltration. It is possible that complex cross signaling is occurring, but although it has been demonstrated in inflammatory models, it has not been confirmed in preclinical studies with PDE5-Is in neurological diseases. For example, elevated levels of cGMP by NO may inhibit PDE3 activity, which leads to increased cAMP levels and PKA activation. PKA inhibits NF-κB transcription activity and, subsequently, the expression of downstream MCP-1 and VCAM-1. ⊣ Inhibition; → activation; ↑ increased expression/activity; ↓ decreased expression/activity.

the hippocampus of Sprague-Dawley rats (injected with aggregated Aβ25-35). NaHS upregulated the expression of peroxisome proliferator-activated receptors (PPAR-α and PPAR-γ), which antagonize the effects of NF-κB [122]. Moreover, the Aβ25-35-injected rats exhibited a decrease in IκB-α degradation and an increase in NF-κB p65 phosphorylation levels, whereas these effects were attenuated by NaHS. NaHS can therefore act as an anti-inflammatory mediator by inhibition of PDE5.

A novel PDE5 inhibitor, Yonkenafil (yonk) (2, 6, or 18 mg/kg i.p.), given daily for 3 months, has been shown to have beneficial effects in APP/PS1 mice through anti-inflammatory mechanisms. Yonk reduced the area of Aβ plaques, increased neurogenesis, and inhibited over-activation of microglia and astrocytes [119]. A recent study by Yin et al. [123] has shown that Icariside II (ICSII), another new PDE5 inhibitor, derived from the Chinese herb *Epimedium brevicornum*, has protective effects on the AD model induced by intracerebroventricular streptozotocin (ICV-STZ) in Sprague-Dawley rats. ICSII (10 mg/kg for 21 days) improved cognitive deficits, attenuated neuronal death, and decreased Aβ levels by suppressing BACE1 and APP expression in the rat hippocampus. In addition, ICSII decreased IL-1β, TNF-α, COX-2, and transforming growth factor-β (TGF-β) levels while increasing IκB-α and decreasing NF-κB activation.

It was demonstrated by Jin et al. [124] that Icariin (ICA), a flavonoid extracted from Chinese herb (*Berberidaceae epimedium* L.), an effective oral agent, is also a PDE5-I. Chronic treatment with ICA (30 and 60 mg/kg, twice a day for 4 months) improved the learning and memory of APP/PS1 transgenic mice, and the levels of APP, Aβ, and PDE5 decreased in the hippocampus and cortex after ICA treatment. Furthermore, ICA-treated mice showed increased expression of three NOS isoforms (nNOS, iNOS, and eNOS), along with increased levels of NO and cGMP. These results suggest that NO itself may be involved in the anti-inflammatory effect of PDE5-Is. NO is an important molecule in supporting neurite outgrowth and synapse remodeling [125, 126]. This study by Jin et al. [124] also showed that the three isoforms of NOS and NO levels decreased in the brain of APP/PS1 mice, reinforcing that NO deficiency may contribute to AD. Thus, ICA has a neuroprotective mechanism, probably due to stimulation of the NO/cGMP signaling pathway through the inhibition of PDE5 activity and coordinated induction of NOS isoform expression. Corroborating this result, Rapôso et al. [89, 127] showed that the absence of iNOS abolished the anti-inflammatory effects of sildenafil in mice brains. Treatment with sildenafil for 4 weeks decreased GFAP, COX-2, and the expression of various pro-inflammatory cytokines in wild-type C57BL/6 mice, although it did not have anti-inflammatory effects in $iNOS^{-/-}$ mice. Also, Nunes et al. [128] reported that eNOS is upregulated following chronic administration of sildenafil. These studies point to the relevance of the physiologic expression of NOS for the anti-inflammatory mechanism of PDE5-Is (**Figure 3B**).

Despite the rich (though recent) literature on the effects of the PDE5 inhibitors on animal models of AD, clinical studies are lacking. However, PCR analysis of postmortem tissue of patients suffering from AD found a considerable increase in PDE5 expression in the temporal cortex of the brain compared to healthy controls of the same age [129]. Also, it was observed that lower levels of cGMP in the cerebrospinal fluid of patients with AD were associated with cognitive decline and amyloid pathology [129]. In addition, a clinical study demonstrated that chronic administration of udenafil (Zydena; available in Korea, Russia, and the Philippines) to 27 patients with ED (100 mg at 3-day intervals for 2 month) has shown to lead to an improvement in cognitive function [130]. This has lead to suggest that sildenafil could improve cognitive function in AD patients.

Thus, the efficacy and safety of treatment with repeated doses of PDE5-Is have been demonstrated in several animal models of AD. Since the side effects of PDE5-Is are widely known and do not preclude its administration to a senile population, and considering the lack of effective treatments for AD, PDE5-Is have been proposed as potential alternatives as cognitive enhancers [99, 131].

4.2. Multiple sclerosis

Multiple Sclerosis (MS), the most common neurological disorder in young adults in the Western world, is a chronic autoimmune/inflammatory disorder characterized by demyelination of the nerve cells, which leads to severe psychomotor impairment [132]. CNS demyelination is frequently associated with acute and chronic inflammatory events involving the recruitment-activation of microglia/macrophages, astrocytes, and leukocytes, with the release of pro-inflammatory cytokines, ROS, and NO (**Figure 2B**) [133, 134]. Neuroinflammatory responses appear to begin before any significant loss of neuronal populations in the progression of MS [135].

It has been demonstrated that NO/cGMP signaling is involved in the regulation of neuroinflammation and myelination [89]. The intracellular accumulation of cGMP in different models of inflammation reduces the production of proinflammatory cytokines and oxidative stress, modulating the inflammatory response [136]. In addition, inhibition of PDEs seems to block the inflammatory response of microglia, reducing myelin sheath changes [137, 138]. Therefore, neuroinflammation mediated by glial cells (astrocytes and microglia) appears to be an important phenomenon that perpetuates neural damage in MS, and since cGMP-mediated pathways regulate inflammatory responses in immune and CNS cells, PDE5-Is are potential tools for treating MS.

In fact, it has been reported that patients suffering from ED, and in parallel MS, showed an improvement in clinical status for both pathologies after treatment with sildenafil [139]. The effect of sildenafil on improving the clinical status of patients with MS was initially attributed to the induction of neurogenesis [140]. However, studies have shown that sildenafil is a modulator of inflammation in the central and peripheral nervous systems and protects the myelin sheath both in pathological and healthy conditions [89, 116, 127, 128, 140–144]. This anti-inflammatory mechanism should better explain the protective effect of PDE5-Is in MS, considering the nature of the disease.

In 2011, Pifarré et al. [142] showed that sildenafil (10 mg/kg, s.c., for 18 days) reduced the clinical signs of experimental autoimmune encephalomyelitis (EAE), a mouse model of MS, developed in female C57BL/6 mice. Sildenafil prevented axonal loss and promoted remyelination. Furthermore, sildenafil decreased CD3+ leukocyte infiltration and microglial/macrophage activation in the spinal cord, while increasing T regulatory cells expressing fork head box transcription factor 3 (Foxp3 Tregs) and decreasing ICAM-1 in the infiltrated cells of the spinal cord. Autoreactive T cells infiltrating the CNS are the initiator and early effector cells in EAE development, but infiltrated macrophages, dendritic cells, and resident microglia constitute the ultimate effector cells that amplify neuroinflammation and tissue injury.

ICAM-1, a type-1 membrane-bound glycoprotein expressed in the majority of leukocyte subtypes, endothelial and CNS glial cells, is involved in leukocyte entry, lymphocyte activation, and other immune responses and plays a central role in the development of MS and EAE [145, 146]. The decrease of ICAM-1 induced by sildenafil was also reported by Rapôso et al. [89]. Pifarré et al. [142] also showed that the presence of astrocytes forming scar-like structures around infiltrates was enhanced by sildenafil, suggesting a possible mechanism for the restriction of the leukocyte dissemination in healthy parenchyma. However, this result does not corroborate other studies showing that PDE5-Is decrease GFAP expression and astrocyte activation [89, 114, 127, 140].

Continuing the investigation, Pifarré et al. [143] demonstrated that sildenafil treatment (10 mg/kg, s.c., for 18 days) preserved axons and myelin and increased the number of remyelinating axons in the EAE model; also, sildenafil protected immature and mature myelinating oligodendrocytes. However, if the protective effect of sildenafil on myelin and axons is secondary to its effect, controlling inflammation remains unknown. In addition, sildenafil upregulated YM-1, a marker of the macrophage/microglial M2 phenotype that has neuroprotective and regenerative properties, while Iba-1, a classical macrophage/microglial activation marker, was downregulated. In vitro analyses of spleen cells from sildenafil-treated animals showed downregulation of Th1/Th2/Th17 responses, while Tregs were upregulated and prevented accumulation of MOG-specific IgG2b in serum. These results suggest that sildenafil has a protective role, modulating central resident and peripheral immune cells.

A sequence of studies has characterized the effects and mechanisms of sildenafil in a cuprizone-induced demyelination and neuroinflammation in rodents, which has been widely used as a model of MS. Nunes et al. [140] and Rapôso et al. [127] demonstrated that sildenafil (25 mg/Kg administrated in the drinking water for 4 weeks) ameliorates cuprizone-induced demyelination in C57BL/6 mice. Sildenafil modulated the neuroinflammatory response (mediated by glial cells), reducing GFAP and Iba-1, IFN-γ, TNF-α, IL-1β, IL-2, and COX-2 expressions. However, the anti-inflammatory effect of sildenafil was abolished in the cuprizone model induced in iNOS$^{-/-}$ mice [127], showing that iNOS plays an important role in the mechanism of PDE5-Is. Sildenafil preserved the myelin and axons' ultrastructure and elevated GST-pi, indicating that sildenafil protects mature oligodendrocytes. However, it is not clear if sildenafil induces oligodendrogenesis or if it inhibits cell death/apoptosis or both. Myelin protection and oligodendrocyte proliferation have also been demonstrated in ischemic models [147, 148], and several studies showed that PDE5-Is inhibit apoptosis in central neurological disease models [122, 148, 149].

Contributing to the understanding of the mechanism by which sildenafil acts in the control of neuroinflammation in MS model, Nunes et al. [128] investigated the involvement of the AMPK/I$\kappa\beta$-α/NF-κB signaling pathway and the eNOS. AMPK, the regulatory protein of the lipid and glucose metabolism, is upregulated in activated astrocytes during reactive gliosis [150], whereas AMPK activators downregulate inflammation in vitro and in vivo in various animal models [151–153], and the loss of AMPK exacerbates the effects of EAE model [154]. The anti-inflammatory activity of AMPK is exerted through multiple signaling pathways, including phosphorylation and activation of eNOS and production of NO. NO may act as an endogenous activator of AMPK, suggesting a reciprocal relationship between AMPK and eNOS [155]. In addition, recent evidence suggests that the activation of AMPK can suppress NF-κB, thus contributing to the regulation of inflammation [71] (**Figure 3A**). Nunes et al. [128] showed that sildenafil treatment (25 mg/Kg administrated in the drinking water for 4 weeks) improved the clinical status of the cuprizone-MS mice model. The treatment reduced unphosphorylated (inactive) AMPK and increased phospho-AMPK (pAMPK, active). Moreover, sildenafil decreased NF-κB p65 expression and increased its inhibitory protein, IKβ-α. However, if AMPK induces NF-κB inhibition and which downstream targets may be involved in this inhibition require further investigation. The same study showed that sildenafil reduced the expression of GFAP, IL-1β, and TNF-α and increased the expression of the anti-inflammatory cytokine IL-10. Besides, the level of eNOS was increased by sildenafil, suggesting reciprocity between AMPK and eNOS. This study then provides evidence that sildenafil has anti-inflammatory effects probably through modulation of AMPK/IKβ-α/NF-κB signaling (**Figure 3A**). However, the involvement of downstream proteins, such as AMPK-SIRT1-NF-κB, and other pathways, such as MAPK-NF-κB, should also be further investigated. In addition, Nunes et al. [128] showed that eNOS may play a role in the sildenafil mechanism. The possible role of NOS in the mechanism of sildenafil corroborates with other studies [89, 124, 127].

The ongoing investigation, in 2016, by Nunes et al. [141] demonstrated that sildenafil increased levels of the chemokine MCP-1 and its receptor, CCR-2, in the cuprizone-induced MS model. This may be part of the anti-inflammatory mechanism, since CCR-2 is a chemokine closely related to the pathology of MS and MS-animal models. In general, during the first weeks of cuprizone exposure, it undergoes a typical overregulation of the chemokine, and both microglia and astrocytes produce CCR-2 [156]. Also, an increase in CCR-2 may be associated with a reduction of macrophage infiltrates after stroke, showing the neuroprotective effects of this receptor [157]. Moreover, mediators in the microenvironment define at what time microglia/macrophages can assume an active and phagocytic phenotype [157]. The expression of MCP-1/CCR-2 by glial cells may promote this change in microglia phenotype in an attempt to repair the injured environment [158]. Sildenafil can, therefore, modulate inflammation by playing a role in the regulation of glial cell morphology and activation through MCP-1/CCR-2 signaling (**Figure 3B**).

Borán et al. [60] estimated that stimulation of cGMP/PKG pathway acts beneficially in microglia, inducing the phagocytic phenotype (M2) and decreasing expression of inflammatory genes, in detriment to the proinflammatory phenotype (M1). The cGMP/PKG pathway stimulated the regulation of microglial cell morphology, inducing a dramatic reorganization of the actin cytoskeleton compatible with a protective phenotype, which is more effective in the removal of dead cells. cGMP-mediated pathways have been implicated in the regulation of the actin cytoskeleton and cell morphology in different cell types, including macrophages and astrocytes [159, 160]. Borán and García [160] demonstrated that the stimulation of the PKG pathway by NO regulates cytoskeleton dynamics and motility in cultured rat astrocytes, and evidence indicates that cGMP is involved in the regulation of astrocyte cytoskeleton through Na^+/K^+-ATPase activity, IP3 receptor (IP3R), and ankyrin B. Ankyrin B, a protein associated with the cytoskeleton, interacts with Na^+/K^+-ATPase and IP3R, connecting the pump to the Ca^{2+} responses from internal cell stores and to the integrity of the cytoskeleton [160] (**Figure 4A**). This suggests

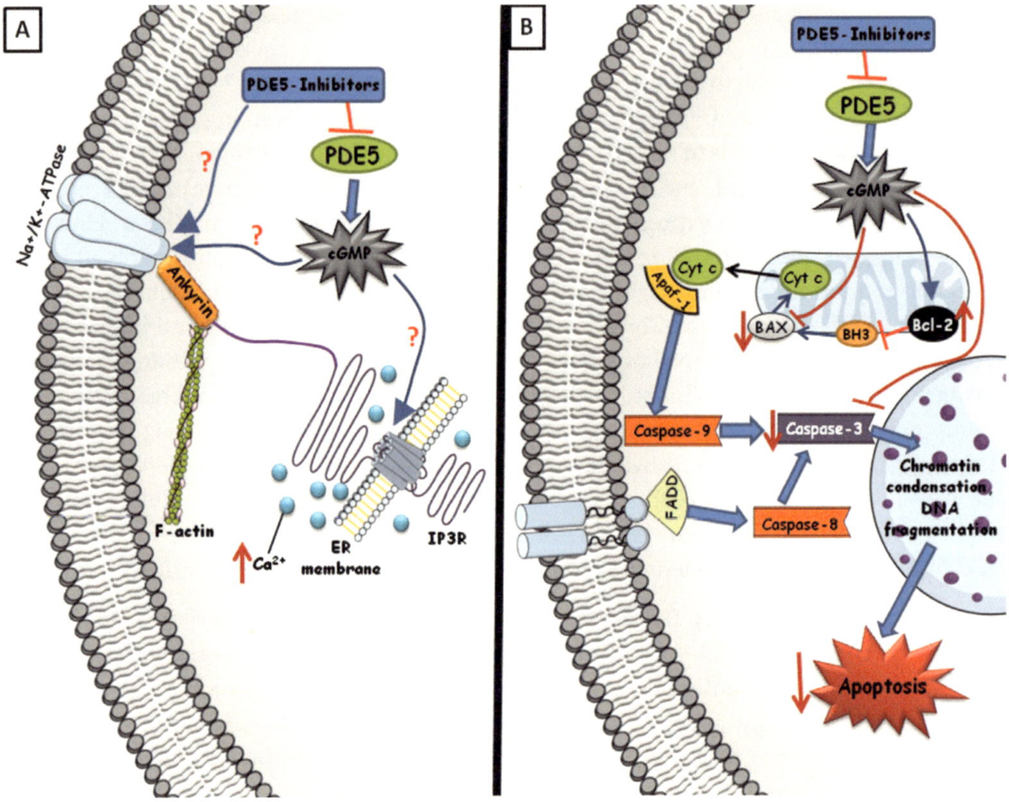

Figure 4. Mechanisms of PDE5-Is in the cytoskeleton and in the apoptosis pathways. (A) PDE5-Is induce Ca^{2+} response and the stabilization of F-actin in astrocytes; however, the mechanism behind this effect is not elucidated. Na^{+}/K^{+}-ATPase interacts with ankyrin B, a cytoskeleton-associated protein, and with the IP3 receptor (IP3R) [coupled to the endoplasmic reticulum (ER) membrane], connecting the pump to the Ca^{2+} responses from internal cell stores and to the integrity of the cytoskeleton. It is possible that this mechanism contributes to the dramatic reorganization of actin cytoskeleton observed in microglia, macrophages, and astrocytes after stimulation of the cGMP/PKG pathway, leading to a more protective phenotype of these inflammatory cells. (B) PDE5-Is have an antiapoptotic effect by enhancing the expression of the antiapoptotic Bcl-2 protein and reducing the proapoptotic BAX and caspase-3 proteins. Whether the PDE5-Is mechanism involves caspase-mediated apoptosis by extrinsic and/or canonical intrinsic pathway is unclear. In the extrinsic pathway, the death receptor-ligand binds to the associated protein with death domain (FADD), which activates the initiator pro-caspase-8. Caspase-8 activates caspase-3, inducing apoptosis. The intrinsic apoptotic pathway is characterized by mitochondrial changes in response to various stress signals, such as severe genetic damage, hypoxia, and oxidative stress, which activate the initiator pro-caspase-9. Proapoptotic mitochondrial proteins, BH3-only members, activate other proapoptotic proteins, such as BAX, and antagonize antiapoptotic proteins, such as Bcl-2. Subsequently, the mitochondrial outer membrane is disrupted, and its permeability increases, resulting in cytochrome-c (Cyt-c) leakage into the cytosol. Cyt-c in the cytosol forms a complex with Apaf-1, called the apoptosome, which assists in auto-activation of initiator pro-caspase-9. Caspase-9 activates caspase-3, leading to apoptosis. ⊣ Inhibition; → activation; ↑ increased expression/activity/level; ↓ decreased expression/activity.

that stress fibers and Ca^{2+} waves could be changed by sildenafil. The involvement of the cytoskeleton in the sildenafil mechanism has been demonstrated by Nunes et al. [116]. Sildenafil induced Ca^{2+} response and a more organized actin fiber pattern in cultured astrocytes, compared to LPS stimulated cells. It is possible that the mechanism behind sildenafil effects in the cytoskeleton involves Na^{+}/K^{+}-ATPase, IP3R, and ankyrin B (**Figure 4A**). In addition, this study showed for the first time that sildenafil has astrocytes as target cells [116], confirming that the control of inflammation is not an indirect effect, secondary to neurogenesis, myelin repair, or improvement of blood flow.

Although there is no clinical report investigating the use of sildenafil chronically in patients with MS, one study has shown the potential of the drug to improve motor impairment. Cocchiarella [161] chronically administrated sildenafil (100 mg per day for 7 month) to a 42-year-old man, who developed a generalized motor deficit with spasticity that made him a quadriplegic (but grew normally, including normal intellectual development). The diagnosis was inconclusive. Physical therapy evaluation for muscle strength and manual measures (scale from 0, no muscle activity whatsoever, to 5, muscle activity with full range of motion and against maximal resistance) by a physical therapist indicated a positive change in muscle activity, following sildenafil administration. After stopping the treatment, the patient kept all gains. The patient experienced common drug-induced events associated with sildenafil treatment, such as erection, headache, and nausea. This study indicates that sildenafil has potential to improve other motor deficiencies, such as MS.

Despite the autoimmune/inflammatory nature of MS that has already been described, the control of the disease through the use of immunosuppressant and immunomodulators has proven to be unsatisfactory. PDE5-Is, being sildenafil the most representative, are widely used and well-tolerated drugs, which may be a useful therapeutic intervention to ameliorate the neuropathology of MS. Therefore, well-designed clinical trials may demonstrate that oral administration of PDE5-Is can be appropriate for individuals with MS and other neuroinflammatory/neurodegenerative diseases, providing additional benefits to current treatments.

4.3. Parkinson's disease and Huntington's disease

Parkinson's disease (PD) is a common, slow-progressing neurological disorder that leads to a constant loss of motor function. Its clinical features include resting tremor, slow movements (bradykinesia), rigidity, impaired balance, difficulty initiating movement (akinesia), and loss of postural reflexes [162]. PD is characterized by the death of dopaminergic neurons in the substantia nigra, which results in the absence of dopamine release in striatum and therefore in motor impairment. The remaining neurons contain intracellular inclusions (Lewy bodies), composed of α-synuclein [163] (**Figure 1C**).

Studies by Uthayathas et al. [164] and by Janis et al. [165] evaluated the use of sildenafil as a neuroprotective agent in the murine model of PD induced by chronic 1-methyl-4-phenyl-1,2,3,6-tetrahydropyridine (MPTP). The hypothesis was that the cGMP accumulation would attenuate the loss of nigrostriatal dopamine neurons induced by the model. The analysis revealed that sildenafil did not prevent neurotoxicity and did not protect against dopamine depletion induced by chronic exposure to MPTP. Also, Uthayathas et al. [164] showed that a single dose of sildenafil (10 mg/kg i.p.) had no effect on fatigue as seen by swimming time. On the other hand, sildenafil did not produce any deleterious effects on nigrostriatal dopamine neuron function, nor did it potentiate the neurotoxic effects of MPTP, suggesting that sildenafil would not accelerate cell loss when used as a treatment of ED in men diagnosed with PD as this drug is used therapeutically to treat sexual dysfunction in PD patients. However, contradictorily, in 2010, a case report by Perkovic et al. [166] described choreoathetotic movements that were most likely induced by sildenafil in a 56-year-old patient with PD. The man presented strange, involuntary movements and anxiety after taking sildenafil 100 mg, 50 min after the last daily dose of levedopa/carbidopa. These adverse effects were considered to be elicited by the administration of sildenafil (drug abuse) in a previously stabilized responder to levedopa therapy. This effect may be a predisposition for pharmacokinetic interaction in short-time interval between levedopa and sildenafil applied in high dosage.

Despite these negative results using a single dose of sildenafil, therapy with the aim of modulating the immune response and neuroinflammation in PD, targeting microglia, astrocytes, and T cells, has recently been proposed [167]. Considerable evidence shows that persistent inflammatory response, T-cell infiltration, and glial cell activation [168, 169] are common features of human patients and animal models of PD and play a crucial role in the degeneration of dopaminergic neurons [170, 171] (**Figure 1C**). As a result, appropriate treatment appears to involve the ability to modulate peripheral and resident immune cells for the purpose of modifying inflammatory response. It is possible that the chronic modulation of neuroinflammation by PDE5-Is may be beneficial for PD. Clinical studies demonstrated that while a single dose of sildenafil does not cause a clear improvement in cognition in healthy adults [172], chronic administration of udenafil has shown to lead to an improvement in cognitive function [130]. This has led some to suggest that the therapeutic benefits of PDE5-Is may be better observed after chronic inhibition rather than after a single dose [173]. However, studies evaluating the anti-inflammatory effects of chronic PDE5-Is in PD models are lacking.

Investigation of the role of cGMP and PDE-Is in Huntington's disease (HD) is also in the beginning. HD is a dominant hereditary neurodegenerative disorder, characterized by progressive impairment of cognitive and motor functions. This disorder is caused by a mutation that encodes an abnormal expansion of CAG-encoded polyglutamine repeats in a protein called huntingtin (htt) [174]. While healthy individuals contain 16–20 repeats, more than 36 are present within the htt gene in HD patients [175]. Toxic protein aggregates are also seen in HD patients, whose brains contain accumulations of mutated HTT protein (**Figure 1D**) [176]. The pathological hallmark of HD involves the loss of neurons in the cortex and striatum that lead to clinical manifestations including involuntary movements known as chorea, behavioral and psychiatric characteristics, and cognitive dysfunction. Mutant huntingtin (mhtt) has been reported to impair cAMP and cGMP/CREB signaling, a transcriptional pathway that has been hypothesized to play a critical role in HD pathology [177, 178].

It was demonstrated by Saavedra et al. [179] that hippocampal cGMP levels were threefold lower in R6/1mice (heterozygous transgenic mice in B6CBA background, expressing exon-1 of mhtt with 145 repeats), when they present deficits in object recognition memory and in passive avoidance learning. nNOS levels were also downregulated, while there were no changes in the levels of PDE5 and PDE9. A single i.p. injection of sildenafil (3 mg/kg), immediately after training, increased cGMP levels and improved memory in R6/1 mice. The same study demonstrated that cGMP levels were also reduced in the human HD hippocampus (six HD patients and five control cases). These results showed that the regulation of hippocampal cGMP levels may be a suitable treatment for cognitive impairment in HD [179]. Other studies have reported decreased levels of nNOS in the caudate of HD patients [180] and in the striatum and cortex of HD mouse models [181, 182]. It has to be investigated whether the mechanism of sildenafil protection in HD neural tissue is via NOS, as demonstrated in other neurological disease models [89, 124, 127, 128].

Puerta et al. [183] demonstrated that the PDE5-Is, sildenafil, and vardenafil (both 1.5 mg/kg p.o., given twice a day for 5 days) protected against 3-nitropropionic acid (3NP), which produces striatal lesions that closely mimic some of the neuropathological features of HD (model induced in male Lewis rats). Rats treated with both sildenafil and vardenafil showed improved neurologic scores and reduced lesion volume. In addition, striatal pCREB levels along with the expression of the downstream target, BDNF, were significantly increased in sildenafil-treated rats, and sildenafil reduced death of GABAergic neurons in the brain tissue. In addition, the activation of calpain (involved in aggregates formation through calpain/p25/CDK5 pathway) was reduced, showing that this drug also can avoid huntingtin N-terminal fragment aggregates. The mechanism demonstrated by Puerta et al. [183] in the HD model is similar to that observed in several studies with AD models.

Also in 2013, Thakur et al. [184] showed that sildenafil was beneficial in the 3NP-HD model induced in Wistar rats, improving cognitive and motor functions. Sildenafil (2 and 4 mg/kg i.p., for 14 days) dose dependently restored body weight and improved memory performance and locomotor activity. The PDE5-I attenuated succinate dehydrogenase activity, balancing the cellular energy deficits induced by 3NP. In addition, as far as we know, this study showed for the first time (and was the only one to show) that sildenafil improves oxidative and nitrosative stress in HD model, indicating that inflammatory parameters may also be the target of this drug in HD.

Despite the lack of studies showing the role of PDE-Is in HD neuroinflammation, several studies carried out on postmortem HD brain tissue and mouse models of HD have found altered expression of immunologically active molecules in the CNS [185–187], and imaging studies indicated increased microglial activity in manifest and premanifest HD gene-expansion carriers [188, 189]. The mhtt leads to activation of microglia and complement, resulting in subsequent production and release of ROS, NO, and cytokines [190]. A study of 20 HD patients, of whom 5 were presymptomatic and 15 were symptomatic, as well as 16 age-matched healthy controls, showed that there were increased levels of IL-6, MMP-9, vascular endothelial growth factor (VEGF), and TGF-β1 in HD patients. These trends were further observed in a murine HD model [191]. Politis and coworkers [192] found an increase in the peripheral plasma levels of the pro-inflammatory cytokine IL-1β in HD gene carriers compared to normal controls; and increased microglial activation in the somatosensory cortex was associated with augmented plasma levels of IL-1β, IL-6, IL8, and TNF-α [193]. In addition, the biomarkers of inflammation were shown to be increased in the plasma of HD gene-expansion carriers, and upregulation was observed up to 16 years prior to expected onset [186, 187, 194], although, in a recent study, these findings were not confirmed [195]. On the other hand, Vinther-Jensen et al. [196] showed that biomarkers of neurodegeneration increased in manifest HD disease, but did not provide evidence of neuroinflammation in early pathogenesis of HD. Therefore, the involvement of neuroinflammation in the HD pathology is not confirmed. However, it is possible that inflammatory events begin years before the onset of the illness. This makes PDE5-Is potential tools to prevent HD development through modulating neuroinflammation, while it is only a speculation and studies need to be developed.

Therefore, despite the important role of neuroinflammation in PD and HD, there is a lack of studies using PDE5-Is to evaluate inflammatory parameters, making this an interesting field for exploration.

4.4. Stroke

Although stroke is the third most common cause of death [197] and the leading cause of permanent disability in adults worldwide [198], the available therapeutic options remain very limited. As vasodilators with good hemodynamic effects, PDE5-Is have been considered potential tools to treat hypoxia and stroke. Due to this obvious effect, these drugs were initially investigated in stroke models considering their mechanisms in cerebral neovascularization and blood flow.

Several studies have shown that administration of sildenafil to animal models of stroke has beneficial effects [147, 199–201]. It was demonstrated that chronic sildenafil elevated cGMP levels in the brain [147], increased angiogenesis in the ischemic border regions, induced capillary-like tube formation, and increased VEGF [199]. Correspondingly, the relative cerebral blood flow in the lesion boundary area has also been improved [147, 200]. Sildenafil also evoked neurogenesis, increased neuronal and oligodendrocyte progenity, and reduced neurological deficits [147, 201]. However, the drug did not alter the size of the lesion [200, 201]. In contrast to these early works, Novitzky et al. [202] reported that sildenafil did not improve the conditions of C57BL/6 mice induced model of occlusion of the middle cerebral artery. However, in this study, sildenafil was given in a single peritoneal dose (Revatio®, Pfizer; 0.8 mg/ml), while in other ones, the drug was administered chronically.

To clarify the mechanism of PDE5-I protection in stroke model, a work by Barros-Miñones et al. [203] showed that sildenafil reduced the activation of calpain and CDK5 and increased the p25/p35 ratio, showing that the protective effects of sildenafil in the ischemia model are, at least in part, by similar mechanism observed in other neurological diseases. As described above, calpain cleaves p35 in its more stable isoform, p25. Cleavage of p35 to p25 and formation of the p25/CDK5 complexes are associated with aggregate formation (**Figure 2B**). As expected, sildenafil prevented tau hyperphosphorylation. This study also showed that sildenafil increased the expression of the antiapoptotic proteins Bcl-2 and Bcl-xL and reduced cell death. The effect of sildenafil on the decrease of apoptosis (through reduction of proapoptotic proteins Bax and caspase-3 expression and increasing the antiapoptotic protein Bcl-2) has also been demonstrated in physiological aging mouse model [149] (**Figure 4B**).

Following the same sequence of investigation of other neurological conditions, more recent studies have shown that the role of sildenafil in promoting stroke recovery is, at least in part, related to the anti-inflammatory mechanism. In 2014, Charriaut-Marlang et al. [148] surgically induced ischemia model in P7 Sprague-Dawley rat pups by occlusion in the right common carotid artery and tested sildenafil. The animals were treated with a single dose of Viagra®

(Pfizer, 10 or 5 mg/kg i.p.). They found that sildenafil increased mean blood flow, reduced brain tissue loss, and decreased apoptosis (demonstrated by TUNEL). In addition, sildenafil increased the index of myelinated fiber density and improved motor capacity. Associated with these beneficial effects, sildenafil had anti-inflammatory effects, reducing astrogliosis and GFAP-positive cell density and decreasing microglial density. A very recent study by Moretti et al. [204] also demonstrated that sildenafil modulates neuroinflammation in the ischemia model induced in C57BL/6 mice P9 pups by permanent middle cerebral artery occlusion. Animals were treated with a single dose of sildenafil (Viagra®, Pfizer, 10 mg/kg i.p., given 5 min after artery occlusion), which provided a reduction of the mean lesion 8 days after ischemia; also, it reduced the number of GFAP-positive cells, decreased microglial density, and modulated the M1 and M2 profiles of microglia/macrophages in the late phase after ischemia. The number of activated microglia/macrophages (M2) increased 72 h after artery occlusion, while it decreased 8 days after ischemia in sildenafil-treated animals. However, despite the clear anti-inflammatory action of sildenafil in ischemic model, the mechanism behind this effect is still unexplained.

A reported clinical study by Silver and coworkers [205] tested the chronic administration of sildenafil (25 mg per day, for 90 days) in ten ischemic stroke patients aged 18 to 80 years, with a score of 2 to 21 (mild to moderately severe stroke; National Institutes of Health Stroke Scale, NIHSS). Sildenafil appeared to be safe in this group of patients, and all of them presented an improvement from baseline NIHSS score. However, despite the success in preclinical and some clinical studies, PDE5-Is have not been more fully investigated in studies with humans and have not moved into clinical practice until now.

5. Conclusion

In conclusion, the relevant role of NO/cGMP signaling in the control of neuroinflammation and in the modulation of glial cell activity has lead researchers to investigate the effects of PDE5 inhibitors on central neurological diseases. These drugs (sildenafil being the most representative and studied among them) have been shown to be safe and effective in the treatment of central neurological disorders, and its mechanisms have been clarified. Modulation of neuroinflammation appears to be a relevant mechanism of PDE-Is, mainly in chronic treatments, whereas it has to be more fully investigated. Despite the safety and benefits of this class of drugs administrated chronically to patients and the success in preclinical studies, there are no Phase I and Phase II clinical trials, which need to be developed to move forward the repositioning of PDE5-Is as therapy to treat neurological diseases.

Acknowledgements

Authors would like to thank the following Brazilian foundations for financial support: Oswaldo Cruz Foundation (FIOCRUZ/PROEP; #1572.2.10/15), Fundação de Amparo à Pesquisa do Estado de São Paulo (the São Paulo Research Foundation) (FAPESP; #2015/04194-0, #2016/15827-6), the Conselho Nacional de Desenvolvimento Científico e Tecnológico (the Brazilian National Council for Scientific and Technological Development) (CNPq; #431465/2016-9, #303514/2015-9), and the Instituto Nacional de Ciência e Tecnologia de Neuroimunomodulação (INCT-NIM; #465489/2014-1).

Author details

Christina A. Peixoto[1*], Ana K.S. Nunes[1] and Catarina Rapôso[2]

*Address all correspondence to: peixoto.christina@gmail.com

1 Laboratory of Ultrastructure, Center of Research Aggeu Magalhães (FIOCRUZ), Recife, Pernambuco, Brazil

2 Department of Structural and Functional Biology, Institute of Biology, State University of Campinas (UNICAMP), Campinas, São Paulo,Brazil

References

[1] Francis SH, Blount MA, Corbin JD. Mammalian cyclic nucleotide phosphodiesterases: Molecular mechanisms and physiological functions. Physiological Reviews. 2011;**91**(2):651-690. DOI: 10.1152/physrev.00030.2010.

[2] Keravis T, Lugnier C. Cyclic nucleotide phosphodiesterase (PDE) isozymes as targets of the intracellular signalling network: Benefits of PDE inhibitors in various diseases and perspectives for future therapeutic developments. British Journal of Pharmacology. 2012;**165**(5):1288-1305. DOI: 10.1111/j.1476-5381.2011.01729.x.

[3] Maurice DH, Ke H, Ahmad F, Wang Y, Chung J, Manganiello VC. Advances in targeting cyclic nucleotide phosphodiesterases. Nature Reviews Drug Discovery. 2014;**13**(4):290-314. DOI: 10.1038/nrd4228.

[4] Gerlo S, Kooijman R, Beck IM, Kolmus K, Spooren A, Haegeman G. Cyclic AMP: A selective modulator of NF-κB action. Cellular and Molecular Life Sciences. 2011;**68**(23):3823-3841. DOI: 10.1007/s00018-011-0757-8.

[5] Aronoff DM, Canetti C, Serezani CH, Luo M, Peters-Golden M. Cutting edge: Macrophage inhibition by cyclic AMP (cAMP): differential roles of protein kinase A and exchange protein directly activated by cAMP-1. The Journal of Immunology. 2015;**174**(2):595-599. DOI: org/10.4049/jimmunol.174.2.595

[6] Bryn T, Mahic M, Enserink JM, Schwede F, Aandahl EM, Tasken K. The cyclic AMP-Epac1-Rap1 pathway is dissociated from regulation of effector functions in monocytes but acquires immunoregulatory function in mature macrophages. The Journal of Immunology. 2006;**176**(12):7361-7370. DOI: 10.4049/jimmunol.176.12.7361.

[7] Hofmann F, Ammendola A, Schlossmann J. Rising behind NO: cGMP-dependent protein kinases. Journal of Cell Science. 2000;**113**(Pt 10):1671-1676.

[8] Corbin JD, Francis SH. Cyclic GMP phosphodiesterase-5: Target of sildenafil. Journal of Biological Chemistry. 1999;**274**(20):13729-32. DOI: 10.1074/jbc.274.20.13729.

[9] Aizawa T, Wei H, Miano JM, Abe J, Berk BC, Yan C. Role of phosphodiesterase 3 in NO/cGMP-mediated antiinflammatory effects in vascular smooth muscle cells. Circulation Research. 2003;**93**(5):406-413. DOI: 10.1161/01.RES.0000091074.33584.F0.

[10] Vandecasteele G, Verde I, Rücker-Martin C, Donzeau-Gouge P, Fischmeister R. Cyclic GMP regulation of the L-type Ca(2+) channel current in human atrial myocytes. Journal of Physiology. 2001;**533**(Pt 2):329-340. DOI: 10.1111/j.1469-7793.2001.0329a.x

[11] Dusse LMS, Cooper AJ, Lwaleed BA. Tissue factor and nitric oxide: A controversial relationship! Journal of Thrombosis and Thrombolysis 2007;23(2):129-133. DOI: 10.1007/s11239-006-0001-9

[12] Puzzo D, Sapienza S, Arancio O, Palmeri A. Role of phosphodiesterase 5 in synaptic plasticity and memory. Neuropsychiatric Disease and Treatment. 2008;**4**(2):371-387.

[13] Ali EMM, Soha HM, Mohamed TM. Nitric oxide synthase and oxidative stress: Regulation of nitric oxide synthase. In: Lushchak V, editor. Oxidative Stress—Molecular Mechanisms and Biological Effects. InTech; 2012. pp. 61-72 ISBN: 978-953-51-0554-1.

[14] Rizzo NO, Maloney E, Pham M, Luttrell I, Wessells H, Tateya S, Daum G, Handa P, Schwartz MW, Kim F. Reduced NO-cGMP signaling contributes to vascular inflammation and insulin resistance induced by high-fat feeding. Arteriosclerosis, Thrombosis, and Vascular Biology. 2010;**30**(4):758-65. DOI: 10.1161/ATVBAHA.109.199893.

[15] Handa P, Tateya S, Rizzo NO, Cheng AM, Morgan-Stevenson V, Han CY, Clowes AW, Daum G, O'Brien KD, Schwartz MW, Chait A, Kim F. Reduced vascular nitric oxide-cGMP signaling contributes to adipose tissue inflammation during high-fat feeding. Arteriosclerosis, Thrombosis, and Vascular Biology. 2011;31(12):2827-35. DOI: 10.1161/ATVBAHA.111.236554.

[16] Spiecker M, Peng HB, Liao JK. Inhibition of endothelial vascular cell adhesion molecule-1 expression by nitric oxide involves the induction and nuclear translocation of IκBα. Journal of Biological Chemistry. 1997;272(49):30969-74.

[17] Matthews JR, Botting CH, Panico M, Morris HR, Hay RT. Inhibition of NF-κB DNA binding by nitric oxide. Nucleic Acids Research. 1996;24(12):2236-42. DOI: 6w0050 [pii].

[18] Grumbach IM, Chen W, Mertens SA, Harrison DG. A negative feedback mechanism involving nitric oxide and nuclear factor κ-B modulates endothelial nitric oxide synthase transcription. Journal of Molecular and Cellular Cardiology. 2005;39(4):595-603. DOI: 10.1016/j.yjmcc.2005.06.012.

[19] Sanz MJ, Hickey MJ, Johnston B, McCafferty DM, Raharjo E, Huang PL, Kubes P. Neuronal nitric oxide synthase (NOS) regulates leukocyte-endothelial cell interactions in endothelial NOS deficient mice. British Journal of Pharmacology. 2001;**134**(2):305-312. DOI: 10.1038/sj.bjp.0704234.

[20] Lefer DJ, Jones SP, Girod WG, Baines A, Grisham MB, Cockrell AS, Huang PL, Scalia R. Leukocyte-endothelial cell interactions in nitric oxide synthase-deficient mice. The American Journal of Physiology. 1999;276(6 Pt 2):H1943-H1950.

[21] Ahluwalia A, Foster P, Scotland RS, McLean PG, Mathur A, Perretti M, Moncada S, Hobbs AJ. Antiinflammatory activity of soluble guanylate cyclase: cGMP-dependent down-regulation of P-selectin expression and leukocyte recruitment. Proceedings of the National Academy of Sciences of the United States of America 2004;**101**(5):1386-1391. DOI: 10.1073/pnas.0304264101.

[22] Gilmore TD. Introduction to NF-κB: Players, pathways, perspectives. Oncogene. 2006; 25(51):6680-6684. DOI: 10.1038/sj.onc.1209954.

[23] Bhaskaran, N, Shukla, S, Srivastava, JK, Gupta, S. Chamomile: An anti-inflammatory agent inhibits inducible nitric oxide synthase expression by blocking RelA/p65 activity. International Journal of Molecular Medicine 2010;**26**(6):935-940.

[24] Arias-Salvatierra D, Silbergeld EK, Acosta-Saavedra LC, Calderon-Aranda, ES. Role of nitric oxide produced by iNOS through NF-κB pathway in migration of cerebellar granule neurons induced by lipopolysaccharide. Cellular Signalling. 2011;**23**(2):425-435. DOI: 10.1016/j.cellsig.2010.10.017.

[25] Minguet S, Huber M, Rosenkranz L, Schamel WWA, Reth M, Brummer T. Adenosine and cAMP are potent inhibitors of the NF-κB pathway downstream of immunoreceptors. European Journal of Immunology 2005;**35**(1):31-41. DOI: 10.1002/eji.200425524.

[26] Wu X, Mahadev K, Fuchsel L, Ouedraogo R, Xu S, Goldstein BJ. Adiponectin suppresses IκB kinase activation induced by tumor necrosis factor-α or high glucose in endothelial cells: Role of cAMP and AMP kinase signaling. American Journal of Physiology, Endocrinology and Metabolism. 2007;**293**(6):1836-1844. DOI: 10.1152/ajpendo.00115.2007.

[27] Kamthong PJ, Wu M. Inhibitor of nuclear factor-κB induction by cAMP antagonizes interleukin-1-induced human macrophage-colony-stimulating-factor expression. The Biochemical Journal. 2001;**356**(Pt 2):525-530.

[28] Chong YH, Shin SA, Lee HJ, Kang JH, Suh YH. Molecular mechanisms underlying cyclic AMP inhibition of macrophage dependent TNF-α production and neurotoxicity in response to amyloidogenic C-terminal fragment of Alzheimer's amyloid precursor protein. Journal of Neuroimmunology. 2002;**133**(1-2):160-74.

[29] Zeiher AM, Fisslthaler B, Schray-Utz B, Busse R. Nitric oxide modulates the expression of monocyte chemoattractant protein 1 in cultured human endothelial cells. Circulation Research. 1995;**76**(6):980-6.

[30] Lee SK, Kim CS, Yang WS, Kim SB, Park SK, Park JS. Exogenous nitric oxide inhibits tumor necrosis factor-α- or interleukin-1-β-induced monocyte chemoattractant protein-1 expression in human mesangial cells. Role of IκB-α and cyclic GMP. Nephron. 2002;**92**(4):780-787.

[31] Desai A, Miller MJ, Huang X, Warren JS. Nitric oxide modulates MCP-1 expression in endothelial cells: implications for the pathogenesis of pulmonary granulomatous vasculitis. Inflammation. 2003;**27**(4):213-223.

[32] Weber NC, Blumenthal SB, Hartung T, Vollmar AM, Kiemer AK. ANP inhibits TNF-α-induced endothelial MCP-1 expression — involvement of p38 MAPK and MKP-1. Journal of Leukocyte Biology. 2003;**74**(5):932-941. DOI: 10.1189/jlb.0603254.1.

[33] Rabender CS, Alam A, Sundaresan G, Cardnell RJ, Yakovlev VA, Mukhopadhyay ND, Graves P, Zweit J, Mikkelsen RB. The role of nitric oxide synthase uncoupling in tumor progression. Molecular Cancer Research. 2015;**13**(6):1034-1043. DOI: 10.1158/1541-7786.MCR-15-0057-T.

[34] Whitt JD, Li N, Tinsley HN, Chen X, Zhang W, Li Y, Gary BD, Keeton AB, Xi Y, Abadi AH, Grizzle WE, Piazza GA. A novel sulindac derivative that potently suppresses colon tumor cell growth by inhibiting cGMP phosphodiesterase and β-catenin transcriptional activity. Cancer Prevention Research (Philadelphia, Pa.) 2012;**5**(6): 822-833.

[35] Zhu B, Vemavarapu L, Thompson WJ, Strada SJ. Suppression of cyclic GMP-specific phosphodiesterase 5 promotes apoptosis and inhibits growth in HT29 cells. Journal of Cellular Biochemistry 2005;**94**(2): 336-350.

[36] Lin S, Wang J, Wang L, Wen J, Guo Y, Qiao W, Zhou J, Xu G, Zhi F. Phosphodiesterase-5 inhibition suppresses colonic inflammation-induced tumorigenesis via blocking the recruitment of MDSC. American Journal of Cancer Research. 2017;**7**(1):41-52. eCollection 2017.

[37] Fiscus RR. Involvement of cyclic GMP and protein kinase G in the regulation of apoptosis and survival in neural cells. Neurosignals 2002;**11**(4):175-190. DOI: 10.1159/000065431.

[38] Nagai-Kusuhara A, Nakamura M, Mukuno H, Kanamori A, Negi A, Seigel GM. cAMP-responsive element binding protein mediates a cGMP/protein kinase G-dependent anti-apoptotic signal induced by nitric oxide in retinal neuro-glial progenitor cells. Experimental Eye Research 2007;**84**(1):152-162. DOI: 10.1016/j.exer.2006.09.010.

[39] Socodato R, Brito R, Portugal CC, de Oliveira NA, Calaza KC, Paes-de-Carvalho R. The nitric oxide-cGKII system relays death and survival signals during embryonic retinal development via Akt-induced CREB1 activation. Cell Death and Differentiation. 2014;**21**(6):915-928. DOI: 10.1038/cdd.2014.11.

[40] Merz K, Herold S, Lie DC. CREB in adult neurogenesis – master and partner in the development of adult-born neurons? European Journal of Neuroscience 2011;**33**(6):1078-1086. DOI: 10.1111/j.1460-9568.2011.07606.x.

[41] Bitner RS. Cyclic AMP response element-binding protein (CREB) phosphorylation: A mechanistic marker in the development of memory enhancing Alzheimer's disease therapeutics. Biochemical Pharmacology. 2012;**83**(6):705-714. DOI: 10.1016/j.bcp.2011.11.009.

[42] Wang L, Zhu ZA. Nitric oxide show its survival role by NO-PKC pathway through cGMP-dependent or independent on the culture of cerebella granular neurons. Neuroscience Letters 2014;**583**:165-169. DOI: 10.1016/j.neulet.2014.06.062.

[43] Das A, Xi L, Kukreja RC. Protein kinase G-dependent cardioprotective mechanism of phosphodiesterase-5 inhibition involves phosphorylation of ERK and GSK3β. Journal of Biological Chemistry. 2008;**283**(43):29572-29585. DOI: 10.1074/jbc.M801547200.

[44] Salloum FN, Chau VQ, Hoke NN, Abbate A, Varma A, Ockaili RA, Toldo S, Kukreja RC. Phosphodiesterase-5 inhibitor, tadalafil, protects against myocardial ischemia/reperfusion through protein-kinase g-dependent generation of hydrogen sulfide. Circulation 2009;**120**(11 Suppl):S31-S36. DOI: 10.1161/CIRCULATIONAHA.108.843979.

[45] Li L, Haider H, Wang L, Lu G, Ashraf M. Adenoviral short hairpin RNA therapy targeting phosphodiesterase 5a relieves cardiac remodeling and dysfunction following myocardial infarction. American Journal of Physiology: Heart and Circulatory Physiology. 2012;**302**(10):H2112-H2121. DOI: 10.1152/ajpheart.00339.2011.

[46] Haider H, Lee YJ, Jiang S, Ahmed RP, Ryon M, Ashraf M. Phosphodiesterase inhibition with tadalafil provides longer and sustained protection of stem cells. American Journal of Physiology: Heart and Circulatory Physiology. 2010;**299**(5):H1395-H1404. DOI: 10.1152/ajpheart.00437.2010.

[47] Glass CK, Saijo K, Winner B, Marchetto MC, Gage FH. Mechanisms underlying inflammation in neurodegeneration. Cell. 2010;**140**(6):918-934. DOI: 10.1016/j.cell.2010.02.016.

[48] Menegazzi M, Di Paola R, Mazzon E, Genovese T, Crisafulli C, Dal Bosco M, Zou Z, Suzuki H, Cuzzocrea S. Glycyrrhizin attenuates the development of carrageenan-induced lung injury in mice. Pharmacological Research. 2008;**58**(1):22-31. DOI: 10.1016/j.phrs.2008.05.012.

[49] Schins RP, McAlinden A, MacNee W, Jimenez LA, Ross JA, Guy K, Faux SP, Donaldson K. Persistent depletion of IκBα and interleukin-8 expression in human pulmonary epithelial cells exposed to quartz particles. Toxicology and Applied Pharmacology. 2000;**167**(2):107-117.

[50] Jensen CJ, Massie A, De Keyser J. Immune players in the CNS: The astrocyte. Journal of Neuroimmune Pharmacology. 2013;**8**(4):824-839. DOI: 10.1007/s11481-013-9480-6.

[51] Parpura V, Verkhratsky A. Homeostatic function of astrocytes: Ca(2+) and Na(+) signalling. Translational Neuroscience. 2012;**3**(4):334-344.

[52] Figley CR, Stroman PW. The role(s) of astrocytes and astrocyte activity in neurometabolism, neurovascular coupling, and the production of functional neuroimaging signals. The European Journal of Neuroscience. 2011;**33**(4):577-588. DOI: 10.1111/j.1460-9568.2010.07584.x

[53] Santello M, Volterra A. TNFα in synaptic function: switching gears. Trends in Neurosciences. 2012;**35**(10):638-47. DOI: 10.1016/j.tins.2012.06.001.

[54] Colodner R, Reznik B, Gal V, Yamazaki H, Hanaki H, Kubo R. Evaluation of a novel kit for the rapid detection of extended-spectrum beta-lactamases. European Journal of Clinical Microbiology and & Infectious Diseases. 2006;**25**(1):49-51.

[55] Stevens CW, Aravind S, Das S, Davis RL. Pharmacological characterization of LPS and opioid interactions at the toll-like receptor 4. British Journal of Pharmacology. 2013 Mar;**168**(6):1421-1429. DOI: 10.1111/bph.12028.

[56] Bsibsi M, Nomden A, van Noort JM, Baron W. Toll-like receptors 2 and 3 agonists differentially affect oligodendrocyte survival, differentiation, and myelin membrane formation. Journal of Neuroscience Research. 2012;**90**(2):388-398. DOI: 10.1002/jnr.22767.

[57] González H, Elgueta D, Montoya A, Pacheco R. Neuroimmune regulation of microglial activity involved in neuroinflammation and neurodegenerative diseases. Journal of Neuroimmunology. 2014;**274**(1-2):1-13. DOI: 10.1016/j.jneuroim.2014.07.012. Review.

[58] Forshammar J, Block L, Lundborg C, Biber B, Hansson E. Naloxone and ouabain in ultralow concentrations restore Na^{+}/K^{+}-ATPase and cytoskeleton in lipopolysaccharide-treated astrocytes. Journal of Biological Chemistry. 2011;**286**(36):31586-31597. DOI: 10.1074/jbc.M111.247767.

[59] Forshammar J, Jörneberg P, Björklund U, Westerlund A, Lundborg C, Biber B, Hansson E. Anti-inflammatory substances can influence some glial cell types but not others. Brain Research 2013 Nov 20;**1539**:34-40. DOI: 10.1016/j.brainres.2013.09.052.

[60] Borán MS, Baltrons MA, García A. The ANP-cGMP-protein kinase G pathway induces a phagocytic phenotype but decreases inflammatory gene expression in microglial cells. Glia. 2008;**56**(4):394-411. DOI: 10.1002/glia.20618.

[61] Wilms H, Sievers J, Rickert U, Rostami-Yazdi M, Mrowietz U, Lucius R. Dimethyl fumarate inhibits microglial and astrocytic inflammation by suppressing the synthesis of nitric oxide, IL-1β, TNF-α and IL-6 in an in-vitro model of brain inflammation. Journal of Neuroinflammation. 2010;**19**(7):30. DOI: 10.1186/1742-2094-7-30

[62] Shin CY, Lee WJ, Choi JW, Choi MS, Ryu JR, Oh SJ, Cheong JH, Choi EY, Ko KH. Down-regulation of matrix metalloproteinase-9 expression by nitric oxide in lipopolysaccharide-stimulated rat primary astrocytes. Nitric Oxide. 2007;**16**(4):425-432. Epub March 24, 2007.

[63] David, S, Kroner, A. Repertoire of microglial and macrophage responses after spinal cord injury. Nature Reviews Neuroscience. 2011;**12**(7):388-399

[64] Streit WJ. Microglial response to brain injury: A brief synopsis. Toxicologic Pathology. 2000;**28**(1):28-30.

[65] Kettenmann H, Hanisch UK, Noda M, Verkhratsky A. Physiology of microglia. Physiological Reviews. 2011;**91**(2):461-553. DOI: 10.1152/physrev.00011.2010. Review.

[66] Jolivalt CG, Hurford R, Lee CA, Dumaop W, Rockenstein E, Masliah E. Type 1 diabetes exaggerates features of Alzheimer's disease in APP transgenic mice. Experimental Neurology. 2010;**223**(2):422-431. DOI: 10.1016/j.expneurol.2009.11.005.

[67] Olson JK. Immune response by microglia in the spinal cord. The Annals of the New York Academy of Sciences 2010;**1198**:271-278. DOI: 10.1111/j.1749-6632.2010.05536.x.

[68] Nagayach A, Patro N, Patro I. Astrocytic and microglial response in experimentally induced diabetic rat brain. Metabolic Brain Disease. 2014;**29**(3):747-761. DOI: 10.1007/s11011-014-9562-z.

[69] Heneka MT, Golenbock DT, Latz E. Innate immunity in Alzheimer's disease. Nature Immunology. 2015;**16**(3):229-36. DOI: 10.1038/ni.3102.

[70] Campbell GR, Kraytsberg Y, Krishnan KJ, Ohno N, Ziabreva I, Reeve A, Trapp BD, Newcombe J, Reynolds R, Lassmann H, Khrapko K, Turnbull DM, Mahad DJ. Clonally expanded mitochondrial DNA deletions within the choroid plexus in multiple sclerosis. Acta Neuropathologica. 2012;**124**(2):209-220. DOI: 10.1007/s00401-012-1001-9.

[71] Zhao S, Zhang L, Lian G, Wang X, Zhang H, Yao X, Yang J, Wu C. Sildenafil attenuates LPS-induced pro-inflammatory responses through down-regulation of intracellular ROS-related MAPK/NF-κB signaling pathways in N9 microglia. International Immunopharmacology. 2011;**11**(4):468-474. DOI: 10.1016/j.intimp.2010.12.017.

[72] Goldman SA, Kuypers NJ. How to make an oligodendrocyte.Development. 2015;**142**(23): 3983-3995. DOI: 10.1242/dev.126409. Review.

[73] Nave KA, Werner HB. Myelination of the nervous system: Mechanisms and functions. Annual Review of Cell and Developmental Biology 2014;**30**:503-533. DOI: 10.1146/annurev-cellbio-100913-013101.

[74] Geva M, Cabilly Y, Assaf Y, Mindroul N, Marom L, Raini G, Pinchasi D, Elroy-Stein O. A mouse model for eukaryotic translation initiation factor 2B-leucodystrophy reveals abnormal development of brain white matter. Brain. 2010;**133**(Pt 8):2448-2461. DOI: 10.1093/brain/awq180.

[75] Matthews PR, Eastwood SL, Harrison PJ. Reduced myelin basic protein and actin-related gene expression in visual cortex in schizophrenia. PLoS One. 2012;**7**(6):e38211. DOI: 10.1371/journal.pone.0038211.

[76] Hayashi Y, Nihonmatsu-Kikuchi N, Hisanaga S, Yu XJ, Tatebayashi Y. Neuropathological similarities and differences between schizophrenia and bipolar disorder: A flow cytometric postmortem brain study. PLoS One. 2012;**7**(3):e33019. DOI: 10.1371/journal.pone.0033019.

[77] Kinnunen KM, Greenwood R, Powell JH, Leech R, Hawkins PC, Bonnelle V, Patel MC, Counsell SJ, Sharp DJ. White matter damage and cognitive impairment after traumatic brain injury. Brain. 2011;**134**(Pt 2):449-463. DOI: 10.1093/brain/awq347

[78] Sievers C, Sämann PG, Dose T, Dimopoulou C, Spieler D, Roemmler J, Schopohl J, Mueller M, Schneider HJ, Czisch M, Pfister H, Stalla GK. Macroscopic brain architec-

ture changes and white matter pathology in acromegaly: A clinicoradiological study. Pituitary. 2009;**12**(3):177-85. DOI: 10.1007/s11102-008-0143-1.

[79] van der Werff SJ, Andela CD, Nienke Pannekoek J, Meijer OC, van Buchem MA, Rombouts SA, van der Mast RC, Biermasz NR, Pereira AM, van der Wee NJ. Widespread reductions of white matter integrity in patients with long-term remission of Cushing's disease. NeuroImage: Clinical. 2014;**4**:659-667. DOI: 10.1016/j.nicl.2014.01.017. eCollection 2014.

[80] Sun J, Fang Y, Ren H, Chen T, Guo J, Yan J, Song S, Zhang L, Liao H. WIN55,212-2 protects oligodendrocyte precursor cells in stroke penumbra following permanent focal cerebral ischemia in rats. Acta Pharmacologica Sinica. 2013;**34**(1):119-128. DOI: 10.1038/aps.2012.141.

[81] Arai K, Lo EL. Experimental models for analysis of oligodendrocyte pathophysiology in stroke. Experimental & Translational Stroke Medicine. 2009;**1**:6. Published online October 24, 2009. DOI: 10.1186/2040-7378-1-6

[82] Ahmed Z, Asi YT, Lees AJ, Revesz T, Holton JL. Identification and quantification of oligodendrocyte precursor cells in multiple system atrophy, progressive supranuclear palsy and Parkinson's disease. Brain Pathology. 2013;**23**(3):263-273. DOI: 10.1111/j.1750-3639.2012.00637.x

[83] Gagyi E, Kormos B, Castellanos KJ, Valyi-Nagy K, Korneff D, LoPresti P, Woltjer R, Valyi-Nagy T. Decreased oligodendrocyte nuclear diameter in Alzheimer's disease and Lewy body dementia. Brain Pathology. 2012;**22**(6):803-810. DOI: 10.1111/j.1750-3639.2012.00595.x.

[84] Desai MK, Mastrangelo MA, Ryan DA, Sudol KL, Narrow WC, Bowers WJ. Early oligodendrocyte/myelin pathology in Alzheimer's disease mice constitutes a novel therapeutic target. The American Journal of Pathology. 2010;**177**(3):1422-1435. DOI: 10.2353/ajpath.2010.100087.

[85] Sims R, Hollingworth P, Moskvina V, Dowzell K, O'Donovan MC, Powell J, Lovestone S, Brayne C, Rubinsztein D, Owen MJ, Williams J, Abraham R. Evidence that variation in the oligodendrocyte lineage transcription factor 2 (OLIG2) gene is associated with psychosis in Alzheimer's disease. Neuroscience Letters. 2009;**461**(1):54-59. DOI: 10.1016/j.neulet.2009.05.051.

[86] Konradi C, Sillivan SE, Clay HB. Mitochondria, oligodendrocytes and inflammation in bipolar disorder: Evidence from transcriptome studies points to intriguing parallels with multiple sclerosis. Neurobiology of Disease. 2012;**45**(1):37-47. DOI: 10.1016/j.nbd.2011.01.025.

[87] Francis GJ, Martinez JA, Liu WQ, Xu K, Ayer A, Fine J, Tuor UI, Glazner G, Hanson LR, Frey WH 2nd, Toth C. Intranasal insulin prevents cognitive decline, cerebral atrophy and white matter changes in murine type I diabetic encephalopathy. Brain. 2008;**131**(Pt 12):3311-3334. DOI: 10.1093/brain/awn288. Retraction in: Brain. 2014 Jun;**137**(Pt 6):e283

[88] Bradl M, Lassmann H. Oligodendrocytes: biology and pathology. Acta Neuropathologica. 2010;**119**(1):37-53. DOI: 10.1007/s00401-009-0601-5

[89] Rapôso C, Luna RL, Nunes AK, Thomé R, Peixoto CA. Role of iNOS-NO-cGMP signaling in modulation of inflammatory and myelination processes. Brain Research Bulletin. 2014;**104**:60-73. DOI: 10.1016/j.brainresbull.2014.04.002

[90] Ramesh G, Benge S, Pahar B, Philipp MT. A possible role for inflammation in mediating apoptosis of oligodendrocytes as induced by the Lyme disease spirochete Borrelia burgdorferi. Journal of Neuroinflammation. 2012;**23**(9):72. DOI: 10.1186/1742-2094-9-72

[91] Carlson NG, Rojas MA, Redd JW, Tang P, Wood B, Hill KE, Rose JW. Cyclooxygenase-2 expression in oligodendrocytes increases sensitivity to excitotoxic death. Journal of Neuroinflammation 2010;**7**:25. DOI: 10.1186/1742-2094-7-25

[92] Nosengo N. Can you teach old drugs new tricks? Nature 2016;**534**:314-316. DOI: 10.1038/534314a

[93] Hartell NA. Inhibition of cGMP breakdown promotes the induction of cerebellar long-term depression. The Journal of Neuroscience 1996;**16**:2881-2890.

[94] Puerta E, Hervias I, Goñi-Allo B, Lasheras B, Jordan J, Aguirre N. Phosphodiesterase 5 inhibitors prevent 3,4-methylenedioxymethamphetamine-induced 5-HT deficits in the rat. Journal of Neurochemistry. 2009;**108**(3):755-766. DOI: 10.1111/j.1471-4159.2008.05825.x

[95] Liu J, Wenzel B, Dukic-Stefanovic S, Teodoro R, Ludwig FA, Deuther-Conrad W, Schröder S, Chezal JM, Moreau E, Brust P, Maisonial-Besset A. Development of a new radiofluorinated quinoline analog for PET imaging of phosphodiesterase5 (PDE5) in brain. Pharmaceuticals (Basel). 2016;**9**(2):E22. DOI: 10.3390/ph9020022

[96] Zhao L, Mason NA, Strange JW, Walker H, Wikins MR. Beneficial effects of phosphodiesterase 5 inhibition in pulmonary hypertension are influenced by natriuretic peptide activity. Circulation. 2002;**107**(2):234-237.

[97] Roustit M, Blaise S, Allanore Y, Carpentier PH, Caglayan E, Cracowski JL. Phosphodiesterase-5 inhibitors for the treatment of secondary Raynaud's phenomenon: Systematic review and meta analysis of randomized trials. Annals of the Rheumatic Diseases. 2013;**72**(10):1696-1699. DOI: 10.1136/annrheumdis-2012-202836

[98] Teich AF, Sakurai M, Patel M, Holman C, Saeed F, Fiorito J, Arancio O. PDE5 exists in human neurons and is a viable therapeutic target for neurologic disease. Journal of Alzheimer's Disease. 2016;**52**(1):295-302. DOI: 10.3233/JAD-151104

[99] Peixoto CA, Nunes AK, Garcia-Osta A. Phosphodiesterase-5 inhibitors: Action on the signaling pathways of neuroinflammation, neurodegeneration, and cognition. Mediators of Inflammation 2015;**2015**:940207. DOI: 10.1155/2015/940207

[100] FDA, 1998. Viagra tablets (sildenafil citrate). Review and evaluation of pharmacology and toxicology data. Report from the Division of Cardio-renal Drug Products (HFD-10). Center for Drug Evaluation and Research. Food and Drug Administration, Washington, DC, pp. 121-122.

[101] Prickaerts J, Sik A, van Staveren WC, Koopmans G, Steinbusch HW, van der Staay FJ, de Vente J, Blokland A. Phosphodiesterase type 5 inhibition improves early memory consolidation of object information. Neurochemistry International. 2004;**45**(6):915-928

[102] Puzzo D, Staniszewski A, Deng SX, Privitera L, Leznik E, Liu S, Zhang H, Feng Y, Palmeri A, Landry DW, Arancio O. Phosphodiesterase 5 inhibition improves synaptic function, memory, and amyloid-beta load in an Alzheimer's disease mouse model. The Journal of Neuroscience. 2009;**29**(25):8075-8086. DOI: 10.1523/JNEUROSCI.0864-09.2009

[103] García-Barroso C, Ricobaraza A, Pascual-Lucas M, Unceta N, Rico AJ, Goicolea MA, Sallés J, Lanciego JL, Oyarzabal J, Franco R, Cuadrado-Tejedor M, García-Osta A. Tadalafil crosses the blood-brain barrier and reverses cognitive dysfunction in a mouse model of AD. Neuropharmacology 2013;**64**:114-123. DOI: 10.1016/j.neuropharm.2012.06.052

[104] Uthayathas S, Karuppagounder SS, Thrash BM, Parameshwaran K, Suppiramaniam V, Dhanasekaran M. Versatile effects of sildenafil: Recent pharmacological applications. Pharmacological Reports. 2007;**59**(2):150-163

[105] Espinoza-Fonseca LM. The benefits of the multi-target approach in drug design and discovery. Bioorganic & Medicinal Chemistry. 2006;**14**(4):896-897

[106] Cuadrado-Tejedor M, Garcia-Barroso C, Sanzhez-Arias J, Mederos S, Rabal O, Ugarte A, Franco R, Pascual-Lucas M, Segura V, Perea G, Oyarzabal J, Garcia-Osta A. Concomitant histone deacetylase and phosphodiesterase 5 inhibition synergistically prevents the disruption in synaptic plasticity and it reverses cognitive impairment in a mouse model of Alzheimer's disease. Clin Epigenetics 2015;**7**:108. DOI: 10.1186/s13148-015-0142-9

[107] Selkoe DJ. Alzheimer's disease is a synaptic failure. Science. 2002;**298**(5594):789-791.

[108] Li XH, Deng YY, Li F, Shi JS, Gong QH. Neuroprotective effects of sodium hydrosulfide against β-amyloid-induced neurotoxicity. International Journal of Molecular Medicine. 2016;**38**(4):1152-1160. DOI: 10.3892/ijmm.2016.2701

[109] Prickaerts J, van Staveren WC, Sik A, Markerink-van Ittersum M, Niewöhner U, van der Staay FJ, Blokland A, de Vente J. Effects of two selective phosphodiesterase type 5 inhibitors, sildenafil and vardenafil, on object recognition memory and hippocampal cyclic GMP levels in the rat. Neuroscience. 2002;**113**(2):351-361.

[110] Tully T, Bourtchouladze R, Scott R, Tallman J. Targeting the CREB pathway for memory enhancers. Nature Reviews Drug Discovery. 2003;**2**(4):267-277.

[111] Cuadrado-Tejedor M, Hervias I, Ricovaraza A, Puerta E, Pérez-Roldán JM, García-Barroso C, Franco R, Aguirre N, García-Osta A. Sildenafil restores cognitive function

without affecting β-amyloid burden in a mouse model of Alzheimer's disease. British Journal of Pharmacology. 2011;**164**(8):2029-2041. DOI: 10.1111/j.1476-5381.2011.01517.x

[112] Hanger DP, Hughes K, Woodgett JR, Brion JP, Anderton BH. Glycogen synthase kinase-3 induces Alzheimer's disease-like phosphorylation of tau: Generation of paired helical filament epitopes and neuronal localisation of the kinase. Neuroscience Letters. 1992;**147**(1):58-62.

[113] Tsai LH, Lee MS, Cruz J. CDK5, a therapeutic target for Alzheimer's disease? Biochimica et Biophysica Acta. 2004;**1697**(1-2):137-142.

[114] Orejana L, Barros-Miñones L, Jordan J, Cedezo-Minguez A, Tordera RM, Aguirre N, Puerta E. Sildenafil decreases BACE1 and cathepsin B levels and reduces APP amyloidogenic processing in the SAMP8 mouse. Journals of Gerontology. Series A, Biological Sciences and Medical Sciences. 2015;**70**(6):675-685. DOI: 10.1093/gerona/glu106

[115] Shi C, Zheng DD, Wu FM, Liu J, Xu J. The phosphatidyl inositol 3 kinase-glycogen synthase kinase 3β pathway mediates bilobalide-induced reduction in amyloid β-peptide. Neurochemical Research. 2012;**37**(2):298-306. DOI: 10.1007/s11064-011-0612-1

[116] Nunes AKS, Rapôso C, Björklund U, Cruz-Höfling MA, Peixoto CA, Hansson E. Sildenafil (Viagra®) prevents and restores LPS-induced inflammation in astrocytes. Neuroscience Letters. 2016;**630**:59-65. DOI: 10.1016/j.neulet.2016.07.029

[117] Zhang J, Guo J, Zhao X, Chen Z, Wang G, Liu A, Wang Q, Zhou W, Xu Y, Wang C. Phosphodiesterase-5 inhibitor sildenafil prevents neuroinflammation, lowers beta-amyloid levels and improves cognitive performance in APP/PS1 transgenic mice. Behavioural Brain Research. 2013;**250**:230-237. DOI: 10.1016/j.bbr.2013.05.017

[118] Terry RD, Peck A, DeTeresa R, Schechter R, Horoupian DS. Some morphometric aspects of the brain in senile dementia of the Alzheimer type. Annals of Neurology. 1981;**10**(2):184-192.

[119] Zhu L, Yang JY, Xue X, Dong YX, Liu Y, Miao FR, Wang YF, Xue H, Wu CF. A novel phosphodiesterase-5 inhibitor: Yonkenafil modulates neurogenesis, gliosis to improve cognitive function and ameliorates amyloid burden in an APP/PS1 transgenic mice model. Mechanisms of Ageing and Development 2015;**150**:34-45. DOI: 10.1016/j.mad2015.07.002

[120] Wang Q, Wu J, Rowan MJ, Anwyl R. Beta-amyloid inhibition of long-term potentiation is mediated via tumor necrosis factor. European Journal of Neuroscience. 2005;**22**(11):2827-2832.

[121] Lyons A, Griffin RJ, Costelloe CE, Clarke RM, Lynch MA. IL-4 attenuates the neuroinflammation induced by amyloid-beta in vivo and in vitro. Journal of Neurochemistry. 2007;**101**(3):771-781.

[122] Ricote M, Glass CK. PPARs and molecular mechanisms of transrepression. Biochimica et Biophysica Acta. 2007;**1771**(8):926-935.

[123] Yin C, Deng Y, Gao J, Li X, Liu Y, Gong Q. Icariside II, a novel phosphodiesterase-5 inhibitor, attenuates streptozotocin-induced cognitive deficits in rats. Neuroscience 2016;**328**:69-79. DOI: 10.1016/j.neuroscience.2016.04.022

[124] Jin F, Gong QH, Xu YS, Wang LN, Jin H, Li F, Li LS, Ma YM, Shi JS. Icariin, a phosphodiesterase-5 inhibitor, improves learning and memory in APP/PS1 transgenic mice by stimulation of NO/cGMP signaling. The International Journal of Neuropsychopharmacology. 2014;**17**(6):871-881. DOI: 10.1017/S1461145713001533

[125] Cooke RM, Mistry R, Challiss RA, Straub VA. Nitric oxide synthesis and cGMP production is important for neurite growth and synapse remodeling after axotomy. The Journal of Neuroscience. 2013;**33**(13):5626-5637. DOI: 10.1523/JNEUROSCI.3659-12.2013

[126] Charriaut-Marlangue C, Bonnin P, Pham H, Loron G, Leger PL, Gressens P, Renolleau S, Baud O. Nitric oxide signaling in the brain: A new target for inhaled nitric oxide? Annals of Neurology. 2013;**73**(4):442448. DOI: 10.1002/ana.23842

[127] Rapôso C, Nunes AKS, Luna RLA, Araújo SM, Cruz-Höfling MA, Peixoto CA. Sildenafil (Viagra) protective effects on neuroinflammation: The role of iNOS/NO system in an inflammatory demyelination model. Mediators of Inflammation 2013;**2013**:321460. DOI: 10.1155/2013/321460

[128] Nunes AKS, Rapôso C, Rocha SW, Barbosa KP, Luna RL, Cruz-Höfling MA, Peixoto CA. Involvement of AMPK, IKβα-NFκB and eNOS in the sildenafil anti-inflammatory mechanism in a demyelination model, Brain Research. 2015;**1627**:119-133. DOI: 10.1016/j.brainres.2015.09.008

[129] Giorgi M, D'Angelo V, Esposito Z, Nuccetelli V, Sorge R, Martorana A, Stefani A, Bernardi G, Sancesario G. Lowered cAMP and cGMP signalling in the brain during levodopa-induced dyskinesias in hemiparkinsonian rats: New aspects in the pathogenetic mechanisms. European Journal of Neuroscience. 2008;**28**(5):941-950. DOI: 10.1111/j.1460-9568.2008.06387.x

[130] Shim YS, Pae CU, Kim SW, Kim HW, Kim, JC, Koh JS. Effects of repeated dosing with Udenafil (Zydena) on cognition, somatization and erection in patients with erectile dysfunction: a pilot study. International Journal of Impotence Research. 2011;**23**(3):109-114.

[131] Umar T, Hoda N. Selective inhibitors of phosphodiesterases: Therapeutic promise for neurodegenerative disorders. Medicinal Chemical Communications 2015;**6**:2063-2080

[132] Noseworthy JH, Lucchinetti C, Rodriguez M, Weinshenker BG. Multiple sclerosis. The New England Journal of Medicine. 2000;**343**(13):938-952.

[133] Block ML, Zecca L, Hong JS. Microglia-mediated neurotoxicity: Uncovering the molecular mechanisms. Nature Review Neuroscience. 2007;**8**(1):57-69.

[134] Trapp BD, Nave KA. Multiple sclerosis: An immune or neurodegenerative disorder? Annual Review of Neuroscience 2008;**31**:247-269. DOI: 10.1146/annurev.neuro.30.051606.094313

[135] Frank-Cannon TC, Alto LT, McAlpine FE, Tansey MG. Does neuroinflammation fan the flame in neurodegenerative diseases? Molecular Neurodegeneration. 2009;**4**:47. DOI: 1186/1750-1326-4-47

[136] Scheiblich H, Roloff F, Singh V, Stangel M, Stern M, Bicker G. Nitric oxide/cyclic GMP signaling regulates motility of a microglial cell line and primary microglia in vitro. Brain Research 2014;**1564**:9-21. DOI: 10.1016/j.brainres.2014.03.048

[137] Paris D, Town T, Parker T, Humphrey J, Mullan M. β-Amyloid vasoactivity and proinflammation in microglia can be blocked by cGMP-elevating agents. Annals of the New York Academy of Sciences. 2000;**903**:446-450.

[138] Wakita H, Tomimoto H, Akiguchi I, Lin JX, Ihara M, Ohtani R, Shibata M. Ibudilast, a phosphodiesterase inhibitor, protect against white matter damage under chronic cerebral hypoperfusion in the rat. Brain Research. 2003;**992**(1):53-59.

[139] Xiao Y, Wang J, Luo H. Sildenafil citrate for erectile dysfunction in patients with multiple sclerosis. Cochrane Database of Systematic Reviews 2012;**4**:CD009427. DOI: 10.1002/14651858.CD009427

[140] Nunes AK, Rapôso C, Luna RL, Cruz-Höfling MA, Peixoto CA. Sildenafil (Viagra®) down regulates cytokines and prevents demyelination in a cuprizone-induced MS mouse model. Cytokine. 2012;**60**(2):540-551. DOI: 10.1016/j.cyto.2012.06.011

[141] Nunes AKS, Rapôso C, Oliveira WH, Thomé R, Verinaud L, Tovar-Moll F, Peixoto CA. Phosphodiesterase-5 inhibition promotes remyelination by MCP-1/CCR-2 and MMP-9 regulation in a cuprizone-induced demyelination model. Experimental Neurology. 2016;**275**(Pt 1):143-153. DOI: 10.1016/j.expneurol.2015.10.013

[142] Pifarré P, Prado J, Baltrons MA, Giralt M, Gabarro P, Feinstein DL, Hidalgo J, Garcia A. Sildenafil (Viagra) ameliorates clinical symptoms and neuropathology in a mouse model of multiple sclerosis. Acta Neuropathologica. 2011;**121**(4):499-508. DOI: 10.1007/s00401-010-0795-6

[143] Pifarré P, Gutierrez-Mecinas M, Prado J, Usero L, Roura-Mir C, Giralt M, Hidalgo J, García A. Phosphodiesterase 5 inhibition at disease onset prevents experimental autoimmune encephalomyelitis progression through immunoregulatory and neuroprotective actions. Experimental Neurology 2014;**251**:58-71. DOI: 10.1016/j.expneurol.2013.10.021

[144] Garcia LA, Hlaing SM, Gutierrez RA, Sanchez MD, Kovanecz I, Artaza JN, Ferrini MG. Sildenafil attenuates inflammation and oxidative stress in pelvic ganglia neurons after bilateral cavernosal nerve damage. International Journal of Molecular Sciences. 2014;**15**(10):17204-17220. DOI: 10.3390/ijms151017204

[145] Bullard DC, Hu X, Schoeb TR, Collins RG, Beaudet AL, Barnum SR. Intercellular adhesion molecule-1 expression is required on multiple cell types for the development of experimental autoimmune encephalomyelitis. The Journal of Immunology. 2007;**178**(2):851-857.

[146] Bynoe MS, Bonorino P, Viret C. Control of experimental autoimmune encephalomyelitis by CD4+ suppressor T cells: Peripheral versus in situ immunoregulation. Journal of Neuroimmunology. 2007;**191**(1-2):61-69.

[147] Zhang R, Wang Y, Zhang L, Zhang Z, Tsang W, Lu M, Zhang L, Chopp M. Sildenafil (Viagra) induces neurogenesis and promotes functional recovery after stroke in rats. Stroke. 2002;**33**(11):2675-2680.

[148] Charriaut-Marlangue C, Nguyen T, Bonnin P, Duy AP, Leger PL, Csaba Z, Pansiot J, Bourgeois T, Renolleau S, Baud O. Sildenafil mediates blood-flow redistribution and neuroprotection after neonatal hypoxia-ischemia. Stroke. 2014;**45**(3):850-856. DOI: 10.1161/STROKEAHA.113.003606

[149] Puzzo D, Loreto C, Giunta S, Musumeci G, Frasca G, Podda MV, Arancio O, Palmeri A. Effect of phosphodiesterase-5 inhibition on apoptosis and beta-amyloid load in aged mice. Neurobiology of Aging. 2014;**35**(3):520-531. DOI: 10.1016/j.neurobiolaging.2013.09.002

[150] Turnley AM, Stapleton D, Mann RJ, Witters LA, Kemp BE, Bartlett PF. Cellular distribution and developmental expression of AMP-activated protein kinase isoforms in mouse central nervous system. Journal of Neurochemistry. 1999;**72**(4):1707-1716.

[151] Davis BJ, Xie Z, Viollet B, Zou MH. Activation of the AMP-activated kinase by antidiabetes drug metformin stimulates nitric oxide synthesis in vivo by promoting the association of heat shock protein 90 and endothelial nitric oxide synthase. Diabetes. 2006;**55**(2):496-505

[152] Nath N, Khan M, Paintlia MK, Singh I, Hoda MN, Giri S. Metformin attenuated the autoimmune disease of the central nervous system in animal models of multiple sclerosis. The Journal of Immunology. 2009;**182**(12):8005-8014. DOI: 10.4049/jimmunol.0803563

[153] Labuzek K, Liber S, Gabryel B, Okopien B. Metformin has adenosine-monophosphate activated protein kinase (AMPK)-independent effects on LPS-stimulated rat primary microglial cultures. Pharmacological Reports. 2010;**62**(5):827-848.

[154] Nath N, Khan M, Rattan R, Mangalam A, Makkar RS, de Meester C, Bertrand L, Singh I, Chen Y, Viollet B, Giri S. Loss of AMPK exacerbates experimental autoimmune encephalomyelitis disease severity. Biochemical and Biophysical Research Communications. 2009:**386**(1):16-20. DOI: 10.1016/j.bbrc.2009.05.106

[155] Zhang J, Xie Z, Dong Y, Wang S, Liu C, Zou MH. Identification of nitric oxide as an endogenous activator of the AMP-activated protein kinase in vascular endothelial cells. Journal of Biological Chemistry. 2008;**283**(41):27452.27461. DOI: 10.1074/jbc.M802578200

[156] Harkness KA, Sussman JD, Davies-Jones GA, Greenwood J, Woodroofe MN. Cytokine regulation of MCP-1 expression in brain and retinal microvascular endothelial cells. Journal of Neuroimmunology. 2003;**142**(1-2):1-9

[157] Rawji KS, Yong VW. The benefits and detriments of macrophages/microglia in models of multiple sclerosis. Clinical and Developmental Immunology 2013;**2013**:948976. DOI: 10.1155/2013/948976

[158] Low QE, Drugea IA, Duffner LA, Quinn DG, Cook DN, Rollins BJ, Kovacs EJ, DiPietro LA. Wound healing in MIP-1α(−/−) and MCP-1(−/−) mice. The American Journal of Pathology. 2001;**159**(2):457-463

[159] Ke X, Terashima M, Nariai Y, Nakashima Y, Nabika T, Tanigawa Y. Nitric oxide regulates actin reorganization through cGMP and Ca(2+)/calmodulin in RAW 264.7 cells. Biochimica et Biophysica Acta. 2001;**1539**(1-2):101-113

[160] Borán MS, Garcia A. The cyclic GMP-protein kinase G pathway regulates cytoskeleton dynamics and motility in astrocytes. Journal of Neurochemistry. 2007;**102**(1):216-230.

[161] Cocchiarella A. Partial motor restoration upon administration of sildenafil: A case study. Developmental Neurorehabilitation. 2012;**15**(1):39-43. DOI: 10.3109/17518423.2011.631947

[162] Jankovic J. Parkinson's disease: Clinical features and diagnosis. Journal of Neurology, Neurosurgery and Psychiatry. 2008;**79**(4):368-376. DOI: 10.1136/jnnp.2007.131045

[163] Eriksen JL, Wszolek Z, Petrucelli L. Molecular pathogenesis of Parkinson disease. Archives of Neurology. 2005;**62**(3):353-357.

[164] Uthayathas S, Karuppagounder SS, Tamer SI, Parameshwaran K, Degim T, Suppiramaniam V, Dhanasekaran M. Evaluation of neuroprotective and anti-fatigue effects of sildenafil. Life Sciences. 2007;**81**(12):988-992.

[165] Janis KL, Brennan RT, Drolet RE, Behrouz B, Kaufman SK, Lookingland KJ, Goudreau JL. Effects of sildenafil on nigrostriatal dopamine neurons in a murine model of Parkinson's disease. Journal of Alzheimer's Disease. 2008;**15**(1):97-107.

[166] Perkovic O, Vitezic D, Rudez J, Vitezic M, Kovacevic M, Mrsic-Pelcic J, Ljubicic D, Jurjevic A. Sildenafil induced choreoathetosis in men with Parkinson's disease. International Journal of Clinical Pharmacology and Therapeutics. 2010;**48**(1):76-78.

[167] von Euler Chelpin M, Vorup-Jensen T. Targets and mechanisms in prevention of Parkinson's disease through immunomodulatory treatments. Scandinavian Journal of Immunology. 2017;**85**(5):321-330.

[168] McGeer PL, Itagaki S, Boyes BE, McGeer EG. Reactive microglia are positive for HLA-DR in the substantia nigra of Parkinson's and Alzheimer's disease brains. Neurology. 1988;**38**(8):1285-1291.

[169] Tansey MG, McCoy MK, Frank-Cannon TC. Neuroinflammatory mechanisms in Parkinson's disease: Potential environmental triggers, pathways, and targets for early therapeutic intervention. Experimental Neurology. 2007;**208**(1):1-25

[170] Gerhard A, Pavese N, Hotton G, Turkheimer F, Es M, Hammers A, Eggert K, Oertel W, Banati RB, Brooks DJ. In vivo imaging of microglial activation with [11C](R)-PK11195PET in idiopathic Parkinson's disease. Neurobiology of Disease. 2006;**21**(2):404-412.

[171] Mosley RL, Hutter-Saunders JA, Stone DK, Gendelman HE. Inflammation and adaptive immunity in Parkinson's disease. Cold Spring Harbor Perspectives in Medicine. 2012;**2**(1):a009381. DOI: 10.1101/chsperspect.a009381

[172] Grass H, Klotz T, Fathian-Sabet B, Berghaus G, Engelmann U, Käferstein H. Sildenafil (Viagra): Is there an influence on psychological performance? International Urology and Nephrology. 2001;**32**(3):409-412.

[173] Reneerkens OA, Sambeth A, Ramaekers JG, Steinbusch HW, Blokland A, Prickaerts J. The effects of the phosphodiesterase type 5 inhibitor vardenafil on cognitive performance in healthy adults: A behavioral-electroencephalography study. Journal of Psychopharmacology. 2013;**27**(7):600-608. DOI: 10.1177/0269881113477747

[174] Zuccato C, Valenza M, Cattaneo E. Molecular mechanisms and potential therapeutical targets in Huntington's disease. Physiological Reviews. 2010;**90**(3):905-981. DOI: 10.1152/physrev.00041.2009

[175] Pringsheim T, Wiltshire K, Day L, Dykeman J, Steeves T, Jette N. The incidence and prevalence of Huntington's disease: A systematic review and meta-analysis. Movement Disorders. 2012;**27**(9):1083-1091. DOI: 10.1002/mds.25075.

[176] Kumar A, Kumar Singh S, Kumar V, Kumar D, Agarwal S, Rana MK. Huntington's disease: An update of therapeutic strategies. Gene. 2015;**556**(2):91-97. DOI: 10.1016/j.gene.2014.11.022

[177] Zuccato C, Ciammola A, Rigamonti D, Leavitt BR, Goffredo D, Conti L, MacDonald ME, Fiedlander RM, Silani V, Havden MR, Timmusk T, Sipione S, Cattaneo E. Loss of huntingtin-mediated BDNF gene transcription in Huntington's disease. Science 2001;**293**:493-498

[178] Choi YS, Lee B, Cho HY, Reyes IB, Pu XA, Saido TC, Hoyt KR, Obrietan K. CREB is a key regulator of striatal vulnerability in chemical and genetic models of Huntington's disease. Neurobiology of Disease. 2009;**36**(2):259-268. DOI: 10.1016/j.nbd.2009.07.014

[179] Saavedra A, Giralt A, Arumí H, Alberch J, Pérez-Navarro E. Regulation of hippocampal cGMP levels as a candidate to treat cognitive deficits in Huntington's disease. PLoS One. 2013;**8**(9):e73664. DOI: 10.1371/journal.pone.0073664

[180] Norris PJ, Waldvogel HJ, Faull RL, Love DR, Emson PC. Decreased neuronal nitric oxide synthase messenger RNA and somatostatin messenger RNA in the striatum of Huntington's disease. Neuroscience. 1996;**72**(4):1037-1047.

[181] Deckel AW, Tang V, Nuttal D, Gary K, Elder R. Altered neuronal nitric oxide synthase expression contributes to disease progression in Huntington's disease transgenic mice. Brain Research. 2002;**939**(1-2):76-86.

[182] Jarabek BR, Yasuda RP, Wolfe BB. Regulation of proteins affecting NMDA receptor-induced excitotoxicity in a Huntington's mouse model. Brain. 2004;**127**(Pt 3):505-516

[183] Puerta E, Hervias I, Barros-Miñones L, Jordan J, Ricobaraza A, Cuadrado-Tejedor M, García-Osta A, Aguirre N. Sildenafil protects against 3-nitropropionic acid neurotoxicity through the modulation of calpain, CREB, and BDNF. Neurobiology of Disease. 2010;**38**(2):237-245. DOI: 10.1016/j.nbd.2010.01.013

[184] Thakur T, Sharma S, Kumar K, Deshmukh R, Sharma PL. Neuroprotective role of PDE4 and PDE5 inhibitors in 3-nitropropionic acid induced behavioral and biochemical toxicities in rats. European Journal of Pharmacology. 2013;714(1-3):515-521. DOI: 10.1016/j.ejphar.2013.06.035

[185] Singhrao SK, Neal JW, Morgan BP, Gasque P. Increased complement biosynthesis by microglia and complement activation on neurons in Huntington's disease. Experimental Neurology 1999;159:362-376.

[186] Björkqvist M, Wild EJ, Thiele J, Silvestroni A, Andre R, Lahiri N, Raibon E, Lee RV, Benn CL, Soulet D, Magnusson A, Woodman B, Landles C, Pouladi MA, Hayden MR, Khalili-Shirazi A, Lowdell MW, Brundin P, Bates GP, Leavitt BR, Möller T, Tabrizi SJ. A novel pathogenic pathway of immune activation detectable before clinical onset in Huntington's disease. Journal of Experimental Medicine. 2008;**205**(8):1869-1877. DOI: 10.1084/jem.20080178

[187] Chang KH, Wu YR, Chen YC, Chen CM. Plasma inflammatory biomarkers for Huntington's disease patients and mouse model. Brain, Behavior, and Immunity 2015;**44**: 121-127. DOI: 10.1016/j.bbi.2014.09.011

[188] Politis M, Pavese N, Tai YF, Kiferle L, Mason SL, Brooks DJ, Tabrizi SJ, Barker RA, Piccini P. Microglial activation in regions related to cognitive function predicts disease onset in Huntington's disease: A multimodal imaging study. Human Brain Mapping 2011;**32**:258-270. DOI: 10.1002/hbm.21008

[189] Tai YF, Pavese N, Gerhard A, Tabrizi SJ, Barker RA, Brooks DJ, Piccini P. Microglial activation in presymptomatic Huntington's disease gene carriers. Brain. 2007;**130**(Pt 7):1759-1766.

[190] Kotrcova E, Jarkovska K, Valekova I, Zizkova M, Motlik J, Gadher SJ, Kovarova H. Challenges of Huntington's disease and quest for therapeutic biomarkers. Proteomics: Clinical Applications. 2015;**9**(1-2):147-158. DOI: 10.1002/prca.201400073

[191] Motta M, Imbesi R, Di Rosa M, Stivala F, Malaguarnera L. Altered plasma cytokine levels in Alzheimer's disease: Correlation with the disease progression. Immunology Letters. 2007;**114**(1):46-51

[192] Politis M, Lahiri N, Niccolini F, Su P, Wu K, Giannetti P, Scahill RI, Turkheimer FE, Tabrizi SJ, Piccini P. Increased central microglial activation associated with peripheral cytokine levels in premanifest Huntington's disease gene carriers. Neurobiology of Disease 2015;**83**:115-121. DOI: 10.1016/j.nbd.2015.08.011

[193] Clark LF, Kodadek T. The immune system and neuroinflammation as potential sources of blood-based biomarkers for Alzheimer's disease, Parkinson's disease, and Huntington's disease. ACS Chemical Neuroscience. 2016;**7**(5):520-527. DOI: 10.1021/acschemneuro.6b0042

[194] Dalrymple A, Wild EJ, Joubert R, Sathasivam K, Björkqvist M, Petersén A, Jackson GS, Isaacs JD, Kristiansen M, Bates GP, Leavitt BR, Keir G, Ward M, Tabrizi SJ. Proteomic profiling of plasma in Huntington's disease reveals neuroinflammatory activation and biomarker candidates. Journal of Proteome Research. 2007;**6**(7):2833-2840.

[195] Silajdzic E, Rezeli M, Végvári Á, Lahiri N, Andre R, Magnusson-Lind A, Nambron R, Kalliolia R, Marko-Varga G, Warner TT, Laurell T, Tabrizi SJ, Björkqvist M. A critical evaluation of inflammatory markers in Huntington's Disease plasma. Journal of Huntington's Disease. 2013;**2**(1):125-134. DOI: 10.3233/JHD-130049

[196] Vinther-Jensen T, Börnsen L, Budtz-Jorgensen E, Ammitzboll C, Larsen IU, Hjermind LE, Sellebjerg F, Nielsen JE. Selected CSF biomarkers indicate no evidence of early neuroinflammation in Huntington disease. Neurology: Neuroimmunology Neuroinflammation. 2016;**3**(6):e287

[197] Lo EH, Dalkara T, Moskowitz MA. Mechanisms, challenges and opportunities in stroke. Nature Review Neuroscience. 2003;**4**(5):399-415

[198] Donnan GA, Fisher M, Macleod M, Davis SM. Stroke. Lancet. 2008;**1**(9624):1612-1623. DOI: 10.1016/S0140-6736(08)60694-7

[199] Zhang R, Wang L, Zhang L, Chen J, Zhu Z, Zhang Z, Chopp M. Nitric oxide enhances angiogenesis via the synthesis of vascular endothelial growth factor and cGMP after stroke in the rat. Circulation Research. 2003;**92**(3):308-313.

[200] Li L, Jiang Q, Zhang L, Ding G, Gang Zhang Z, Li Q, Ewing JR, Lu M, Panda S, Ledbetter KA, Whitton PA, Chopp M. Angiogenesis and improved cerebral blood flow in the ischemic boundary area detected by MRI after administration of sildenafil to rats with embolic stroke. Brain Research. 2007;**1132**(1):185-192.

[201] Zhang RL, Chopp M, Roberts C, Wei M, Wang X, Liu X, Lu M, Zhang ZG. Sildenafil enhances neurogenesis and oligodendrogenesis in ischemic brain of middle-aged mouse. PLoS One. 2012;**7**(10):e48141. DOI: 10.1371/journal.pone.0048141

[202] Novitzky I, Marianayagam NJ, Weiss S, Muhsinogly O, Fridman M, Leibovitch TA, Goldenberg-Cohen N, Michowiz S. Comparison of neuroprotective effect of bevacizumab and sildenafil following induction of stroke in a mouse model. BioMed Research International. 2016;**2016**:3938523, DOI: 10.1155/2016/3938523

[203] Barros-Miñones L, Martín-de-Saavedra D, Perez-Alvarez S, Orejana L, Suquía V, Goñi-Allo B, Hervias I, López MG, Jordan J, Aguirre N, Puerta E. Inhibition of calpain-regulated p35/cdk5 plays a central role in sildenafil-induced protection against chemical hypoxia produced by malonate. Biochimica et Biophysica Acta. 2013;**1832**(6):705-717. DOI: 10.1016/j.bbadis.2013.02.002

[204] Moretti R, Leger PL, Besson VC, Csaba Z, Pansiot J, Di Criscio L, Gentili A, Titomanlio L, Bonnin P, Baud O, Charriaut-Marlangue C. Sildenafil, a cyclic GMP phosphodiesterase inhibitor, induces microglial modulation after focal ischemia in the neonatal mouse brain. Journal of Neuroinflammation. 2016;**13**(1):95. DOI: 10.1186/s12974-016-0560-4

[205] Silver B, McCarthy S, Lu M, Mitsias P, Russman AN, Katramados A, Morris DC, Lewandowski CA, Chopp M. Sildenafil treatment of subacute ischemic stroke: A safety study at 25-mg daily for 2 weeks. Journal of Stroke and Cerebrovascular Diseases. 2009;**18**(5):381-383.

Section 4

Neuroinflammation and Disease

Chapter 9

Roles of Pro- and Anti-inflammatory Cytokines in Traumatic Brain Injury and Acute Ischemic Stroke

Rachelle Dugue, Manan Nath, Andrew Dugue and Frank C. Barone

Additional information is available at the end of the chapter

http://dx.doi.org/10.5772/intechopen.70099

Abstract

This chapter will introduce the reader to the pathophysiology of two devastating neurologic events, traumatic brain injury (TBI) and acute ischemic stroke (AIS). Here we focus on the role of key pro-inflammatory and anti-inflammatory cytokines. Several experimental interventions have been found to modulate cytokine production and brain injury after AIS or TBI. Here minocycline, biological response modifiers, hormonal therapies, omega-3 fatty acids, N-acetylcysteine, and cannabinoids will be discussed. In addition, the role of cytokine-induced inflammasomes in both TBI and AIS will be addressed and followed by discussion of pro-inflammatory cytokines (e.g., TNF-α, IL-1β, IL-18, and IFN-γ). Finally, the main anti-inflammatory cytokines, IL-33, IL-10, IL-6, and IL-4, will be discussed in the context of both TBI and AIS. It should be noted that the role of these cytokines is diverse and the dichotomization of classically pro-versus anti-inflammatory cytokines is being re-examined, as many of these cytokines have been found to play dual roles in TBI and AIS brain injury.

Keywords: traumatic brain injury, ischemic stroke, cytokines, interleukins, inflammasome

1. Pathophysiology of traumatic brain injury

Traumatic brain injury (TBI) is a major cause of death and disability worldwide [1, 2]. It is one of the most commonly diagnosed neurological disorders in the United States, impacting people of a variety of ages and segments of society [3]. In Europe, the economic cost of

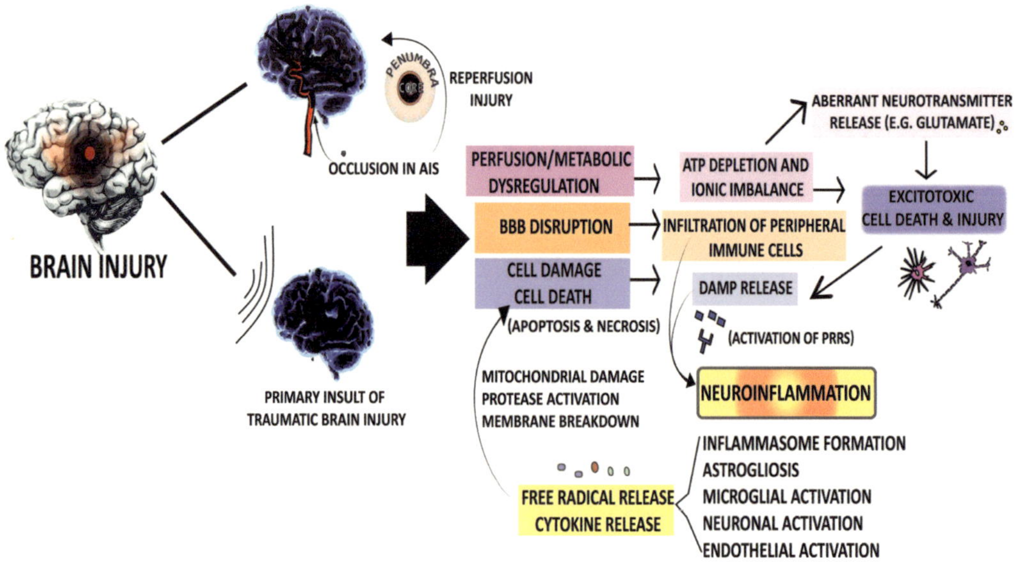

Figure 1. AIS and TBI pathophysiology. The pathophysiology of AIS and TBI share common mechanisms. The initial insult in AIS, an occlusion of blood flow resulting in a core infarct zone surrounded by a poorly perfused penumbra, versus the initial primary physical impact in TBI both result in perfusion and metabolic dysregulation leading to decreased glucose delivery and resultant adenosine triphosphate (ATP) depletion. The depletion of ATP prevents ATP-dependent ion pumps from regulating ionic gradients across cell membranes. As a result, there is aberrant neurotransmitter release and fluxes of ions like calcium causing excitotoxic cell death and cell injury via the activation of downstream molecules, like proteases. Cell damage leads to the release of damage-associated molecular patterns (DAMPs) which bind to pattern recognition receptors (PRRs) to exacerbate neuroinflammation via inflammasome formation, and astroglial, microglial, neuronal, and endothelial cell activation; these cells orchestrate the release of numerous cytokines, both pro-and anti-inflammatory. Blood-brain barrier disruption also occurs following the initial brain injury in TBI and AIS, permitting the influx of peripheral immune cells that exacerbate the inflammatory response through cytokine release, free radical release, and complement cascade activation. Further oxygen free radical production and reperfusion cellular injury occurs due to re-establishment of blood flow after its blockade in AIS. **Abbreviations**: AIS, acute ischemic stroke; ATP, adenosine triphosphate; BBB, blood-brain barrier; DAMP, Damage-associated molecular patterns; PRRs, pattern recognition receptors; TBI, traumatic brain injury.

TBI is over 33 billion euros per year [4]. Continued surveillance and research is being done to reduce primary and secondary TBI [as well as acute ischemic stroke(AIS)]–induced brain injury [1].

The pathophysiology of TBI begins with the initial brain trauma (i.e., the primary injury). This primary injury results from mechanical damage that disrupts the blood-brain barrier (BBB), alters the vasculature and damages brain tissue. The resulting injured glia and neurons release their intracellular contents (i.e., damage-associated molecular patterns; (DAMPs)) into the extracellular space and activate neighboring glia and neurons. Activated glia and neurons then produce molecular signals that can both exacerbate and mend the acute injury and contribute to long-term recovery [5–9]. These downstream molecular and cellular processes (i.e., the secondary injury in TBI) are the focus of many pre-clinical and clinical therapeutic studies. Secondary injury in TBI involves a host of molecular and cellular responses to the primary impact including: (a) an influx of peripheral inflammatory cells through the disrupted BBB leading to the release of reactive oxygen species (ROS), cytokines, chemokines, and free radicals; (b) the excessive release of excitatory neurotransmitters in response to ion imbalance across the cell membrane following adenosine triphosphate (ATP) depletion and metabolic dysregulation; and (c) significant increases in intracellular calcium concentration that contribute to protease, nuclease and lipase/phosphatase activation [10]. All of these factors culminate in cellular dysfunction and cell death/loss via rapid necrotic and more delayed (e.g., apoptotic) cell death pathways (See **Figure 1**).

The spatiotemporal distribution of pro- and anti-inflammatory cytokine production in secondary injury is a key feature of TBI pathophysiology and the development of post-TBI acute, sub-acute and chronic disability and recovery. By examining the role of individual cytokines in these processes, we can expect to identify novel approaches to TBI intervention/therapy.

2. Pathophysiology of ischemic stroke

Stroke is the fifth leading cause of death worldwide. Each year it affects approximately 800,000 people [11, 12]. Of all the people affected by stroke, two-thirds either die or are disabled [13]. Ischemic stroke constitutes 87% of all stroke cases [14]. The initial acute insult occurs when a thrombus or embolus lodges in one of the cerebral arteries. This blockage produces cellular and chemical changes in the ischemic core and the ischemic penumbra (the periphery of the lesion which receives some collateral blood flow from other arteries). The lack of perfusion to the ischemic core causes brain cells to die and release their intracellular contents due to a lack of ATP. The intracellular contents act as DAMPs to trigger neuroinflammatory cascades, while decreased perfusion in the ischemic penumbra leads to aberrantly functioning brain cells [15]. Macrophage scavenger receptor 1 and other macrophage receptors clear DAMPs and when deleted in a mouse model of AIS exacerbated neurologic deficits and infarct size [16]. Congruently, increased expression of *Mafb*, a transcription factor that promotes the expression of macrophage scavenger receptor 1, decreased the severity of post-AIS deficits [16].

Glutamate is also released in AIS and interacts with glutamate receptors in the penumbra resulting in excitotoxicity. This along with a state of energy depletion increases influx of sodium and calcium into the cells, resulting in membrane and cytoskeletal disintegration, enzyme activation, and eventual cell death [17]. Neuroinflammation, driven by cytokine production and complement activation, leads to the recruitment and adhesion of leukocytes into the CNS and endothelial surface and increases BBB disruption [15]. Subsequent reperfusion, although essential to protect brain tissue from further ischemic injury, is responsible for "reperfusion injury" by initiating additional inflammatory cascades; cytokines, free radicals and degradation enzyme activation as well as recruitment of leukocytes from the periphery further aggravate these processes [18]. This additionally causes mitochondrial damage, phospholipid membrane breakdown, cytoskeletal disintegration and cell death (See **Figure 1**) [18].

There is increasing emphasis on the importance of ongoing inflammatory processes in the pathophysiology of stroke. Neuroinflammation is central to ischemic stroke pathophysiology from the initial endothelial activation within minutes to hours post-insult to the post-injury reparative phases occurring over days to months [8, 15]. Cytokine signaling plays an especially extensive role in the pathophysiology of stroke and in the reparative mechanisms and residual deficits detected post-stroke. They also contribute to behavioral changes following AIS that include post-stroke depression, apathy, fatigue, as well as post-traumatic stress and anxiety (i.e., related to the presence of various cytokines and neuroinflammatory changes) [19–25].

3. The role of cytokines in central nervous system injury

3.1. What are cytokines?

Cytokines are small, secreted proteins released by many brain parenchymal cells and infiltrating immune cells (i.e., via autocrine, paracrine or endocrine actions) that influence the interaction and communication between cells. Historically, cytokines have been defined as lymphokines (when secreted by lymphocytes), monokines (when secreted by monocytes), chemokines (having chemotactic/attractant properties) and interleukins (cytokines made by one leukocyte that act on other leukocytes) [26]. Importantly, many brain cells (i.e., other cell types) can release cytokines. Cytokines have been broadly classified based on their receptor homology, their overall action as pro-versus anti-inflammatory, or their membership into the tumor necrosis factor, lymphokine, interleukin (IL-) and interferon (IFN-) families [9]. Cytokine receptor classes include the tumor necrosis factor receptor family, interleukin-1 receptor family, Class-II cytokine receptor family which includes interferon receptors and the IL-10 receptor, and Class-I or hematopoietin cytokine receptors which includes receptors of the IL-2, IL-3, and IL-6 family, as well as homodimeric receptors [9, 27–30].

Similar to their effects in the periphery, CNS cytokines are known to regulate the production of other cytokines. They can also alter the BBB, recruit inflammatory cells and influence neurotransmitter metabolism (monoamines, serotonin, dopamine and glutamate) [31–33]. In AIS and TBI, activated glial and neuronal cells both produce and respond to anti- and pro-inflammatory cytokines, influencing reparative and destructive mechanisms after brain injury has occurred. The balance of these reparative and destructive processes influences post-stroke and post-TBI outcomes.

3.2. Pro-inflammatory cytokines

In AIS and TBI, tissue injury and hypoxia activate microglia, the endogenous brain immune cells and a major source of pro-inflammatory cytokines in the CNS [8]. Pattern recognition receptors (PRRs) on microglia detect DAMPs triggering microglia to transition to various phenotypes, some of which promote the production of pro-inflammatory cytokines or anti-inflammatory cytokines. Classically, microglia have been characterized as M1 (i.e., pro-inflammatory) versus M2 (anti-inflammatory) phenotypes [34]. However, the classic nomenclature is under scrutiny, as many studies have demonstrated results incongruent with the simple categorization of M1 versus M2. Microglia are dynamic cells, continuously changing and responding to local stimuli. The M1/M2 polarization scheme does not necessarily fully capture the versatility of microglia behavior along a pro- to anti-inflammatory continuum [35]. Microglia contribute to neurodegeneration through the release of pro-inflammatory cytokines such as IL-1β, TNF-α, and IFN-γ, and via promotion of cytotoxic levels of ROS, reactive nitrogen species, nitric oxide, glutamate, and histamine [27, 34, 36]. Additionally, other CNS effector cells such as astrocytes, neurons, oligodendrocytes, CNS-derived macrophages and mast cells contribute to the pro-inflammatory cytokine milieu post-injury [37–39]. The pro-inflammatory cytokines TNF-α and IL-1β, as well as IL-6, are also involved in the initiation of sickness behaviors and may be related to post-AIS and post-TBI recovery responses [40].

Post-AIS and post-TBI inflammatory changes may be deleterious or beneficial. Several studies show that the inflammatory response in AIS relates to infarct volume and the inflammatory response in TBI to injury severity and contusion volume. While some studies consistently demonstrate deleterious roles of cytokines such as TNF-α, others are inconsistent in polarizing cytokines as pro-versus anti-inflammatory [41–48]. Thus, the roles of cytokines in TBI and AIS are still unclear and while categorization of cytokines as pro-versus anti-inflammatory is helpful, it is not definitive in all cases.

3.3. The inflammasome and pro-inflammatory cytokine release

Inflammasomes play a major role in the release of pro-inflammatory cytokines and the induction of cell death in TBI and AIS. Multiple molecules join together due to the activation of PRRs by DAMPs to form inflammasomes specific to their PRR. Inflammasomes can be formed in the cytoplasm of a variety of cells (neurons, microglia, macrophages, brain endothelial cells) [49] and upregulate cytokines that augment the inflammatory response [50]. The standard inflammasome is composed of a PRR in the cell cytosol connected to the protease caspase-1 by an adaptor protein. In TBI and AIS, NLRP1 and NLRP3 inflammasomes are formed in microglia and neurons in response to DAMPs [51, 52]. NLRP1 and NLRP3 are both formed via cytosolic NOD-like PRRs (i.e. NLR) with a carboxy-terminal leucine-rich repeat, nucleotide-binding domain, and pyrin domain; these components permit interactions with an adaptor apoptosis-associated speck-like protein (ASC) which contains a caspase activation and recruitment domain to permit the activation of caspase-1 (See **Figure 2**, Key concepts box) [50, 53]. Activated caspase-1 goes on to activate cytokines IL-1β and IL-18 while triggering apoptotic cell death. The NLRP1 inflammasome can additionally recruit various cell molecular responses including the membrane channel pannexin-1, the X-linked inhibitor of apoptosis protein (XIAP), caspase-5, caspase-11, and P2X purinoreceptor 7 to guide its activation and actions in various cell types [50].

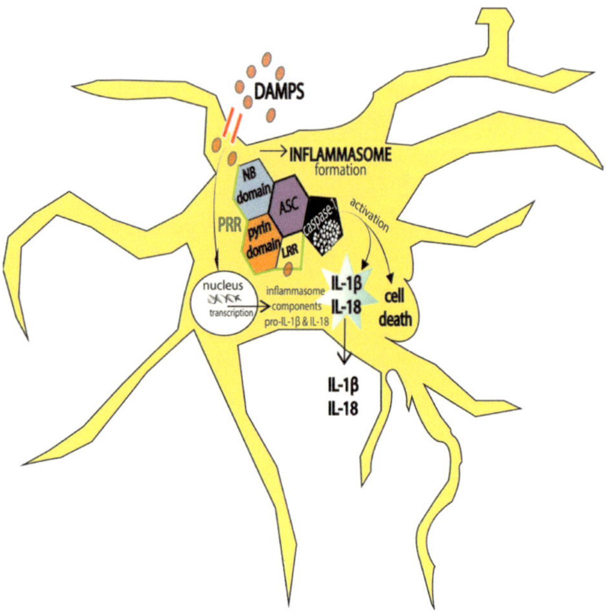

Figure 2. The Inflammasome. Inflammasome complexes form in response to activation via DAMPs or cell signaling molecules produced in states of cell stress and injury. Cytoplasmic or transmembrane PRRs recognize DAMPs and initiate the assembly of the inflammasome complex and the transcription of cytokine precursors. The typical inflammasome complex is composed of a PRR connected via an adaptor protein to caspase-1. Through PRR activation by DAMPs, caspase-1 is activated and initiates an inflammatory cascade involving the activation of the cytokines IL-18 and IL-1β as well as cell death mechanisms. The inflammasome depicted above is representative of the NLRP3 inflammasome of the NLR family of pattern recognition receptors. The NOD-like receptor pattern recognition receptor is a cytoplasmic receptor complex containing a leucine rich repeat, pyrin domain, and nucleotide-binding domain. It is activated by DAMPs/molecular pattern signals to activate caspase-1 which it is connected to via the apoptosis-associated speck-like protein, an adaptor protein. Activated caspase-1 cleaves pro- IL-18 and IL-1β to their active forms to promote neuroinflammation and cell death mechanisms. **Abbreviations**: ASC, apoptosis-associated speck-like protein; DAMP, Damage-associated molecular patterns; LRR, carboxy-terminal leucine-rich repeat, NB domain, nucleotide-binding domain; NLR, NOD-like receptor; PRR, pattern recognition receptor. See Key Concept Box.

Key Concept Box:

Key components of the inflammatory response in AIS and TBI

DAMPs (**Damage-associated molecular patterns**)-intracellular contents and products released from damaged cells that act as molecular signals to trigger neighboring and infiltrating cells to respond, thus promoting inflammation. DAMPs interact with PRRs on cells to recruit additional cells and organize an inflammatory response

PRRs (**Pattern recognition receptors**)-a receptor that recognizes the molecular signatures associated with damage or pathogen invasion to activate downstream signal transduction and the formation of the inflammasome complex. DAMPs or pathogen-associated molecular patterns (PAMPs) bind to their respective PRR, triggering the downstream inflammatory response.

Inflammasome-large multiprotein complexes named after their respective PRR (e.g. NLRP1, named for the NOD-like receptor, NLR). These complexes have been observed in astrocytes, microglia, and neurons. The standard inflammasome is composed of a PRR attached to an adaptor protein linking it to a protease, classically, caspase-1, which goes on to cleave and activate cytokines IL-1β and IL-18. Cell death is triggered via activation of these cytokines and pyropoptosis.

Cytokines-small proteins secreted by immune cells both centrally and peripherally to relay information between cells and trigger immune responses and cell interactions to be protective or damaging. Cytokine actions include the recruitment of immune cells, alteration of the BBB, alteration of neurotransmitter metabolism, angiogenesis, astrogliosis, the promotion of other cytokines, protease activation, activation of apoptotic cell death mechanisms, and many more.

NLRP3 inflammasomes were found in astrocytes, microglia and cortical neurons in a weight-drop model of TBI in rats [54]. Protein levels of NLRP3, active caspase-1, and IL-18 all gradually increased over the course of 7 days in cortical tissue ipsilateral to the contusion, while levels of IL-1β rose at 6 h post-injury and declined over the course of 7 days to sham levels [54]. In support of the role of NLRP3 in TBI, another animal study showed that the expression of NLRP3, caspase-1, and thioredoxin-interacting protein (TXNIP), a regulator of NLRP3 activity, were all increased in the cerebral cortex of rats at 12 and 24 h post-blast injury [55]. In a fluid-percussion model of TBI in rats, NLRP1 inflammasome complexes containing ASC, caspase-1, caspase-11, XIAP, and pannexin-1 with resultant caspase-1 activation and XIAP cleavage were present in injured cortical lysate at 4 h post-injury. These complexes were also localized to cortical neurons [52]. Thus, the NLRP3 inflammasome is implicated in multiple mechanisms of brain injury ranging from diffuse blast injury to localized fluid percussion injury in animal models and may translate to patients with different mechanisms of brain injury as well.

A single immediate intracerebroventricular post-TBI dose of anti-ASC antibody, an antibody targeting the ASC component of the NLRP1 and NLRP3 inflammasome complex, decreased the activation of caspase-1, IL-1β and XIAP cleavage at 24 h post-injury. This same intracerebroventricular dose followed by booster anti-ASC antibody injections intraperitoneally (i.p.) at 24 and 48 h post-TBI significantly decreased the lesion volume at 3 days post-injury [52]. In contrast, a study using the controlled-cortical impact (CCI) TBI model in NLRP1 knockout mice and ASC knockout mice found no differences in the recovery of motor function up to 14 days post-injury in wild-type injured mice versus knockout mice; there were also no differences in lesion volume or the number of dead cells in the cortex or dentate gyrus ipsilateral to the injury at 3 days post-injury, despite an observed decrease in IL-1β at 1 day post-injury. Interestingly, the level of IL-6 also decreased in NLRP1 knockouts [56]. These findings suggest a role for additional inflammatory mediators in determining histological and behavioral outcomes post-injury. The baseline versus injury-induced inflammatory environment may influence post-injury outcomes, dictating the amount and type of cytokines necessary to produce a certain outcome. Knockout animals have a completely different baseline inflammatory environment with potentially alternate mechanisms of immune activation.

In humans, higher cerebrospinal fluid (CSF) levels of inflammasome complex components caspase-1, ASC, and NACHT leucine rich repeat protein-1 (NALP-1) were associated with significantly poorer outcomes as determined by unfavorable versus favorable Glasgow outcome scores at 5 months post-injury in moderate-severe TBI patients [57]. Similiarly, increased levels of inflammasome proteins, NLRP1, NLRP3, as well as caspase-1 and IL-1β have been detected in ipsilateral brain tissue samples of stroke patients [58].

Preclinically, in a rodent and neuronal culture model of AIS, Fann et al. showed an upregulation of NLRP3, NLRP1, caspase-1, IL-18 and IL-1β. The authors then used a caspase-1 inhibitor to thwart detrimental post-ischemia effects, reducing neuronal cell death in the culture model and functional deficits and infarct volumes in the mouse model [58]. These findings showcase the role of caspase-1 in post-ischemic deficits, a downstream component of many inflammasome complexes.

The NLRP1 inflammasome also plays a role in AIS. In a study by Abulafia et al. using a thromboembolic mouse model of stroke, NLRP1 was detected in microglia post-stroke as early as

6 h as compared to sham mice (NLRP1 was expressed in neurons and astrocytes, but not in microglia in sham mice). Despite this finding, the overall concentration of NLRP1 in cortical lysates was no different than shams [51]. In this same study, intracerebroventricular injection of anti-NLRP1 antibody 15 min post-thromboembolic stroke reduced caspase-1 and IL-1β activation at 24 h, but did not affect infarct volume. These results are similar to the results from the NLRP1 knockout mice studies in TBI. While the reduction in caspase-1 and IL-1β activation via anti-NLRP1 in Abulafia's study evidences the role of NLRP1 in inflammasome formation post-stroke, it does not distinguish NLRP1's relative importance to other inflammasomes formed post-stroke. In a rodent model of stroke, the NLRC4 (NLR family, CARD domain containing 4) and AIM2 (absent in melanoma 2) inflammasomes were shown to contribute to brain injury without NLRP3 involvement (i.e., without this inflammasome commonly involved in brain injury) [58–61]. Furthermore, knock-out mice ($NLRC4^{-/-}$, $AIM2^{-/-}$, $ASC^{-/-}$) studies all show an improvement in function following AIS with decreased microglia activation, decreased leukocyte recruitment and decreased infarct volume [59]. These discoveries identify the NLRC4 and AIM2 inflammasomes in addition to the NLRP3 inflammasome as potential therapeutic targets for stroke and provide new insights into how the inflammatory response is regulated post-stroke.

3.4. Inflammatory cytokine–tissue necrosis factor-α (TNF-α)

TNF-α can interact with two receptor subtypes: TNF receptor type 1 (TNFR1) or type 2 (TNFR2). TNF-α binds to TNFR1 or TNFR2 triggering the formation of intracellular complexes (complex 1, 2a, 2b, and 2c in TNFR1 and complex 1 in TNFR2) to promote inflammation, apoptosis, neurodegeneration, necroptosis, as well as some aspects of cell survival and proliferation through respective signal transduction pathways [62]. TNFR1 activation is classically associated with the exacerbation of cell injury and the promotion of cell death, while TNFR2 is associated with cell survival and proliferation, but has also been associated with inflammation and apoptosis [62–64].

TNF-α is among the first cytokines upregulated following TBI and AIS and is involved in the regulation of microglia activation as well as glutamatergic synaptic and glial signaling [64, 65]. Two biologically active forms of TNF-α, a soluble form and a transmembrane form, can be released primarily by microglia in inflammatory conditions, in addition to astrocytes, endothelial cells, and neurons. Many studies in a variety of animal models of mild to severe TBI have detected increased levels of TNF-α post-injury [66–69].

3.5. TNF-α in TBI

In TBI patients, increased levels of TNF-α have been detected in the CSF for up to 22 days after injury and have been noted in varying degrees in post-mortem tissue from TBI brain samples taken early post-injury (less than 17 min survival time) versus late post-injury (6–122 h survival time) [70, 71]. Tissue from the cortex ipsilateral to injury in both the early group and late group showed higher levels of TNF-α than controls. Specifically, the late group had TNF-α concentrations approximately five times higher than the early group, and higher levels of TNF-α in the contralateral cortex as compared to controls [71].

In animal models of TBI, TNF-α inhibition has resulted in protective effects. The lipophilic analog of thalidomide, 3,6′ dithiothalidomide, an inhibitor of TNF-α synthesis, ameliorated Y-maze spatial memory deficits and deficits in novel object recognition at 7 days post-injury when dosed up to 12 h post-mild TBI injury in mice [69]. Another TNF-α synthesis inhibitor, pentoxifylline, and a TNF-α activity inhibitor, TNF-α binding protein, improved edema at 24 h and motor deficits at up to 14 days post-injury as measured by rats' neurologic severity score in a closed head injury weight drop model of TBI in the rat [72]. The effect of pentoxifylline on motor recovery being reversible with administration of recombinant TNF-α [72].

TNF-α has demonstrated dual effects based on timing post-injury. In a study examining motor function and lesion severity in TNF-α knockout mice at 48 h post-injury, TNF-α knockouts had better motor function [73]. However, at 2 and 4 weeks post-injury, TNF-α knockouts had worse motor function and more cortical tissue loss than wildtype mice [73]. In another study, mice lacking the mitogen activated protein kinase (MAPK), p38α, a downstream signaling mechanism in microglia known to promote TNF-α and IL-1β cytokine release (p38α knockout mice) were examined in a model of diffuse TBI using fluid percussion injury causing massive microglia activation. Interestingly, in the TBI-injured p38α knockout mice, TNF-α levels were actually higher than wildtype TBI-injured mice at 6 h post-injury and returned to baseline levels by 7 days post-injury, alongside the reversal of motor deficits on rotarod and a decrease in activated microglia morphology in p38α knockout TBI-injured mice [74]. These findings support additional sources of TNF-α post-TBI and contrast the role of other microglia-induced cytokines to TNF-α in aspects of functional recovery post-TBI.

In a closed head injury model of TBI in mice, the expression of the complement system's C5a receptor was examined in TNF/lymphotoxin-α knockout mice. C5a is an anaphylatoxin involved in neutrophil and glial cell chemotaxis to the site of injury as well as neuronal apoptosis [75, 76]. The TNF/lymphotoxin-α knockout TBI mice experienced high levels of C5a receptor in neurons, neuroglia, and neutrophils at 24 and 72 h, similar to wild-type TBI mice, but displayed lower C5a receptor levels than the wild-type TBI mice by 7 days post-injury; sham-injured knockout mice had low levels of C5a receptors [77]. These findings emphasize the importance of the timing of cytokines in the regulation of the immune response post-TBI, as lack of TNF-α decreased C5a receptor expression at only 7 days post-TBI.

3.6. TNF-α in AIS

In AIS patients, TNF-α has been demonstrated in neurons and astrocytes in brain tissue within the first 24 h and for up to 18 days post-stroke; TNF-α immunoreactivity overlapped many TUNEL stained dying cells in the infarct core and peri-infarct region within the first days post-stroke, spreading as far as the contralateral hemisphere by 1.6 days in one case [78]. In patients, TNF-α was also found to be a good marker of ischemia in peripheral blood at 24 h post-stroke [79]. Peripheral TNF-α can induce the production of MCP1/CCL2 which not only help to recruit monocytes into the CNS [80], but also induce leukocyte rolling and adhesion to cerebral vasculature via E- and P-selectins [81].

In a pre-clinical study by Botchkina et al. examining AIS and TNF-α expression, TNF-α was increased locally in astrocytes, microglia, choroid plexus cells, endothelial cells, and in infiltrating polymorphonuclear cells; neurons expressed maximal levels of TNF-α by 6 h post-stroke, and were surrounded by activated microglia. TNF-α regulates microglial activation as well as glutamatergic glial and synaptic transmission [82]. Apoptotic neurons were also found to express TNF-α at 24 h post-stroke [83]. TNF-α expression in AIS results in the upregulation of MMP-9 and other metalloproteinases that increase BBB permeability; the increased BBB permeability permits entry of leukocytes, proteases, immunoglobulins and thrombin into the CNS, facilitating cell injury [84–86]. Higher baseline peripheral levels of MMP-9 were correlated with larger lesion volumes in stroke patients [79].

Higher levels of TNF-α are generally related to worse outcomes in AIS. Mice genetically modified to overexpress TNF-α have larger infarct volumes post-stroke, as well as increased neuronal apoptosis [87]. Barone et al. showed that administration of TNF-α prior to AIS resulted in worse functional deficits and larger infarcts that were reversed via neutralization with anti-TNF-α antibody. The pre- and post-stroke intracerebroventricular administration of anti-TNF-α antibody or soluble TNF-receptor I also decreased infarct size in this study [88]. The soluble TNFR1 receptors sequester the TNF-α that has already been released due to AIS, thus helping reduce ischemic injury. Additional studies administering TNF-α neutralizing antibodies or soluble TNF-α receptor post-stroke result in smaller lesion volumes and less cerebral edema [86, 89]. A study by Pan et al. on TNF-α trafficking across the BBB post-stroke found that mice who underwent AIS had higher levels of TNF-α transported across the BBB on day 5 post-stroke in both hemispheres, cortically and subcortically without an increase in overall BBB permeability. This finding was substantiated by a peak number of TNFR1 and TNFR2 receptors in endothelial cells ipsilateral to the ischemic site at 5 days post-stroke that would permit this selective uptake across the BBB. However, interestingly, these increases in TNF-α transport peaked while functional deficits began to improve [90]. Thus, the observed time course of increased TNF-α levels in this study may additionally implicate TNF-α in post-stroke repair and neuroplasticity. Further evidence of TNF-α's potential benefit is seen via its ability to activate the formation of the TNFR1-TRADD (TNF receptor associated protein death domain) complex to induce NF-κB mediated transcription of anti-apoptotic proteins, contributing to cell survival. However, TNF-α can also induce cell death via recruitment of caspases and proteins like Fas-associating protein with a death domain (FADD)[64].

3.7. TNF-α polymorphisms

In both AIS and TBI, single-nucleotide polymorphisms (SNPs) in TNF-α have been correlated to different risk profiles for disease severity [91–93]. A meta-analysis on AIS risk in individuals with TNF-α-308G/A gene versus-238G/A gene polymorphisms, both of which lead to high TNF-α production, suggests differences in AIS risk associated with these SNPs in Caucasians versus Asians; the TNF-α-308G/A gene polymorphism was protective in Asians, while the TNF-α-238G/A gene polymorphism was associated with a higher risk of AIS in Caucasians [92]. In a study of the TNF-α-308G/A gene polymorphism in TBI patients, those with this polymorphism had worse clinical outcomes as measured by the Glasgow outcome scale at 6 months post-injury [93].

3.8. Inflammatory cytokine–interleukin-1β

IL-1β is an essential mediator in the neuroinflammatory response, is constitutively expressed in the CNS, and is upregulated minutes after a neuronal insult [94]. As previously mentioned, pro- IL-1β is cleaved by caspase-1 into its active form [94]. The transcription and translation of pro-IL-1β is modulated by molecules that are altered in neuronal injury and infection, such as prostaglandins, lipopolysaccharide, and glucocorticoids; glucocorticoids decrease the production of pro-IL-1β, while lipopolysaccharides and prostaglandins, as well as intercellular adhesion molecules increase it [94].

The type 1 IL-1 receptor (IL-1R1) and type 2 IL-1 receptor (IL-1R2) bind to active IL-1β to regulate cytokine concentration. IL-1R2 acts as a decoy receptor, as it does not induce downstream effects upon binding to IL-1β [94]. In contrast, the type 1 IL-1 receptor induces signal transduction pathways in multiple cell types (endothelial cells, oligodendrocytes, neurons, astrocytes, microglia, leukocytes). For example, when IL-1β binds to IL-1R1 on microglia, cytoplasmic GTPases signal to MAPK p38α downstream to induce the transcription and release of other cytokines, such as TNF-α and the phagocytosis of axonal and cellular debris; IL-1β also induces the expression and secretion of heat shock proteins that activate other PRRs and expand the neuroinflammatory response [95, 96]. IL-1 receptors can also circulate in a soluble form to bind and impact the concentrations of IL-1 cytokines [94, 95]. The IL-1 receptor antagonist, IL-1Ra, is an innate competitive antagonist to other IL-1 receptors and does not induce a downstream biological response [94, 95].

3.9. Inflammatory IL-1β in TBI

Numerous studies demonstrate the rapid rise of IL-1β post-injury associated with increased cell death. The exogenous addition of IL-1β or increased production of IL-1β post-TBI is associated with an exacerbation of injury [97–100]. For example, Lu et al. observed increased levels of hippocampal IL-1β as early as 3 h, peaking at 12 h and remaining for 48 h post-injury in a weight drop model of TBI in rats associated with severe hippocampal neuronal loss [101]. Lawrence et al. demonstrated an exacerbation of neuronal loss in the cortex when IL-1β was co-administered into the ipsilateral or contralateral striatum with excitotoxin infusion in the cortex. These studies provide examples of IL-1β's global influence on cell death post-injury [102].

Accordingly, studies ablating the expression of IL-1β or inhibiting its biological effect via anti-IL-1β antibodies, upregulation of the endogenous IL-1β receptor antagonist, IL-1Ra, or interleukin-1 receptor antagonists show improvements in TBI outcomes in rat models [103–105]. Injury-induced neuron loss in the rat hippocampus was also significantly improved with pre-injury intracerebroventricular administration of IL-1β antibody [101]. Post-CCI i.p. administration of anti-IL-1β antibody decreased edema at 48 h post-injury, as well as microglia activation, lesion size, and visuospatial learning deficits in the Morris water maze (MWM) task (decreased latency to the hidden platform on 2 out of 4 training days, but did not improve memory probe trial performance) at up to 20 days post-injury [106]. Anti-IL-1β antibody administration via osmotic minipump in this same CCI model resulted in decreased neutrophil and activated T cell penetration across the BBB into the cortex at 7 days post-injury [107].

IL-1β neutralizing antibodies were also tested in a central fluid percussion injury mouse model of diffuse axonal TBI; IL-1β neutralizing antibodies were administered i.p. 30 min post-injury, improving the latency to hidden platform times in the probe trial (long-term memory) of the MWM task at 21 days post-injury to near sham-injured levels [108]. Decreases in the number of stereotypies in a multivariate concentric square field test were also seen in IL-1β neutralizing antibody-treated mice 2 and 9 days post-injury. Histologically, the number of microglia and macrophages were unchanged in treated mice [108]. The difference in IL-1β neutralizing antibodies' effect on cognitive outcomes post-TBI in these models could be related to the different injury models used.

The genetic overexpression of the endogenous receptor antagonist to IL-1β, IL-1Ra in a closed head injury mouse model of TBI resulted in an improved neurologic severity score, lower cortical levels of harmful TNF-α, and a delayed rise in IL-1β and IL-6 at 6 versus 4 h post-injury in wildtype mice [104]. However, in a study examining the use of the recombinant human IL-1Ra (i.e, anakinra), in patients with severe TBI, treatment, while safe without serious adverse effects, was found to induce a shift in cytokine levels towards an unexpected phenotypically M1 microglial response in comparison to non-treated controls [109, 110]. These findings evidence a more broadly defined role for IL-1Ra in TBI and the effect of IL-1Ra on microglial activation.

In a study of post-mortem TBI cortical tissue ipsilateral and contralateral to the lesion site, IL-1β levels were significantly higher in brains from patients with survival times ranging from 6 to 122 h post-injury, signifying a later peak of action [71]. IL-1β CSF samples were higher than extracellular plasma levels of IL-1β and IL-1Ra following severe TBI in 12 patients, with peaks occurring 1 day and 2 days post-injury, respectively [111].

3.10. Inflammatory IL-1β in AIS

IL-1β is released from activated microglia within 30 min of ischemic stroke and appears to be the main IL-1 agonist induced in the brain in response to systemic or local insults [112, 113]. In the acute phase of injury, IL-1β interacts with its receptors to enhance microglial activation, stimulate astrocytic production of vascular endothelial growth factor (VEGF), and MMP-9 from NG2-oligodendrocyte precursor cells (NG2-OPC) [114, 115]. Evidence from human culture systems suggests that hypoxia itself induces the production of IL-1β in endothelial cells, which then upregulates leukocyte adhesion molecules by an autocrine mechanism [116]. Additional preclinical studies have further clarified IL-1β participation in AIS pathophysiology noting that neither IL-1β nor IL-1Ra influence glutamate release or reuptake [117, 118].

A study by Clausen et al. showed that IL-1β and TNF-α are produced by largely segregated populations of microglia and macrophages after AIS in mice, providing evidence of the functional diversity among microglia and macrophages induced post-stroke [119]. This information may inform the design and characterization of anti-inflammatory therapies in stroke. The mRNA of the natural receptor antagonist, IL-1Ra was also much higher at 12 h after permanent middle cerebral artery occlusion and remained elevated for up to 5 days post-stroke in the ischemic cortex and may reflect its effort to dampen the influence of IL-1β in the acute phase of AIS [120]. Multiple laboratories have examined IL-1Ra as a therapy in preclinical models of AIS in mice. In a multicenter international project examining the short- and long-term effects of IL-1Ra therapy in preclinical models of AIS, consistent decreases in lesion size on days 1 and 7 were noted via histology and MRI after treatment with subcutaneous IL-1Ra [121]. Improvements in neurologic deficits/function ("sensorimotor asymmetry") for up to 28 days post-treatment were also noted in this study across AIS models [121].

The potentially noxious role of IL-1β in AIS is supported by the finding that inhibition of IL-1β converting enzyme (ICE) decreases infarct volumes in mice [122] and rats [123]. Moreover, transgenic mice with a mutant ICE gene developed smaller infarcts, fewer neurological deficits, lower IL-1β levels and decreased DNA fragmentation after transient and permanent middle cerebral artery occlusion [124, 125]. Furthermore, many studies testing therapeutics in animal models of AIS correlate declines in IL-1β levels post-drug administration to improved functional and histologic outcomes post-stroke [115, 126, 127]. Thus, levels of IL-1β and IL-1Ra can be important predictors of the degree of neuroinflammation following ischemic stroke, as increased levels of IL-1β worsened AIS whereas IL-1Ra provided brain protection [114].

Clinically, a longitudinal study of patients with ischemic stroke revealed acutely increased mRNA levels of IL-1β, IL-8, and IL-17 in peripheral blood samples, with IL-1β and IL-8 correlating with Scandinavian stroke scale scores [128]. IL-1β levels were higher in those with more severe neurologic impairment [128]. Increased intrathecal production of several cytokines, including interleukins IL-1β, IL-6, IL-8, IL-10, TNF-α, and granulocyte-macrophage colony-stimulating factor, has also been demonstrated in patients with AIS [42, 129, 130]. In a clinical study involving 30 stroke patients, an early increase in intrathecal, but not systemic levels of IL-1β were observed post-stroke [42]. Ormstad et al. noted an association between high acute serum levels of glucose and IL-1β, and low IL-1Ra and IL-9 to post-stroke fatigue [21]. These findings support the involvement of cytokines in fatigue after stroke [21].

3.11. Inflammatory cytokine–interleukin-18

IL-18 (previously known as IFN-γ inducing factor) is a pro-inflammatory cytokine of the IL-1 family, namely produced by microglia in the CNS [131]. IL-18 also regulates IFN-γ signaling in T-cells and Natural Killer (NK) cells [60, 76]. As previously mentioned, IL-18 can be activated through caspase-1 cleavage via inflammasome formation in addition to other proteases such as proteinase-3[94]. Activated IL-18 binds to IL-18 receptors on a variety of cell types to trigger downstream signal transduction pathways; the release of glutamate at the synapse as well as the upregulation of postsynaptic AMPA receptors in hippocampal neurons is induced via IL-18 and has been shown to inhibit long-term potentiation in the dentate gyrus [132]. IL-18 can also induce apoptotic pathways (Fas-Fas ligand binding via induction of FasL expression on glia), cytotoxic immune cell activation, the extravasation of polymorphonuclear cells, their respiratory burst response and degranulation, as well as the release of matrix metalloproteinases and cytokines like TNF-α, IL-1β and IFN-γ [131].

3.12. Inflammatory IL-18 in TBI

IL-18 is heavily involved in neuroinflammation and neurodegeneration in TBI and AIS. IL-18 levels were found to be elevated for up to 10 days post-TBI in the CSF of patients who had experienced a severe head injury [133] and have been associated with more severe disability [134]. In a study examining serum levels of IL-18 in TBI patients, plasma IL-18 levels were elevated at 7 days, 3 months, and 6 months post-injury and were noted to decrease over time in parallel to cognitive improvement as measured by the mini mental state examination (MMSE). Those with higher MMSE scores had lower levels of IL-18 at all time points [135]. In mice, IL-18 was elevated above control levels at 7 days post-weight drop TBI. The administration of the IL-18 inhibitor, IL-18-binding protein, at 1 h post-injury improved injury-induced deficits involving motor function, reflexes, and normal behaviors tallied via a neurologic severity score at 7 days, but did not improve cerebral edema or behavioral deficits acutely at 24 h post-injury [133]. This evidences a role for IL-18 in the later phase of inflammation post-injury.

3.13. Inflammatory IL-18 in AIS

IL-18 shows a delayed rise (24–48 h) and peak (7–14 days) following ischemic stroke in mice [136]. However, IL-18 knockout mice showed no difference in infarct size at 24 or 48 h post-AIS, suggesting its limited effect on lesion severity early post-AIS [137, 138].

However, examination of human atherosclerotic plaques from carotid arteries show higher levels of IL-18, IL-18 receptor and caspase-1 expression, with IL-18 levels highest near macrophages and higher in ulcerating, unstable plaques [139]. This supports a pathogenic role for IL-18 early in the pathophysiology of AIS, at stages of thrombus formation. In AIS patients, plasma IL-18 levels obtained from blood samples taken by venous access at 48 h following AIS in 217 patients were significantly higher than in control groups. Patients with high IL-18 had significantly higher incidences of 90-day recurrent stroke and death. Thus, plasma IL-18 levels could be a major independent inflammatory predictor of 90-day morbidity and mortality in AIS patients [140]. However, these observations are incongruent with a larger study in 2008 where IL-6, IL-18 and TNF-α levels were examined in relation to recurrent stroke risk. The data was obtained from the perindopril protection against recurrent stroke study (PROGRESS) study. It was found that IL-6 and TNF-α, but not IL-18, were associated with risk of recurrent ischemic stroke independent of conventional risk markers [141].

Yang et al. explored IL-18 as a potential marker for post-AIS depression. It was observed that serum IL-18 levels on both days 1 and 7 post-AIS were significantly higher in post-stroke depression patients and non-post-stroke depression patients than in non-stroke controls. Serum IL-18 on day 7 was significantly higher in post-stroke depression patients than in non-post-stroke depression patients, suggesting a role for IL-18 in post-AIS changes in mood [25].

3.14. Inflammatory cytokine–interferon-γ

Interferon-γ is a classic pro-inflammatory cytokine released peripherally by activated T cells and natural killer cells to activate macrophages, monocytes, and microglia [33]. In any type of brain injury, compromise of the BBB permits the influx of peripheral T cells and NK cells, subjecting CNS cells to the effects of IFN-γ. IFN-γ may exacerbate BBB permeability to peripheral immune cells post-injury through the upregulation of vascular cell adhesion molecule in astrocytes of the BBB [142]. IFN-γ then directs microglia to express neuroprotective versus cytotoxic features depending on the cytokines' concentration [143]. Microglia activated by low levels of IFN-γ can actually induce neurogenesis and oligodendrogenesis [143]. IFN-γ was also recently discovered to be released by microglia in response to IL-12 or IL-18 [144].

3.15. Inflammatory interferon-γ in TBI

In biopsies from the brains of severely injured patients, IFN-γ was detected within the first 24 h post-injury and was found to be higher than IL-4 and IL-6 at 3–5 days post-injury, indicating a robust pro-inflammatory response at up to 5 days post-TBI [145]. Post-mortem TBI brain analyses show significantly increased levels of IFN-γ in brains with survival times less than 17 min with even higher levels in tissue ipsilateral and contralateral to the injury in brains with survival times ranging from 6 to 122 h post-injury [71]. In a study examining cytokine levels in patients with severe TBI with post-traumatic hypoxia, the duration of elevated IFN-γ levels was longer, persisting 5 days post-TBI, as compared to severe TBI patients without hypoxia, indicating more persistent neuroinflammation in TBI patients with hypoxia [146]. Experimental models of TBI have also investigated the time course of IFN-γ expression post-injury and have detected variations according to the injury type and sex. A penetrating ballistic injury model of TBI in male rats demonstrated rises in IFN-γ within 4 h post-injury, while a post-craniotomy weight drop model of TBI in female rats did not detect IFN-γ by post-injury day 2 [147–149]. CCI injury versus craniotomy alone in mice also showed significant increases in IFN-γ expression with different cytokine expression time courses, supporting the impact of injury severity on cytokine expression; the mild injury via craniotomy resulted in a shorter lived cytokine response, while the severe CCI injury resulted in a response persisting for at least 21 days. IFN-γ expression peaked at 3 and 7 days post-injury in CCI-injured and craniotomy mice, respectively, with CCI-injured mice expressing higher peak levels of IFN-γ [150].

3.16. Inflammatory interferon-γ in AIS

IFN-γ has been strongly detected in autopsied human brains for up to 28 days post-ischemic stroke and is substantially expressed by inflammatory glia [151]. However, the rise of IFN-γ post-stroke may be largely facilitated by infiltrative lymphocytes, like $CD4^+$ and $CD8^+$ T cells, as IFN-γ is not present in normal brain tissue [152]. A study by Yilmaz et al. utilized the transient middle cerebral artery occlusion model of AIS in mice and knockout mice lacking various lymphocyte populations to assess the role, interaction, and contribution of lymphocytes and IFN-γ to infarct severity and functional deficits post-stroke. AIS-induced increases in platelet and leukocyte adhesion were significantly attenuated in CD4+ T cell knockout mice and CD8+ T cell knockout mice. Leukocyte adhesion also decreased in neutrophil deficient mice. Similarly, lymphocyte deficient mice ($Rag^{-/-}$ mice) and IFN-γ knockout mice had significantly lower levels of leukocyte and platelet adhesion post-stroke. Ischemic infarct volume was also lower in IFN-γ knockout mice and lymphocyte deficient ($Rag1^{-/-}$) mice. In contrast, neurologic deficits were only improved in lymphocyte deficient $Rag1^{-/-}$ mice [152]. These effects were reversed when splenocytes were added to restore lymphocytes in $Rag^{-/-}$ mice [152]. While the absence of IFN-γ alone was enough to significantly impact infarct volume post-AIS, it was not sufficient to significantly change outcomes in neurologic deficits post-AIS [152].

IFN-γ mRNA expression is also systemically increased in blood monocytes, splenocytes, and lymph node cells in AIS [153]. In a study by Li et al., systemic IFN-γ mRNA expression was increased as early as 1 h and remained elevated at 6 days, while expression levels in the ischemic hemisphere had a more delayed onset, rising at 12 h and remaining elevated at 6 days post-stroke in rats; the expression levels correlated with the infarct size [153].

IFN-γ employs the induction of adhesion molecule expression, stimulation of NADPH oxidase and activation of microglial cells and other immune cells to promote neuroinflammation [154–156]. Furthermore, IFN-γ may directly induce arteriosclerosis, increasing the risk of ischemic stroke. A study by Tellides et al. using porcine and human artery grafts transplanted into immunodeficient mice showed that arteriosclerotic changes could be induced by IFN-γ administration alone through its interaction with vascular smooth muscle cells, without the presence of immune cells [157]. IFN-γ may therefore be a chief mediator of inflammatory and thrombogenic responses in the microvasculature.

3.17. Anti-inflammatory cytokines in traumatic brain injury and ischemic stroke

The pro-inflammatory response of effector cells in the CNS to tissue injury is opposed by cytokine-induced anti-inflammatory effects that initiate repair processes and curb excessive inflammation. Some examples are provided below.

3.18. Anti-inflammatory cytokine interleukin-10

IL-10 binds to IL-10 receptors (IL-10R) which contain two receptor subunits, IL-10R- α and IL-10R-β [158]. Through activation of its receptor, IL-10 induces the JAK/STAT pathway to decrease inflammation and the PI3K/Akt pathway, to decrease apoptosis through the upregulation of anti-apoptotic factors and downregulation of caspase-3 expression [159]. Astrocytes, neurons and microglia generate IL-10 in the CNS, while lymphopoietic cells are responsible for its production outside of the CNS [160–162]. Regulatory T-cells produce IL-10 to decrease the activity of other T-cells and are involved in suppressing the immune response contributing to CNS injury [40]. IL-10 is involved in astroglial activation and microglia suppression to promote anti-inflammatory and immunosuppressive actions; microglia stimulated via TLR activation produce IL-10 and can have enhanced production in the presence of other signaling molecules like adenosine [163]. IL-10 inhibits macrophage production of NO and ROS [70] and also inhibits leukocyte adhesion to the endothelium [164]. It also decreases macrophage and lymphocyte production of IL-1, IL-6, IL-8, TNF-α, and IFN-γ [165, 166]. Furthermore, IL-10 curbs inflammatory processes such as T cell generation and MHC class II antigen upregulation [167, 168].

3.19. Anti-inflammatory IL-10 in TBI

In the context of TBI, IL-10 is demonstrably higher intrathecally and has been shown to activate the anti-inflammatory subtype of microglia (phenotypically referred to as M2 microglia) involved in matrix formation and the remodeling of tissue [169–171]. In a study examining IL-10 in TBI, Knoblach et al. administered intravenous IL-10 at 30 min prior to and 1 h after lateral fluid percussion TBI in rats. IL-10 administration improved motor function at 7 and 14 days post-injury and decreased TBI-related cortical TNF-α and IL-1 expression, as well as hippocampal IL-1 expression at 4 h post-injury [165]. In contrast, intracerebroventricularly administered IL-10 did not result in the same improvements, highlighting the systemic involvement of IL-10 on TBI pathophysiology [165]. Furthermore, the higher intracerebroventricularly administered dose trended towards a lower survival rate than the lower dose and control groups [165].

In a 21-day analysis of cytokine expression post-CCI in mice, IL-10 was modestly elevated by day one post-injury with peak expression at 3 days post-CCI [150]. A weight drop model of TBI in rats showed an acute rise of IL-10 brain levels beginning 2 h post-injury followed by a progressive rise beginning at 4 h post-TBI; mRNA expression of IL-10 peaked within minutes post-injury followed by an acute drop and rebound that progressively declined over the remaining 24 h [98]. These findings demonstrate variability in the degree of the cytokine response in relation to the mechanism of injury.

Clinically, in pediatric TBI patients, IL-10 was detectable in CSF on days 1–3 post-injury [172]. High IL-10 levels were associated with increased mortality and with children under 4 years old [172]. High serum levels of IL-10 in adult patients with severe TBI were also associated with increased mortality and a worse GCS [173]. Csuka et al. monitored CSF and plasma IL-10 levels in severe TBI patients, noting that CSF levels of IL-10 were generally higher than serum levels, with a first peak around days 0–2 post-injury followed by a smaller peak at 7–9 days post-injury with some individual patient variation; these levels did not correlate with BBB dysfunction, but correlated with different cytokines (IL-6, TNF-α) in some patients [70].

3.20. Anti-inflammatory IL-10 in AIS

In AIS, IL-10 can be released by microglia via IL-33/ST2 signaling [174]. IL-10 and IL-10R mRNA levels increase post-AIS with IL-10Rs noted on astrocytes in the infarct zone where astrocytes attempt to wall off the lesion site from viable surrounding tissue [175]. IL-10 plays an important role in neuroprotection post-stroke, as IL-10 knockout mice do not improve histologically with administration of the anti-inflammatory cytokine IL-33 post-AIS (158). Furthermore, IL-10 knockout mice have an exacerbated, delayed inflammatory response with higher mRNA levels of TNF-α, IL-1β, MMP-9, and COX-2 at day 4 post-AIS, whereas wild-type mice express high IL-10 and IL-10R levels at this time point [175]. Studies show that decreased levels of IL-10 are associated with poor stroke outcomes and that administration of IL-10 post-stroke helps to reduce poor histological and behavioral outcomes [17, 175–179]. However, IL-10 knockout mice have been shown to induce a degree of immunosuppression post-AIS with higher levels of T-cell inhibitory CTLA-4 mRNA, phagocytic macrophages, and the M2 microglia marker arginase-1 at day 4 post-stroke [175].

In a clinical study, assessing the presence of IL-10 and IL-4 in AIS in relation to clinical worsening, significantly lower concentrations of IL-10 were found in patients with neurological worsening within the first 48 h after stroke onset versus IL-4 levels which were similar in patients both with and without neurologic deterioration [180]. Lower plasma concentrations of IL-10 were only independently associated with clinical worsening in patients with subcortical or lacunar strokes [180]. Thus, IL-10 is associated with the acute neuroinflammatory response in AIS, especially in those with cerebral microvascular disease or subcortical infarcts [180].

Another clinical study assessed the relationship between stroke severity and the serum levels of IL-1β, IL-2, and IL-10 in 26 patients with AIS, analyzing neurological outcome and interleukin levels at 72 h post-AIS. In this study, patients with lower IL-10 levels deteriorated neurologically within the first 72 h. Thus, IL-10 may be involved in protective mechanisms during the acute phase of AIS [181]. However, IL-10's role in AIS and post-stroke recovery may be influenced by additional patient characteristics, such as sex. Conway et al. noted that sex may interact with IL-10 levels on stroke outcomes since female patients with higher IL-10 levels at 24 h post-stroke were noted to have a higher incidence of post-stroke urinary tract infections and poorer overall outcomes [182]. However, these levels did not independently predict outcome, suggesting the involvement of other interacting factors such as age, stroke risk, stroke severity and baseline IL-10 levels pre-stroke in addition to sex [182].

Interestingly, pre-clinically, spontaneously hypertensive rats have been shown to have lower baseline IL-10 levels and a decrease in IL-10 levels within the ischemic hemisphere at 24 h post-AIS [183]. This contrasts with the cytokine response in normal rats who have an increase in IL-10 levels at 24 h post-AIS [183]. Spontaneously hypertensive rats have generally poorer outcomes with larger infarcts and degrees of edema [184]. These findings emphasize the influence of baseline cytokine levels and stroke risk factors, such as hypertension, in dictating cytokine responses, as well as stroke severity and recovery.

3.21. Anti-inflammatory cytokine interleukin-33

IL-33, a cytokine belonging to the IL-1 family, is constitutively expressed in oligodendrocytes and astrocytes, as well as endothelial cells [185]. IL-33 undergoes activating cleavage by caspase-1 and interacts with a host of immune cells to shift the neuroinflammatory response towards neuroprotective, anti-inflammatory microglial and Th2 cell phenotypes, increasing the release of anti-inflammatory cytokines IL-4, IL-5, and IL-10, while decreasing the release of pro-inflammatory cytokines like TNF-α [186, 187]. IL-33 binds to suppression of tumorigenicity 2 (ST2) receptor, a receptor that can either be expressed on the membranes of astrocytes and microglia to increase microglia phagocytosis or as a soluble receptor [188].

3.22. Anti-inflammatory IL-33 in TBI

In a study examining the effects of IL-33 in a culture model of the CNS, incubation of cells with IL-33 resulted in microglial proliferation and triggered mRNA expression of pro-inflammatory markers TNF-α and IL-1β, as well as the anti-inflammatory cytokine IL-10 [188]. In IFN-γ stimulated microglia, IL-33 induced iNOS mRNA expression, a demonstrated neuroprotectant in TBI [189], demonstrating the interaction of various cytokines on microglia phenotype [188]. More studies need to be conducted on the role of IL-33 in TBI.

3.23. Anti-inflammatory IL-33 in AIS

In a recent study by Yang et al., mice deficient in the IL-33 transmembrane ST2 receptor had worse outcomes with a shift in the post-AIS response towards pro-inflammatory microglial behavior accompanied by larger infarcts with higher levels of neuronal cell death and poor behavioral performance at 7 days post-AIS, as well as higher mortality rates [174]. These findings showcase ST2 signaling as an important neuroprotective factor post-AIS. Under normal conditions, transmembrane ST2 receptors are primarily expressed on microglia and astrocytes. However, following AIS, ST2 receptor expression increases in these cells, as well as in macrophages and neutrophils. Post-stroke IL-33 levels increase in parallel, mainly from oligodendrocyte and astrocyte production [174].

Administration of IL-33 in in-vivo and in-vitro models of AIS is associated with improved neurologic scores, smaller infarct volumes, as well as improvements in the level of cerebral edema and neuronal survival with a shift towards protective microglia phenotypes [174, 186, 187]. IL-33's protective effects, mediated via its ST2 transmembrane receptor, are thought to be partially mediated by IL-10, as IL-33 is known to induce IL-10 production by microglia and IL-10 knockout mice did not experience the protective, infarct shrinking effects of IL-33 administration post-AIS [174]. IL-33 administration in AIS also resulted in changes in concentrations of IL-4 post-stroke. Korhonen et al. showed that decreases in lesion size with post-stroke IL-33 administration was associated with increases in IL-4 levels in the penumbra post-AIS and that these improvements diminished with the administration of anti-IL-4 antibody [186]. These observations demonstrate the interaction of IL-4 in the neuroprotective cascade induced by IL-33 [186].

Clinically, Korhonen et al. demonstrated that the soluble ST2 receptor, a decoy receptor that inhibits the actions of IL-33, was higher in the plasma of patients with poorer outcomes as measured by the modified Rankin score at 3 months post-AIS, while lower levels of this IL-33 inhibiting receptor were associated with better outcomes [186]. In agreement with these findings, serum IL-33 levels have also been found to be significantly higher in patients with AIS compared with healthy controls, with higher levels of IL-33 associated with smaller infarct volumes amongst those in the AIS group [190]. Serum IL-33 was also significantly higher in the patients with mild stroke as compared to the patients with severe stroke. Furthermore, serum IL-33 levels in AIS patients were higher in those with better functional outcomes at 3 months [190]. In a smaller study by Liu et al. serum IL-33 levels were also increased in AIS patients in comparison to controls, but IL-33 levels were noted to be positively correlated with infarction volume [191]. These findings suggest a role for IL-33 in the pathophysiology of AIS and a potential use for serum IL-33 levels for diagnostic and prognostic purposes post-stroke.

3.24. Anti-inflammatory cytokine Interleukin-4

IL-4 is generated by eosinophils, mast cells, basophils, and Th2 cells and plays a role in apoptosis, gene expression, the Th2 immune response and cell proliferation [192]. IL-4 produced by T-cells has shown involvement in the formation of memories and learning; mice lacking IL-4 as well as T-cell depleted mice have spatial memory impairments in the MWM task, reversed by transfer of IL-4 producing T-cells [193]. IL-4 knockout mice actually express higher levels of pro-inflammatory TNF-α mRNA [192]. In a cell culture experiment, astrocytic BDNF production, induced by IL-4, partially ameliorated the pro-inflammatory cytokine induced reduction in astrocytic BDNF [192]. Furthermore, IL-4 receptor complexes (type 1 and type 2) mediate IL-4 signaling through downstream JAK/STAT pathways to induce M2-like microglia, Th2 cell proliferation, and growth factor release, as well as cell growth and survival via the downstream PI3K/Akt and PKB/mTOR pathways, evidencing its neuroprotective role [194].

3.25. Anti-inflammatory IL-4 in TBI

In pre-clinical models of TBI, IL-4 gene and protein expression peaks at 24 h post-TBI in the injured hippocampus of CCI–injured rats, with a largely pro-inflammatory M1 response initiated more acutely within 2 h post-injury and peaking between 2 and 6 h post-injury [195]. IL-4 and IL-13 can activate the M2a polarization state of microglia, an anti-inflammatory microglia subtype and may be an avenue for potential therapy post-TBI [169, 171]. Clinically, in patients undergoing surgery post-severe TBI, IL-4 expression levels were increased in the first 24 h post-injury in brain tissue samples, while lower IL-4 levels were present in patients undergoing surgery on days 3–5 post-injury; in the late group, IL-4 levels were also significantly lower than IL-1β and IFN-γ levels [145].

3.26. Anti-inflammatory IL-4 in AIS

IL-4 is beneficial post-AIS via a variety of mechanisms. It increases the number of astrocytes with BDNF expression, acts on microglia to decrease their release of TNF-α, and increases anti-inflammatory M2 microglia; in conjunction with TGF-β2, IL-4 also activates these microglia [196, 197].

A preclinical study examining the effect of IL-4 on long-term recovery and microglia/macrophage polarization utilized two well-established models of stroke in wild-type and IL-4 knockout mice [198]. In this study, IL-4 deficiency worsened neuronal loss within 5 days post-stroke but had no impact on neuronal tissue loss at 14 or 21 days post-stroke, suggesting a key role for IL-4 in earlier phases of stroke pathophysiology and recovery [198]. Lack of IL-4 promoted the expression of M1 microglia and macrophage markers and dampened the expression of M2 markers at 5 and 14 days post-stroke [198]. Functionally, IL-4 knockout mice exhibited an exacerbation of stroke-induced sensorimotor deficits as early as 5 days post-stroke and impaired long-term cognitive function at 21 days post-stroke [198]. Congruently, a week-long infusion of IL-4 into the cerebral ventricles of wildtype mice post-AIS reversed the effects shown in the deficient IL-4 knockout mice, improving long-term sensorimotor and cognitive recovery [198]. Thus, IL-4 may help to improve long-term neurological outcomes after stroke through anti-inflammatory microglia phenotypes. Additionally, a clinical study by García-Berrocoso et al. demonstrated the utility of the IL-4 receptor as an early biomarker of poor post-stroke outcomes [199].

3.27. Mixed inflammatory and anti-inflammatory cytokine interleukin-6

Interleukin-6 (IL-6) is involved in neuroprotective and neuroinflammatory mechanisms. IL-6 can bind to its membrane-bound IL-6 receptor (IL-6R) or soluble IL-6 receptor (sIL-6R), both of which can induce transcription through the Janus kinase/signal transducer and activator of transcription (i.e. JAK/STAT) pathway [200–202]. The JAK/STAT pathway is crucial to NMDA receptor triggered-long term depression and could possibly support synapse elimination. Conversely, the cytokine-activated phosphatidylinositol-3-kinase/protein kinase B (i.e. PI3K/Akt) pathway, may support synapse survival through long term potentiation triggered by NMDA receptors [7, 203].

IL-6 also acts as an agonist of VEGF, which modifies tight junction proteins to disturb the integrity of the BBB and interferes with NO production [33, 200, 201]. Concurrently, IL-6 can decrease IL-1 and TNF-α synthesis in activated monocytes and may increase the production of IL-1Ra and soluble TNF receptors to decrease the influence of these largely pro-inflammatory cytokines [204, 205]. IL-6's neuroprotective effects have been shown to be mediated via the upregulation of adenosine A1 receptors on cells [206]. IL-6 also potentially aids in tissue remodeling and recovery through the initiation of astrogliosis and angiogenesis after injury [202, 207, 208].

In a hypoxic environment, such as those created by TBI or AIS, neurons undergo oxidative stress, excitotoxicity, and apoptosis [201]. IL-6 exerts a protective effect during these biochemical processes. As part of the early response to hypoxia, neutrophils, which abundantly express sIL-6R, extravasate to CNS parenchyma [202]. Damaged parenchymal cells' production of cytokines, including IL-6, facilitate leukocyte migration to the hypoxic site. IL-6 inhibits TNF-α, dampening post-injury pro-inflammatory and pro-apoptotic cascades [202]. In the late phase of the hypoxic response, IL-6 inhibits neutrophils and recruits monocytes and T-cells for the initiation of the late inflammatory response [160].

3.28. IL-6 in TBI

IL-6 is upregulated in many models of TBI and demonstrates both protective and inflammatory effects. IL-6 knockout mice show higher levels of oxidative stress, compromised activation of neuroglia, an impaired inflammatory response, diminished recruitment of lymphocytes and restricted healing and recovery rates [66, 209–215]. Corresponding to the results seen in IL-6 knockout mice, GFAP-IL-6 mice, which overexpress IL-6 in the CNS, showed faster recovery and healing after TBI [215, 216]. Transcriptome analyses of IL-6 knockout versus wildtype [217] and GFAP-IL-6 mice [218] post-TBI via cryoinjury, showed that multiple pathways involving inflammation, apoptosis and oxidative stress were affected by IL-6. For example, IL-6 knockouts had lower expression of the gene producing suppressor of cytokine signaling (SOCS), an inhibitory protein transcribed by the JAK/STAT pathway after IL-6 activation [217]. IL-6 knockouts also expressed fewer neurotrophic genes (i.e. brain-derived neurotrophic factor, early growth response 1) post-injury [217]. Injured GFAP-IL-6 mice expressed higher levels of complement component 4 and other inflammatory mediator genes in addition to lower levels of select pro-apoptotic genes and oxidative stress-related genes in comparison to injured wildtype mice [218].

In a study of post-mortem TBI cortical tissue, IL-6 levels were significantly higher in brains from patients with both short survival times of less than 17 min and late survival times ranging from 6 to 122 h post-injury [71]. In biopsies from contused brains in a study by Holmin and Höjeberg, IL-6 expression was lower than IFN-γ and IL-1 in the late patient group (biopsies taken 3–5 days post-TBI) with higher expression early, at 3–24 h post-injury [145], while a weight drop TBI rat model study by the same authors showed delayed IL-6 expression at 4–6 days post-injury [147]. In a study of TBI patients, plasma IL-6 levels were used to predict infectious complications and patient prognoses; higher IL-6 levels at 1-day post-injury predicted poorer outcomes [219]. McClain et al. observed that plasma IL-6 levels decreased more rapidly in patients with higher GCS scores on admission [220]. However, it must be stated that these correlations do not imply causality, as high IL-6 levels may not have induced poorer healing, but may have been simultaneously elevated in response to the severity of injury or pro-inflammatory response. Additional co-morbidities, such as coronary artery disease can also elevate plasma IL-6 levels, influencing detected levels post-injury [221]. The IL-6 polymorphism (-174C/G) is also associated with fatalities in severe TBI patients [222].

3.29. IL-6 in AIS

IL-6 levels rise within 7 h post-stroke in multiple experimental animal models. This is slightly delayed in comparison to the rapid rise of the pro-inflammatory cytokines, IL-1β and TNF-α [223]. Intracerebroventricular administration of IL-6 in the rat pre- and post-stroke resulted in significantly smaller lesions [224], while IL-6 knockout mice had significantly larger lesions and higher mortality when body temperature was regulated [225], supporting the protective role of IL-6 in stroke.

IL-6 has also demonstrated a role in angiogenesis post-stroke. An experiment utilizing IL-6 knockout mice showed exacerbation of lesion volumes and a reduction in angiogenesis and regional cerebral perfusion at 4 weeks post-stroke [208]. In-vitro models of ischemia after IL-6 administration, resulted in increased IL-6 mRNA expression in neurons, glial cells, and endothelial cells, as well transcription of genes associated with neovascularization [208]. However, a clinical study by Smith et al. correlated peak IL-6 levels in the first week post-AIS with worse outcomes as measured by the modified Rankin score at 3 months and larger ischemic volumes [45]. A study by Acalovschi et al. showed that the post-AIS inflammatory response due to IL-6 expression is influenced by genetic variation and that the induction of the inflammatory response by IL-6 might be enhanced by a transient downregulation of the potential IL-6 antagonist sgp130 [44].

4. Cytokine modulation as therapeutic interventions

Various agents have been used to decrease the pro-inflammatory response and augment the anti-inflammatory response post-TBI and post-AIS. Antibiotics, steroids, anesthetics, immunomodulating therapies, non-steroidal anti-inflammatory agents, as well as hormonal therapies and nutritional supplements have been shown to impact the immune response post-brain injury in pre-clinical and some clinical studies. However, findings in animal models pre-clinically do not always translate clinically. For example, cytokines have been detected in the CSF of TBI patients for up to 1 year post-injury while detected more transiently in animal models of TBI [92].

Furthermore, cytokine modulation does not always correlate with positive functional outcomes, as treatments may need to be tailored to injury severity and mechanism, patient genotype and sex, immune response time course, and particular cytokine targets, details of which may be obtained through cytokine biomarker identification and monitoring. Currently, there are no acceptable therapeutics for TBI, as management is limited to skull fracture repair, control of increased intracranial pressure and stabilization of the primary injury [10]. The only FDA-approved agent for AIS is intravenous tissue plasminogen activator (tPA) which dissolves clots up to 4.5 h post-stroke symptom onset. FDA-approved retrievable stent devices are also now recommended to physically remove clots in large vessels within an acute time window of up to 6 h post-stroke symptom onset in eligible patients [17, 226].

4.1. The antibiotic minocycline in AIS and TBI

The tetracycline antibiotic minocycline alters inflammatory cytokine production post-TBI and post-AIS, thus improving functional and histological outcomes. Bye et al. examined minocycline in a closed head injury model of TBI in mice and observed that administration of minocycline acutely decreased lesion volume and functional deficits at 1 day post-injury [227]. In a study by Yang et al. examining minocycline administration post-AIS in spontaneously hypertensive rats, infarct size and degree of tissue loss/damage in the ischemic hemispheres were reduced as seen via magnetic resonance imaging and apparent diffusion coefficient mapping at two and 4 weeks post-AIS [228]. Minocycline treatment also reduced AIS-induced levels of TNF-α and IL-1β, and increased levels of TGF-β, IL-10, anti-inflammatory M2 microglia/macrophage markers, as well as cerebral perfusion [228]. Small clinical studies of minocycline in AIS have shown a decrease in IL-6 levels at 24 h post-AIS [229] and have proven safety in AIS patients both with and without tPA administration [230]. Lampl et al. showed improvements in functional recovery as measured by the NIH stroke scale (NIHSS), modified Rankin scale (mRS) and Barthel index(BI), in patients started on 200 mg of minocycline for 5 days within 6–24 h of stroke onset [231]. Srivastava et al., utilizing the same treatment paradigm as Lampl et al., found improved mRS and BI scores at 3 months post-AIS in those treated with minocycline [232]. The same treatment paradigm was also utilized by Amiri-Nikpour et al. who reported improved NIHSS scores at 30, 60 and 90 days post-AIS in male patients receiving minocycline [233]. Kohler et al. utilized lower doses of minocycline (five 100 mg doses) and saw no improvement in NIHSS at 7 days nor in the mRS or BI at 90 days post-AIS [234].

Minocycline administration in multiple adult animal models of TBI has been shown to decrease activation of microglia, improve functional behavioral deficits such as spatial memory deficits and post-TBI anxiety [235], and decrease caspase activation and markers of neuroinflammation and damage [236]. In a study examining the use of minocycline in a blast injury model of TBI in rats, researchers noted a decrease in post-TBI anxiety via the elevated plus maze at 46 days post-injury accompanied by decreased corticosterone levels and improvements in spatial memory via Barnes maze testing post-injury as late as 47 days post-TBI [237]. Minocycline administration also decreased inflammatory and neuron and glial injury-associated markers c-reactive protein, monocyte-chemotactic protein-1, neuron-specific enolase, S100 β, tau, and neurofilament H in this study [237].

In contrast to findings in adult TBI models examining minocycline, in a neonatal model of TBI, minocycline did not improve functional deficits and actually worsened microglial activation and neurodegeneration, highlighting the influence of age on TBI pathophysiology and therapeutic selection [238]. In contrast, in a study of minocycline in neonatal ischemia, microglial activation was not affected, but lesion volume was reduced [239]. Minocycline was also shown to reduce apoptosis and excitotoxicity in neonatal hypoxic-ischemic injury in rats, suggesting a more extensive use for minocycline in ischemic pathologies [240].

To establish the use of minocycline in focal embolic stroke with comorbidities, Type 1 diabetic rats underwent embolic stroke and were given minocycline with or without tPA. It was observed that compared with treatments of saline or tPA alone, minocycline plus tPA combination therapy significantly reduced brain infarction, intracerebral hemorrhage, and hemispheric swelling at 24 h after stroke. The combination also significantly suppressed stroke-induced elevations in plasma levels of MMP-9 and IL-1β up to 24 h after stroke (57).

4.2. Biological response modifiers in TBI and AIS

IL-1R antagonists are currently being examined in AIS and TBI both pre-clinically as discussed above and clinically. A meta-analysis analyzing IL-1R antagonists in rodent models of stroke, reported an overall decrease in infarct volumes and an improvement in functional outcomes [241]. A recent cross-laboratory study of subcutaneous IL-1R antagonist treatment in AIS also found consistent decreases in neurologic deficits and lesion volume across preclinical models of AIS in multiple laboratories [121]. Pradillo et al. demonstrated that post-AIS subcutaneous administration of IL-1Ra in old rats with comorbidities and in young rats increased neurogenesis and functional outcomes in both populations [242]. IL-1R antagonists have also been proven pre-clinically to reach therapeutic levels via intranasal administration, decreasing IL-1β and TNF-α levels post-stroke in a rat model [243]. IL-1R antagonists compete with IL-1β and IL-1α for IL-1R binding, preventing downstream pro-inflammatory cascades from being activated, thus exerting a neuroprotective effect. Emsley et al. showed the safety of a recombinant human IL-1R antagonist administered post-AIS which also incidentally showed lower levels of IL-6 and peripheral inflammation, in addition to improved clinical outcomes [244]. A phase II clinical trial examining the use of subcutaneous IL-1R antagonist, anakinra, initially administered within 6 h post-stroke with repeat dosing every 12 h for a total of 6 injections over 72 h (ISRCTN74236229) has recently been completed. In TBI, as previously stated, Helmy et al. showed the safety of IL-1R antagonists, but actually reported an increase in the pro-inflammatory M1 microglia phenotype, acknowledging the variation in the immune response depending on the mechanism of injury [109]. The off-label perispinal administration of the anti-TNF-α monoclonal antibody, etanercept in post-stroke cognitive dysfunction and TBI have demonstrated benefit as well [245]. Studies by Chio et al. have demonstrated that post-TBI i.p. administration of etanercept in the fluid percussion model of brain injury in the rat improves motor deficits at 7 days and increases markers of neurogenesis [246], decreases acute TBI-induced rises in glutamate, the lactate/pyruvate ratio, and improves injury-induced motor deficits [247], cognitive deficits in the passive avoidance task [248], and the severity of ischemia at 3 days post-injury [247, 248]. A major barrier to the efficacy of etanercept as a TNF-α inhibitor for AIS and TBI is its poor BBB permeability due to its large size. Therefore, formulations of TNF decoy receptors with better BBB penetrance have been designed and tested in both TBI and AIS. Sumbria et al. show the utility of cTfRMAb-TNFR fusion protein (carboxy terminal transferrin receptor monoclonal antibody-TNF receptor), a genetically engineered monoclonal antibody against the mouse transferrin receptor found in the BBB linked to the TNF receptor to achieve whole molecule transfer into the brain, post-AIS. The administration of intravenous cTfRMAb-TNFR at 45 min post-AIS in mice resulted in significant decreases in subcortical, cortical, and hemispheric stroke volume, in addition to a 54% reduction in neurologic deficits at 24 h and 7 days post-AIS [249]. Clausen et al. examined the use of a dominant-negative inhibitor of soluble TNF called XPro1595 versus etanercept which inhibits both soluble and transmembrane TNF, in a mouse model of AIS. While infarct size was not affected, XPro1595 administration resulted in a decrease in granulocyte influx into the infarct, and improvements in motor and somatosensory function as measured by symmetrical grip strength, rotarod performance, and horizontal rod slip testing [250]. Simultaneously, the acute phase response in the liver was decreased by etanercept administration, indicating the importance of transmembrane TNF-α on the peripheral immune response [250]. TNF-α inhibitors, 3,6′ dithiothalidomide, TNF-α binding protein, and pentoxifylline have also been explored to achieve adequate TNF-α inhibition post-brain injury [69, 72, 251] and post-AIS [252–255], demonstrating improved histologic and behavioral outcomes. More recently, a third generation thalidomide, pomalidomide, was also shown to decrease neuronal cell death and curb neuroinflammation via a large decrease in TNF-α concentration, in addition to improving motor and sensory functional deficits when administered as late as 5 h post-TBI in rats [256]. Additional biologic TNF-α inhibitors, such as infliximab and adalimumab, currently approved for the treatment of inflammatory and autoimmune diseases, such as rheumatoid arthritis, may prove beneficial in AIS and TBI. B-cells have been detected in the brain post-injury due to increased BBB permeability, permitting their infiltration into the brain parenchyma, and have been shown to mediate inflammation in an animal model of stroke resulting in delayed post-stroke cognitive impairment [257]. An analog of the biologic B-cell inhibitor drug, Rituximab, has been shown to decrease B-cell infiltration across the BBB and improve post-stroke cognitive impairment when administered to mice at 5 days post-stroke with biweekly doses for 7 weeks [257].

4.3. Hormonal modulation

Hormonal intervention also impacts post-injury cytokine expression and has been examined in AIS and TBI. Pre-clinically, progesterone administration post-TBI and post-AIS has been shown to decrease edema, lesion size, excitotoxicity, apoptosis, free radical production, microglial activation and pro-inflammatory cytokines like TNF-α and IL-1β, while promoting remyelination and short-term functional preservation [258, 259]. However, these benefits have not been able to translate clinically. While the pilot phase II ProTECT trial (progesterone for traumatic brain injury, experimental clinical treatment) and a randomized controlled trial of progesterone in severe TBI in China showed improved outcomes and decreased mortality in TBI patients, the larger phase III SyNAPSe trial (study of a neuroprotective agent, progesterone in severe traumatic brain injury) and phase III PROTECT trial showed no benefit [260–263]. Progesterone has not been tested clinically in AIS patients.

4.4. Omega-3 fatty acids

Administration of omega-3 fatty acids in pre-clinical animal studies of TBI and AIS have been demonstrated to decrease post-injury neuronal death, curb increases in pro-inflammatory cytokine IL-1β and caspase-1 and functional deficits post-TBI [264]. In TBI, pre-injury administration of omega-3 fatty acids in rats' diet and via gavage resulted in decreases in neuronal cell death, edema, lesion volume, caspase-1, IL-18, IL-6 and IL-1β, as well as functional deficits in MWM and beam balance; these effects were largely mediated via G-protein coupled receptor 40 (GPR40), as blockage of this receptor reversed these benefits [264]. In patients, fish consumption has been correlated to decreased cerebrovascular disease risk, but omega-3 fatty acid supplementation alone has not been associated with decreased risk [265]. However, in a study of spontaneously hypertensive rats at increased risk for stroke, glucose utilization and cerebral perfusion were improved with omega-3 fatty acid administration [266]. A clinical trial in Japan examining statin therapy in combination with the omega-3 fatty acid, eicosapentaenoic acid, versus statin therapy alone, demonstrated a decreased incidence of recurrent stroke of 20% within 5 years [267].

4.5. N-acetylcysteine

N-acetylcysteine has been shown to have anti-inflammatory and antioxidant actions, increasing glutathione synthesis to scavenge ROS, decreasing IL-1β and TNF-α levels in brain injury, decreasing caspase-3 levels, and shifting microglia towards M2 anti-inflammatory phenotypes [268–271].

A pre-clinical experiment evaluating the modulation of oxidative stress with N-acetylcysteine and selenium treatments in TBI demonstrated that use of these treatments affected the oxidant and antioxidant, pro- and anti-inflammatory cytokines balance in rats by both down-regulating IL-1β, a pro-inflammatory cytokine, and up-regulating IL-4, an anti-inflammatory cytokine [272]. N-acetylcysteine administered 30 min post-TBI in rats resulted in improved MWM performance to near sham-injured levels [273]. When administered 60 min post-weight drop injury in mice, functional deficits in novel object recognition and Y-maze were significantly improved [273]. In combination with minocycline, N-acetylcysteine has been shown to act synergistically to reduce TBI-induced demyelination, augment M2 microglia activation in white matter and modulate TBI-induced neuroinflammation, increasing microglial activation yet decreasing the number of injury-induced phagocytic CD68+ macrophages in the corpus callosum. The combination also improves learning and long-term retention in the active place avoidance task [274]. Clinically, N-acetylcysteine has been tested in a double-blind, placebo controlled study of blast-induced mild TBI; mild TBI symptoms included balance dysfunction, headache, hearing loss, neurocognitive dysfunction and confusion. Patients receiving N-acetylcysteine within 24 h of blast injury had fewer to none of these symptoms on day 7 post-treatment with 86% of treated patients experiencing complete symptom resolution by day 7 versus 42% in those receiving placebo [275].

N-acetylcysteine has also shown efficacy in AIS. In a rat model of AIS, N-acetylcysteine administration reduced infarct volume, apoptosis, as well as TNF-α, IL-1β, and iNOS expression [276]. Functionally, rats receiving N-acetylcysteine had improved motor function [275]. Additional studies showed reduced levels of AIS-induced hippocampal cell death with N-acetylcysteine administration [277] and decreased ischemia evoked levels of Nuclear factor kappaB [271].

4.6. Cannabinoids

In a closed head injury model of TBI in rats, Dexanabinol (HU-211), a synthetic cannabinoid that inhibits TNF-α as well as NMDA receptors and free radical proliferation has been shown to reduce BBB breakdown, edema, and functional deficits [278]. Dexanabinol has also been shown to improve deficits in animal models of AIS [279]. In TBI patients, a phase II clinical trial examining the administration of i.v Dexanabinol within 6 h post-injury was observed to improve rises in intracranial pressure 2–3 days post-injury with non-significant increases in Glasgow outcome scores at 6 months in patients with more severe injuries at presentation [280]. However, in the larger phase III trial of Dexanabinol for severe TBI, no benefits were seen, indicating the need for larger sample sizes and well-defined exclusion criteria and outcome measures to detect true effects [281]. Despite the failure of Dexanabinol, other cytokine-modulating cannabinoids continue to be evaluated and show potential utility in TBI and AIS. The endocannabinoid, 2-arachidonoylglycerol, has been shown to decrease pro-inflammatory cytokine expression, decrease breakdown of the BBB and post-injury edema pre-clinically in a closed head injury model of TBI [282, 283].

5. Brain inflammation and brain injury–conclusions

This chapter has focused on the role of select cytokines in the pathophysiology of TBI and AIS. By reviewing pre-clinical and clinical studies from the TBI and AIS literature, one can identify hypotheses that have been successfully confirmed in patient populations and identify gaps in the translation of pre-clinical observations to the hospital wards. In translating concepts from preclinical studies one must be cognizant of the variability in the patient populations examined. For example, the impact of the TNF-α polymorphisms identified in Caucasians and Asians would likely impact the efficacy of TNF-α targeting treatments in these populations. Common cytokine gene polymorphisms should continue to be studied in detail to understand variations in the AIS and TBI-induced inflammatory responses in different patient groups [284]. Various mechanisms of TBI ranging from blunt injury to blast versus penetrating injury also induce distinct cytokine responses as described above. Therefore pre-clinical trials of therapeutics as well as the spatiotemporal characterization of cytokine expression should examine multiple modalities of injury and ischemic insults (embolic versus thrombotic). Effects noted consistently across multiple models of TBI and AIS are more likely to translate clinically.

The pathophysiology of AIS and TBI have significant overlap with similar cytokine roles post-injury. Using genetic knockout studies, the particular role of cytokines in these conditions has

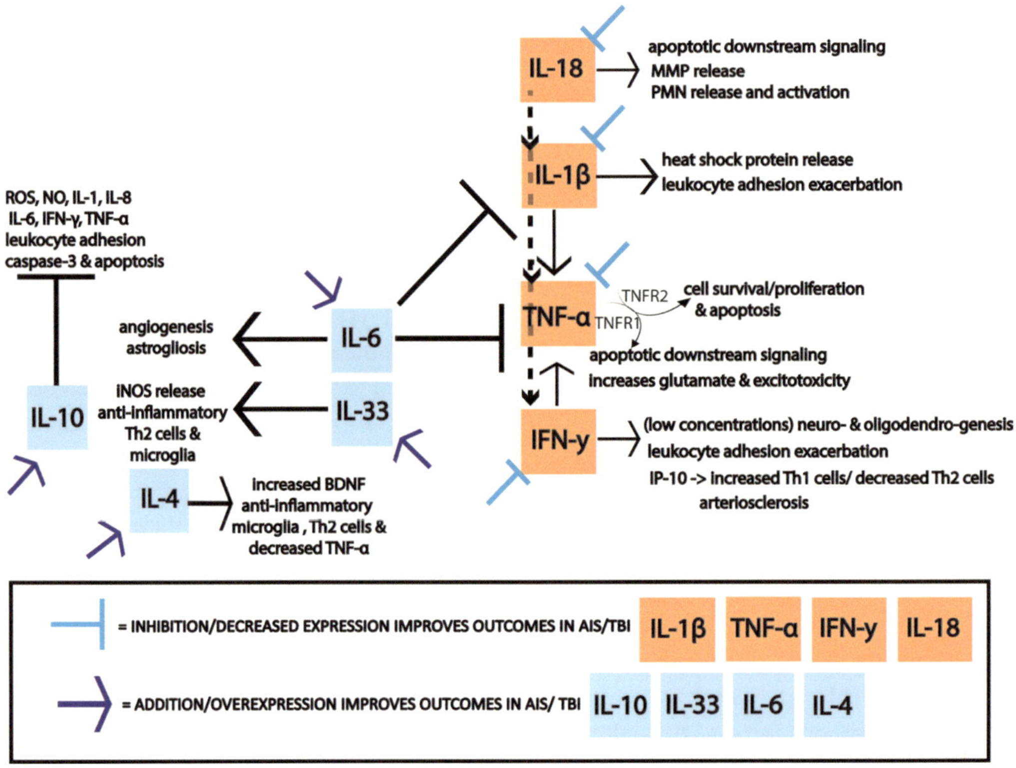

Figure 3. Summary of cytokines reviewed. Knockout or inhibition of TNF-α, IL-1β, IFN-γ, and IL-18 improved outcomes in AIS and TBI. TNF-α can induce cell survival and proliferation, but has been demonstrated to also induce apoptosis via TNFR2 and TNFR1. IFN-γ can induce neuro- and oligodendro-genesis at low concentrations, while higher concentrations cause leukocyte adhesion, arteriosclerosis, and increase the ratio of Th1:Th2 cells via upregulation of IP-10. IFN-γ, IL-18, and IL-1β promote TNF-α expression. IL-18 causes apoptosis, MMP and PMN release and activation, while IL-1β promotes heat shock protein release and leukocyte adhesion. In contrast, addition or overexpression of IL-10, IL-33, IL-6, and IL-4 improves outcomes. IL-6 decreases TNF-α and IL-1β, while promoting angiogenesis and astrogliosis. IL-33 leads to iNOS release and anti-inflammatory Th2 cells and microglia, in addition to the promotion of IL-10 and IL-4. IL-10 decreases brain injury and the cytokines IL-1, IL-8, IL-6, TNF-α, and IFN-γ, while inhibiting nitric oxide, reactive oxygen species, and leukocyte adhesion, as well as apoptosis and caspase-3. IL-4 increases BDNF, anti-inflammatory microglia, and decreases TNF-α expression. Abbreviations: BDNF, brain-derived neurotrophic factor, IP-10, interferon gamma-induced protein 10 (i.e. C-X-C motif chemokine 10), iNOS, inducible nitric oxide synthase, MMP, metalloproteinase, NO, nitric oxide, PMN, polymorphonuclear cells, Th1 cell, T-helper cell type 1, Th2 cell, T-helper cell type 2, TNFR2, TNF-α receptor 2, TNFR1, TNF-α receptor 1, ROS, reactive oxygen species.

been well defined. However, modulation of cytokine expression just prior to injury, rather than from conception is more informative to the molecule's role in AIS and TBI. Knockout or inhibition of TNF-α, IL-1β, IFN-γ, and IL-18 improved outcomes (see **Figure 3**). In contrast, addition or overexpression of IL-10, IL-33, IL-6, and IL-4 improves AIS and TBI outcomes (see **Figure 3**).

Treatments blocking pro-inflammatory and upregulating anti-inflammatory cytokines through receptor inhibition, synthesis inhibition versus induction, neutralizing antibodies, and inflammatory response modulators have shown promise. The ratio of pro-versus anti-inflammatory cytokines, as well as baseline cytokine levels may allow one to gauge the overall progression of injury in AIS and TBI to better intervene or establish prognoses. Computational modeling of cytokine patterns and interactions in AIS and TBI of different severities with or without co-morbidities or genetic predispositions may help to further predict how changing one or more variables can impact overall pathophysiology and prognosis.

Author details

Rachelle Dugue, Manan Nath, Andrew Dugue and Frank C. Barone*

*Address all correspondence to: frank.barone@downstate.edu

Departments of Neurology and Physiology & Pharmacology, SUNY Downstate Medical Center, Brooklyn, NY, USA

References

[1] Thurman DJ, Sniezek JE, Johnson D, Greenspan A, Smith SM. Guidelines for surveillance of central nervous system injury. Atlanta, GA: US Department of Health and Human Services, Public Health Service, CDC; 1995

[2] Norton R, Kobusingye O. Injuries. New England Journal of Medicine. 2013;**368**:1723-1730

[3] Corrigan JD, Selassie AW, Orman JAL. The epidemiology of traumatic brain injury. The Journal of Head Trauma Rehabilitation. 2010;**25**:72-80

[4] Olesen J, Gustavsson A, Svensson M, Wittchen H-U, Jönsson B. The economic cost of brain disorders in Europe. European Journal of Neurology. 2012;**19**:155-162

[5] Kigerl KA, de Rivero Vaccari JP, Dietrich WD, Popovich PG, Keane RW. Pattern recognition receptors and central nervous system repair. Experimental Neurology. 2014;**258**:5-16

[6] Amor S, Peferoen LA, Vogel D, Breur M, Valk P, Baker D, Noort JM. Inflammation in neurodegenerative diseases: An update. Immunology. 2014;**142**:151-166

[7] Heneka MT, Rodriguez JJ, Verkhratsky A. Neuroglia in neurodegeneration. Brain Research Reviews. 2010;**63**:189-211

[8] Dugue R, Barone FC. Ischemic, traumatic and neurodegenerative brain inflammatory changes. Future Neurology. 2016;**11**:77-96

[9] Dinarello CA. Historical insights into cytokines. European Journal of Immunology. 2007;**37**:S34-S45

[10] Werner C, Engelhard K. Pathophysiology of traumatic brain injury. British Journal of Anaesthesia. 2007;**99**:4-9

[11] Feigin VL, Forouzanfar MH, Krishnamurthi R, Mensah GA, Connor M, Bennett DA, Moran AE, Sacco RL, Anderson L, Truelsen T. Global and regional burden of stroke during 1990-2010: Findings from the Global Burden of Disease Study 2010. The Lancet. 2014;**383**:245-255

[12] Mozaffarian D, Benjamin EJ, Go AS, Arnett DK, Blaha MJ, Cushman M, Das SR, de Ferranti S, Després J-p, Fullerton HJ. Executive summary: Heart disease and stroke statistics-2016 update: A report from the American Heart Association. Circulation. 2016; **133**:447

[13] Corbyn Z. A growing global burden. Nature. 2014;**510**:S2

[14] Feigin VL, Lawes CM, Bennett DA, Anderson CS. Stroke epidemiology: A review of population-based studies of incidence, prevalence, and case-fatality in the late 20th century. The Lancet Neurology. 2003;**2**:43-53

[15] Iadecola C, Anrather J. The immunology of stroke: From mechanisms to translation. Nature Medicine. 2011;**17**:796-808

[16] Shichita T, Ito M, Morita R, Komai K, Noguchi Y, Ooboshi H, Koshida R, Takahashi S, Kodama T, Yoshimura A. MAFB prevents excess inflammation after ischemic stroke by accelerating clearance of damage signals through MSR1. Nature Medicine. 2017;**23**:723-732

[17] Deb P, Sharma S, Hassan K. Pathophysiologic mechanisms of acute ischemic stroke: An overview with emphasis on therapeutic significance beyond thrombolysis. Pathophysiology. 2010;**17**:197-218

[18] Garden D, Granger D. Pathophysiology of ischemia-reperfusion injury. The Journal of Pathology. 2000;**190**:255

[19] Swardfager W, Herrmann N, Andreazza A, Swartz R, Khan M, Black S, Lanctôt K. Poststroke neuropsychiatric symptoms: Relationships with IL-17 and oxidative stress. BioMed Research International. Article ID: 245210 2014;**2014**:1-6

[20] Swardfager W, Winer DA, Herrmann N, Winer S, Lanctôt KL. Interleukin-17 in post-stroke neurodegeneration. Neuroscience & Biobehavioral Reviews. 2013;**37**:436-447

[21] Ormstad H, Aass HCD, Amthor K-F, Lund-Sørensen N, Sandvik L. Serum cytokine and glucose levels as predictors of poststroke fatigue in acute ischemic stroke patients. Journal of Neurology. 2011;**258**:670-676

[22] Pascoe MC, Crewther SG, Carey LM, Crewther DP. Inflammation and depression: Why poststroke depression may be the norm and not the exception. International Journal of Stroke. 2011;**6**:128-135

[23] Wohleb ES, Patterson JM, Sharma V, Quan N, Godbout JP, Sheridan JF. Knockdown of interleukin-1 receptor type-1 on endothelial cells attenuated stress-induced neuroinflammation and prevented anxiety-like behavior. Journal of Neuroscience. 2014;**34**:2583-2591

[24] Spalletta G, Cravello L, Imperiale F, Salani F, Bossú P, Picchetto L, Cao M, Rasura M, Pazzelli F, Orzi F. Neuropsychiatric symptoms and interleukin-6 serum levels in acute stroke. The Journal of Neuropsychiatry and clinical Neurosciences. 2013;**25**:255-263

[25] Yang L, Zhang Z, Sun D, Xu Z, Zhang X, Li L. The serum interleukin-18 is a potential marker for development of post-stroke depression. Neurological Research. 2010;**32**:340-346

[26] Zhang J-M, An J. Cytokines, inflammation and pain. International Anesthesiology Clinics. 2007;**45**:27

[27] Ransohoff RM, Brown MA. Innate immunity in the central nervous system. The Journal of Clinical Investigation. 2012;**122**:1164-1171

[28] Turvey SE, Broide DH. Innate immunity. Journal of Allergy and Clinical Immunology. 2010;**125**:S24-S32

[29] Shastri A, Bonifati DM, Kishore U. Innate immunity and neuroinflammation. Mediators of inflammation. Article ID: 342931 2013;**2013**:1-19

[30] Ormstad H, Aass HCD, Lund-Sørensen N, Amthor K-F, Sandvik L. Serum levels of cytokines and C-reactive protein in acute ischemic stroke patients, and their relationship to stroke lateralization, type, and infarct volume. Journal of Neurology. 2011;**258**: 677-685

[31] Miller AH, Haroon E, Raison CL, Felger JC. Cytokine targets in the brain: Impact on neurotransmitters and neurocircuits. Depression and Anxiety. 2013;**30**:297-306

[32] Ghirnikar RS, Lee YL, Eng LF. Inflammation in traumatic brain injury: Role of cytokines and chemokines. Neurochemical Research. 1998;**23**:329-340

[33] Ransohoff RM, Benveniste EN. Cytokines and the CNS. Boca Raton: CRC Press, Taylor & Francis Group, 2006

[34] Orihuela R, McPherson CA, Harry GJ. Microglial M1/M2 polarization and metabolic states. British journal of Pharmacology. 2016;**173**:649-665

[35] Ransohoff RM. A polarizing question: Do M1 and M2 microglia exist? Nature Neuroscience. 2016;**19**:987-991

[36] Kingham P, Cuzner M, Pocock J. Apoptotic pathways mobilized in microglia and neurones as a consequence of chromogranin A-induced microglial activation. Journal of Neurochemistry. 1999;**73**:538-547

[37] Hernandez-Ontiveros DG, Tajiri N, Acosta S, Giunta B, Tan J, Borlongan CV. Microglia activation as a biomarker for traumatic brain injury. Frontiers in Neurology. Article:30 2013;**4**:30:1-9

[38] Skaper SD, Facci L, Giusti P. Mast cells, glia and neuroinflammation: Partners in crime? Immunology. 2014;**141**:314-327

[39] Mosser DM. The many faces of macrophage activation. Journal of Leukocyte Biology. 2003;**73**:209-212

[40] Filiano AJ, Gadani SP, Kipnis J. How and why do T cells and their derived cytokines affect the injured and healthy brain? Nature Reviews Neuroscience. 2017;**18**:375-384

[41] Fassbender K, Rossol S, Kammer T, Daffertshofer M, Wirth S, Dollman M, Hennerici M. Proinflammatory cytokines in serum of patients with acute cerebral ischemia: Kinetics of secretion and relation to the extent of brain damage and outcome of disease. Journal of the Neurological Sciences. 1994;**122**:135-139

[42] Tarkowski E, Rosengren L, Blomstrand C, Wikkelsö C, Jensen C, Ekholm S, Tarkowski A. Intrathecal release of pro- and anti-inflammatory cytokines during stroke. Clinical & Experimental Immunology. 1997;**110**:492-499

[43] Vila N, Castillo J, Dávalos A, Chamorro A. Proinflammatory cytokines and early neurological worsening in ischemic stroke. Stroke. 2000;**31**:2325-2329

[44] Acalovschi D, Wiest T, Hartmann M, Farahmi M, Mansmann U, Auffarth GU, Grau AJ, Green FR, Grond-Ginsbach C, Schwaninger M. Multiple levels of regulation of the interleukin-6 system in stroke. Stroke. 2003;**34**:1864-1869

[45] Smith CJ, Emsley HC, Gavin CM, Georgiou RF, Vail A, Barberan EM, Del Zoppo GJ, Hallenbeck JM, Rothwell NJ, Hopkins SJ. Peak plasma interleukin-6 and other peripheral markers of inflammation in the first week of ischaemic stroke correlate with brain infarct volume, stroke severity and long-term outcome. BMC Neurology. 2004;**4**:2

[46] Di Napoli M, Schwaninger M, Cappelli R, Ceccarelli E, Di Gianfilippo G, Donati C, Emsley HC, Forconi S, Hopkins SJ, Masotti L. Evaluation of C-reactive protein measurement for assessing the risk and prognosis in ischemic stroke. Stroke. 2005;**36**: 1316-1329

[47] Sotgiu S, Zanda B, Marchetti B, Fois ML, Arru G, Pes GM, Salaris F, Arru A, Pirisi A, Rosati G. Inflammatory biomarkers in blood of patients with acute brain ischemia. European Journal of Neurology. 2006;**13**:505-513

[48] Smith CJ, Emsley HC, Vail A, Georgiou RF, Rothwell NJ, Tyrrell PJ, Hopkins SJ. Variability of the systemic acute phase response after ischemic stroke. Journal of the Neurological Sciences. 2006;**251**:77-81

[49] Nagyőszi P, Nyúl-Tóth Á, Fazakas C, Wilhelm I, Kozma M, Molnár J, Haskó J, Krizbai IA Regulation of NOD-like receptors and inflammasome activation in cerebral endothelial cells. Journal of Neurochemistry. 2015;**135**:551-564

[50] Walsh JG, Muruve DA, Power C. Inflammasomes in the CNS. Nature Reviews Neuroscience. 2014;**15**:84-97

[51] Abulafia DP, de Rivero Vaccari JP, Lozano JD, Lotocki G, Keane RW, Dietrich WD. Inhibition of the inflammasome complex reduces the inflammatory response after thromboembolic stroke in mice. Journal of Cerebral Blood Flow & Metabolism. 2009;**29**:534-544

[52] de Rivero Vaccari JP, Lotocki G, Alonso OF, Bramlett HM, Dietrich WD, Keane RW. Therapeutic neutralization of the NLRP1 inflammasome reduces the innate immune response and improves histopathology after traumatic brain injury. Journal of Cerebral Blood Flow & Metabolism. 2009;**29**:1251-1261

[53] Schroder K, Tschopp J. The inflammasomes. Cell. 2010;**140**:821-832

[54] Liu H-D, Li W, Chen Z-R, Hu Y-C, Zhang D-D, Shen W, Zhou M-L, Zhu L, Hang C-H. Expression of the NLRP3 inflammasome in cerebral cortex after traumatic brain injury in a rat model. Neurochemical Research. 2013;**38**:2072-2083

[55] Ma J, Xiao W, Wang J, Wu J, Ren J, Hou J, Gu J, Fan K, Yu B. Propofol inhibits NLRP3 inflammasome and attenuates blast-induced traumatic brain injury in rats. Inflammation. 2016;**39**:2094-2103

[56] Brickler T, Gresham K, Meza A, Coutermarsh-Ott S, Williams TM, Rothschild DE, Allen IC, Theus MH. Nonessential role for the NLRP1 inflammasome complex in a murine model of traumatic brain injury. Mediators of Inflammation. Article ID: 6373506 2016;**2016**:1-11

[57] Adamczak S, Dale G, de Rivero Vaccari JP, Bullock MR, Dietrich WD, Keane RW. Inflammasome proteins in cerebrospinal fluid of brain-injured patients as biomarkers of functional outcome: Clinical article. Journal of Neurosurgery. 2012;**117**:1119-1125

[58] Fann DY-W, Lee S, Manzanero S, Tang S-C, Gelderblom M, Chunduri P, Bernreuther C, Glatzel M, Cheng Y-L, Thundyil J. Intravenous immunoglobulin suppresses NLRP1 and NLRP3 inflammasome-mediated neuronal death in ischemic stroke. Cell Death & Disease. 2013;**4**:e790

[59] Kinoshita T, Imamura R, Kushiyama H, Suda T. NLRP3 mediates NF-κB activation and cytokine induction in microbially induced and sterile inflammation. PloS One. 2015;**10**:e0119179

[60] Denes A, Coutts G, Lénárt N, Cruickshank SM, Pelegrin P, Skinner J, Rothwell N, Allan SM, Brough D. AIM2 and NLRC4 inflammasomes contribute with ASC to acute brain injury independently of NLRP3. Proceedings of the National Academy of Sciences. 2015;**112**:4050-4055

[61] Alexander JJ, Anderson AJ, Barnum SR, Stevens B, Tenner AJ. The complement cascade: Yin-Yang in neuroinflammation-neuro-protection and -degeneration. Journal of Neurochemistry. 2008;**107**:1169-1187

[62] Kalliolias GD, Ivashkiv LB. TNF biology, pathogenic mechanisms and emerging therapeutic strategies. Nature Reviews Rheumatology. 2016;**12**:49-62

[63] Depuydt B, Van Loo G, Vandenabeele P, Declercq W. Induction of apoptosis by TNF receptor 2 in a T-cell hybridoma is FADD dependent and blocked by caspase-8 inhibitors. Journal of Cell Science. 2005;**118**:497-504

[64] Smith JA, Das A, Ray SK, Banik NL. Role of pro-inflammatory cytokines released from microglia in neurodegenerative diseases. Brain Research Bulletin. 2012;**87**:10-20

[65] Ziebell JM, Morganti-Kossmann MC. Involvement of pro-and anti-inflammatory cytokines and chemokines in the pathophysiology of traumatic brain injury. Neurotherapeutics. 2010;**7**:22-30

[66] Taupin V, Toulmond S, Serrano A, Benavides J, Zavala F. Increase in IL-6, IL-1 and TNF levels in rat brain following traumatic lesion: Influence of pre-and post-traumatic treatment with Ro5 4864, a peripheral-type (p site) benzodiazepine ligand. Journal of Neuroimmunology. 1993;**42**:177-185

[67] Shohami E, Novikov M, Bass R, Yamin A, Gallily R. Closed head injury triggers early production of TNF-α and IL-6 by brain tissue. Journal of Cerebral Blood Flow & Metabolism. 1994;**14**:615-619

[68] Knoblach SM, Fan L, Faden AI. Early neuronal expression of tumor necrosis factor-α after experimental brain injury contributes to neurological impairment. Journal of Neuroimmunology. 1999;**95**:115-125

[69] Baratz R, Tweedie D, Rubovitch V, Luo W, Yoon JS, Hoffer BJ, Greig NH, Pick CG. Tumor necrosis factor-α synthesis inhibitor, 3, 6′-dithiothalidomide, reverses behavioral impairments induced by minimal traumatic brain injury in mice. Journal of Neurochemistry. 2011;**118**:1032-1042

[70] Csuka E, Morganti-Kossmann MC, Lenzlinger PM, Joller H, Trentz O, Kossmann T. IL-10 levels in cerebrospinal fluid and serum of patients with severe traumatic brain injury: Relationship to IL-6, TNF-α, TGF-β1 and blood-brain barrier function. Journal of Neuroimmunology. 1999;**101**:211-221

[71] Frugier T, Morganti-Kossmann MC, O'Reilly D, McLean CA. In situ detection of inflammatory mediators in post mortem human brain tissue after traumatic injury. Journal of Neurotrauma. 2010;**27**:497-507

[72] Shohami E, Bass R, Wallach D, Yamin A, Gallily R. Inhibition of tumor necrosis factor alpha (TNF-α) activity in rat brain is associated with cerebroprotection after closed head injury. Journal of Cerebral Blood Flow & Metabolism. 1996;**16**:378-384

[73] Scherbel U, Raghupathi R, Nakamura M, Saatman KE, Trojanowski JQ, Neugebauer E, Marino MW, McIntosh TK. Differential acute and chronic responses of tumor necrosis factor-deficient mice to experimental brain injury. Proceedings of the National Academy of Sciences. 1999;**96**:8721-8726

[74] Bachstetter AD, Rowe RK, Kaneko M, Goulding D, Lifshitz J, Van Eldik LJ. The p38α MAPK regulates microglial responsiveness to diffuse traumatic brain injury. Journal of Neuroscience. 2013;**33**:6143-6153

[75] Pavlovski D, Thundyil J, Monk PN, Wetsel RA, Taylor SM, Woodruff TM. Generation of complement component C5a by ischemic neurons promotes neuronal apoptosis. The FASEB Journal. 2012;**26**:3680-3690

[76] Van Beek J, Bernaudin M, Petit E, Gasque P, Nouvelot A, MacKenzie ET, Fontaine M. Expression of receptors for complement anaphylatoxins C3a and C5a following permanent focal cerebral ischemia in the mouse. Experimental Neurology. 2000;**161**:373-382

[77] Stahel PF, Kariya K, Shohami E, Barnum SR, Eugster H-P, Trentz O, Kossmann T, Morganti-Kossmann MC. Intracerebral complement C5a receptor (CD88) expression is regulated by TNF and lymphotoxin-α following closed head injury in mice. Journal of Neuroimmunology. 2000;**109**:164-172

[78] Sairanen T, Carpén O, Karjalainen-Lindsberg M-L, Paetau A, Turpeinen U, Kaste M, Lindsberg PJ. Evolution of cerebral tumor necrosis factor-α production during human ischemic stroke. Stroke. 2001;**32**:1750-1758

[79] Montaner J, Rovira A, Molina CA, Arenillas JF, Ribó M, Chacón P, Monasterio J, Alvarez-Sabín J. Plasmatic level of neuroinflammatory markers predict the extent of diffusion-weighted image lesions in hyperacute stroke. Journal of Cerebral Blood Flow & Metabolism. 2003;**23**:1403-1407

[80] D'Mello C, Le T, Swain MG. Cerebral microglia recruit monocytes into the brain in response to tumor necrosis factor-α signaling during peripheral organ inflammation. Journal of Neuroscience. 2009;**29**:2089-2102

[81] Carvalho-Tavares J, Hickey MJ, Hutchison J, Michaud J, Sutcliffe IT, Kubes P. A role for platelets and endothelial selectins in tumor necrosis factor-α-induced leukocyte recruitment in the brain microvasculature. Circulation Research. 2000;**87**:1141-1148

[82] Santello M, Bezzi P, Volterra A. TNFα controls glutamatergic gliotransmission in the hippocampal dentate gyrus. Neuron. 2011;**69**:988-1001

[83] Botchkina G, Meistrell 3rd M, Botchkina I, Tracey K. Expression of TNF and TNF receptors (p55 and p75) in the rat brain after focal cerebral ischemia. Molecular Medicine. 1997;**3**:765

[84] Rosenberg GA, Cunningham LA, Wallace J, Alexander S, Estrada EY, Grossetete M, Razhagi A, Miller K, Gearing A. Immunohistochemistry of matrix metalloproteinases in reperfusion injury to rat brain: Activation of MMP-9 linked to stromelysin-1 and microglia in cell cultures. Brain Research. 2001;**893**:104-112

[85] Seo JH, Miyamoto N, Hayakawa K, Pham L-DD, Maki T, Ayata C, Kim K-W, Lo EH, Arai K. Oligodendrocyte precursors induce early blood-brain barrier opening after white matter injury. The Journal of Clinical Investigation. 2013;**123**(2):782-786

[86] Hosomi N, Ban CR, Naya T, Takahashi T, Guo P, Song XR, Kohno M. Tumor necrosis factor-α neutralization reduced cerebral edema through inhibition of matrix metalloproteinase production after transient focal cerebral ischemia. Journal of Cerebral Blood Flow & Metabolism. 2005;**25**:959-967

[87] Pettigrew LC, Kindy MS, Scheff S, Springer JE, Kryscio RJ, Li Y, Grass DS. Focal cerebral ischemia in the TNFalpha-transgenic rat. Journal of Neuroinflammation. 2008;**5**:47

[88] Barone F, Arvin B, White R, Miller A, Webb C, Willette R, Lysko P, Feuerstein G. Tumor necrosis factor-α. Stroke. 1997;**28**:1233-1244

[89] Nawashiro H, Martin D, Hallenbeck JM. Neuroprotective effects of TNF binding protein in focal cerebral ischemia. Brain Research. 1997;**778**:265-271

[90] Pan W, Ding Y, Yu Y, Ohtaki H, Nakamachi T, Kastin AJ. Stroke upregulates TNFα transport across the blood-brain barrier. Experimental Neurology. 2006;**198**:222-233

[91] Um J-Y, An N-H, Kim H-M. TNF-α and TNF-β gene polymorphisms in cerebral infarction. Journal of Molecular Neuroscience. 2003;**21**:167-171

[92] Kumar P, Misra S, Kumar A, Pandit AK, Chakravarty K, Prasad K. Association between tumor necrosis factor-α (-238G/A and-308G/A) gene polymorphisms and risk of ischemic stroke: A meta-analysis. Pulse. 2015;**3**:217-228

[93] Waters RJ, Murray GD, Teasdale GM, Stewart J, Day I, Lee RJ, Nicoll JA. Cytokine gene polymorphisms and outcome after traumatic brain injury. Journal of Neurotrauma. 2013;**30**:1710-1716

[94] Allan SM, Tyrrell PJ, Rothwell NJ. Interleukin-1 and neuronal injury. Nature Reviews Immunology. 2005;**5**:629

[95] Dinarello CA. Biologic basis for interleukin-1 in disease. Blood. 1996;**87**:2095-2147

[96] Swaroop S, Sengupta N, Suryawanshi AR, Adlakha YK, Basu A. HSP60 plays a regulatory role in IL-1β-induced microglial inflammation via TLR4-p38 MAPK axis. Journal of Neuroinflammation. 2016;**13**:27

[97] Rooker S, Jander S, Reempts JV, Stoll G, Jorens PG, Borgers M, Verlooy J. Spatiotemporal pattern of neuroinflammation after impact-acceleration closed head injury in the rat. Mediators of Inflammation. Article ID:90123 2006;**2006**: 1-6

[98] Kamm K, VanderKolk W, Lawrence C, Jonker M, Davis AT. The effect of traumatic brain injury upon the concentration and expression of interleukin-1β and interleukin-10 in the rat. Journal of Trauma and Acute Care Surgery. 2006;**60**:152-157

[99] Knoblach SM, Faden AI. Cortical interleukin-1β elevation after traumatic brain injury in the rat: No effect of two selective antagonists on motor recovery. Neuroscience Letters. 2000;**289**:5-8

[100] Fan L, Young PR, Barone FC, Feuerstein GZ, Smith DH, McIntosh TK. Experimental brain injury induces expression of interleukin-1β mRNA in the rat brain. Molecular Brain Research. 1995;**30**:125-130

[101] Lu K-T, Wang Y-W, Yang J-T, Yang Y-L, Chen H-I. Effect of interleukin-1 on traumatic brain injury-induced damage to hippocampal neurons. Journal of Neurotrauma. 2005;**22**:885-895

[102] Lawrence CB, Allan SM, Rothwell NJ. Interleukin-1β and the interleukin-1 receptor antagonist act in the striatum to modify excitotoxic brain damage in the rat. European Journal of Neuroscience. 1998;**10**:1188-1195

[103] Yang G-Y, Zhao Y-J, Davidson BL, Betz AL. Overexpression of interleukin-1 receptor antagonist in the mouse brain reduces ischemic brain injury. Brain Research. 1997;**751**:181-188

[104] Tehranian R, Andell-Jonsson S, Beni SM, Yatsiv I, Shohami E, Bartfai T, Lundkvist J, Iverfeldt K. Improved recovery and delayed cytokine induction after closed head injury in mice with central overexpression of the secreted isoform of the interleukin-1 receptor antagonist. Journal of Neurotrauma. 2002;**19**:939-951

[105] Toulmond S, Rothwell N. Interleukin-1 receptor antagonist inhibits neuronal damage caused by fluid percussion injury in the rat. Brain Research. 1995;**671**:261-266

[106] Clausen F, Hånell A, Israelsson C, Hedin J, Ebendal T, Mir AK, Gram H, Marklund N. Neutralization of interleukin-1β reduces cerebral edema and tissue loss and improves late cognitive outcome following traumatic brain injury in mice. European Journal of Neuroscience. 2011;**34**:110-123

[107] Clausen F, Hånell A, Björk M, Hillered L, Mir AK, Gram H, Marklund N. Neutralization of interleukin-1β modifies the inflammatory response and improves histological and cognitive outcome following traumatic brain injury in mice. European Journal of Neuroscience. 2009;**30**:385-396

[108] Ekmark-Lewén S, Flygt J, Fridgeirsdottir GA, Kiwanuka O, Hånell A, Meyerson BJ, Mir AK, Gram H, Lewén A, Clausen F. Diffuse traumatic axonal injury in mice induces complex behavioural alterations that are normalized by neutralization of interleukin-1β. European Journal of Neuroscience. 2016;**43**:1016-1033

[109] Helmy A, Guilfoyle MR, Carpenter KL, Pickard JD, Menon DK, Hutchinson PJ. Recombinant human interleukin-1 receptor antagonist promotes M1 microglia biased cytokines and chemokines following human traumatic brain injury. Journal of Cerebral Blood Flow & Metabolism. 2016;**36**:1434-1448

[110] Helmy A, Guilfoyle MR, Carpenter KL, Pickard JD, Menon DK, Hutchinson PJ. Recombinant human interleukin-1 receptor antagonist in severe traumatic brain injury: A phase II randomized control trial. Journal of Cerebral Blood Flow & Metabolism. 2014;**34**:845-851

[111] Helmy A, Carpenter KL, Menon DK, Pickard JD, Hutchinson PJ. The cytokine response to human traumatic brain injury: Temporal profiles and evidence for cerebral parenchymal production. Journal of Cerebral Blood Flow & Metabolism. 2011;**31**:658-670

[112] Rothwell NJ, Luheshi G, Toulmond S. Cytokines and their receptors in the central nervous system: Physiology, pharmacology, and pathology. Pharmacology & Therapeutics. 1996;**69**:85-95

[113] Cunningham A, Murray C, O'Neill L, Lynch M, O'Connor J. Interleukin-1β(IL-1β) and tumour necrosis factor (TNF) inhibit long-term potentiation in the rat dentate gyrus in vitro. Neuroscience Letters. 1996;**203**:17-20

[114] Rothwell N, Allan S, Toulmond S. The role of interleukin 1 in acute neurodegeneration and stroke: Pathophysiological and therapeutic implications. Journal of Clinical Investigation. 1997;**100**:2648

[115] Park MJ, Sohrabji F. The histone deacetylase inhibitor, sodium butyrate, exhibits neuroprotective effects for ischemic stroke in middle-aged female rats. Journal of Neuroinflammation. 2016;**13**:300

[116] Pearson VL, Rothwell NJ, Toulmond S. Excitotoxic brain damage in the rat induces interleukin-1β protein in microglia and astrocytes: Correlation with the progression of cell death. Glia. 1999;**25**:311-323

[117] Boxer PA, Bigge CF. Mechanisms of neuronal cell injury/death and targets for drug intervention. Drug Discovery Today. 1997;**2**:219-228

[118] Allan S, Lawrence C, Rothwell N. Interleukin-1β and interleukin-1 receptor antagonist do not affect glutamate release or calcium entry in rat striatal synaptosomes. Molecular Psychiatry. 1998;**3**:178-182

[119] Clausen BH, Lambertsen KL, Babcock AA, Holm TH, Dagnaes-Hansen F, Finsen B. Interleukin-1beta and tumor necrosis factor-alpha are expressed by different subsets of microglia and macrophages after ischemic stroke in mice. Journal of Neuroinflammation. 2008;**5**:46

[120] Shreeniwas R, Koga S, Karakurum M, Pinsky D, Kaiser E, Brett J, Wolitzky B, Norton C, Plocinski J, Benjamin W. Hypoxia-mediated induction of endothelial cell interleukin-1 alpha. An autocrine mechanism promoting expression of leukocyte adhesion molecules on the vessel surface. Journal of Clinical Investigation. 1992;**90**:2333

[121] Maysami S, Wong R, Pradillo JM, Denes A, Dhungana H, Malm T, Koistinaho J, Orset C, Rahman M, Rubio M. A cross-laboratory preclinical study on the effectiveness of interleukin-1 receptor antagonist in stroke. Journal of Cerebral Blood Flow & Metabolism. 2016;**36**:596-605

[122] Relton JK, Rothwell NJ. Interleukin-1 receptor antagonist inhibits ischaemic and excitotoxic neuronal damage in the rat. Brain Research Bulletin. 1992;**29**:243-246

[123] Hara H, Friedlander RM, Gagliardini V, Ayata C, Fink K, Huang Z, Shimizu-Sasamata M, Yuan J, Moskowitz MA. Inhibition of interleukin 1β converting enzyme family proteases reduces ischemic and excitotoxic neuronal damage. Proceedings of the National Academy of Sciences. 1997;**94**:2007-2012

[124] Loddick SA, MacKenzie A, Rothwell NJ. An ICE inhibitor, z VAD DCB attenuates isch aemic brain damage in the rat. Neuroreport. 1996;7:1465-1468

[125] Friedlander RM, Gagliardini V, Hara H, Fink KB, Li W, MacDonald G, Fishman MC, Greenberg AH, Moskowitz MA, Yuan J. Expression of a dominant negative mutant of interleukin-1β converting enzyme in transgenic mice prevents neuronal cell death induced by trophic factor withdrawal and ischemic brain injury. Journal of Experimental Medicine. 1997;**185**:933-940

[126] Lin R, Cai J, Kostuk EW, Rosenwasser R, Iacovitti L. Fumarate modulates the immune/inflammatory response and rescues nerve cells and neurological function after stroke in rats. Journal of Neuroinflammation. 2016;**13**:269

[127] Sheu J-R, Chen Z-C, Jayakumar T, Chou D-S, Yen T-L, Lee H-N, Pan S-H, Hsia C-H, Yang C-H, Hsieh C-Y. A novel indication of platonin, a therapeutic immunomodulating medicine, on neuroprotection against ischemic stroke in mice. Scientific Reports. Article:42277 2017;**7**:1-14

[128] Kostulas N, Pelidou SH, Kivisäkk P, Kostulas V, Link H. Increased IL-1β, IL-8, and IL-17 mRNA expression in blood mononuclear cells observed in a prospective ischemic stroke study. Stroke. 1999;**30**:2174-2179

[129] Beamer NB, Coull BM, Clark WM, Hazel JS, Silberger JR. Interleukin-6 and interleukin-1 receptor antagonist in acute stroke. Annals of Neurology. 1995;**37**:800-805

[130] Tarkowski E, Rosengren L, Blomstrand C, Wikkelsö C, Jensen C, Ekholm S, Tarkowski A. Early intrathecal production of interleukin-6 predicts the size of brain lesion in stroke. Stroke. 1995;**26**:1393-1398

[131] Dinarello C, Novick D, Kim S, Kaplanski G. Interleukin-18 and IL-18 binding protein. Frontiers in Immunology. Article: 289 2013;**4**:1-10

[132] Cumiskey D, Pickering M, O'Connor JJ. Interleukin-18 mediated inhibition of LTP in the rat dentate gyrus is attenuated in the presence of mGluR antagonists. Neuroscience Letters. 2007;**412**:206-210

[133] Yatsiv I, Morganti-Kossmann MC, Perez D, Dinarello CA, Novick D, Rubinstein M, Otto VI, Rancan M, Kossmann T, Redaelli CA. Elevated intracranial IL-18 in humans and mice after traumatic brain injury and evidence of neuroprotective effects of IL-18-binding protein after experimental closed head injury. Journal of Cerebral Blood Flow & Metabolism. 2002;**22**:971-978

[134] Ciaramella A, Della Vedova C, Salani F, Viganotti M, D'Ippolito M, Caltagirone C, Formisano R, Sabatini U, Bossu P. Increased levels of serum IL-18 are associated with the long-term outcome of severe traumatic brain injury. Neuroimmunomodulation. 2014;**21**:8-12

[135] Sun C, He W, Xu X, Yuhui J, Wang G, Zhang J. Serum level of IL-1 beta and IL-18 in patients with traumatic brain injury and their effects on cognitive impairment. International Journal of Clinical and Experimental Pathology. 2016;**9**:1975-1981

[136] Jander S, Schroeter M, Stoll G. Interleukin-18 expression after focal ischemia of the rat brain: Association with the late-stage inflammatory response. Journal of Cerebral Blood Flow & Metabolism. 2002;**22**:62-70

[137] Braeuninger S, Kleinschnitz C, Stoll G. Interleukin-18 does not influence infarct volume or functional outcome in the early stage after transient focal brain ischemia in mice. Experimental & translational stroke medicine. 2010;**2**:1

[138] Wheeler RD, Boutin H, Touzani O, Luheshi GN, Takeda K, Rothwell NJ. No role for interleukin-18 in acute murine stroke-induced brain injury. Journal of Cerebral Blood Flow & Metabolism. 2003;**23**:531-535

[139] Mallat Z, Corbaz A, Scoazec A, Besnard S, Lesèche G, Chvatchko Y, Tedgui A. Expression of interleukin-18 in human atherosclerotic plaques and relation to plaque instability. Circulation. 2001;**104**:1598-1603

[140] Yuen C-M, Chiu C-A, Chang L-T, Liou C-W, Lu C-H, Youssef AA, Yip H-K. Level and value of interleukin-18 after acute ischemic stroke. Circulation Journal. 2007;**71**:1691-1696

[141] Welsh P, Lowe GD, Chalmers J, Campbell DJ, Rumley A, Neal BC, MacMahon SW, Woodward M. Associations of proinflammatory cytokines with the risk of recurrent stroke. Stroke. 2008;**39**:2226-2230

[142] Rosenman SJ, Shrikant P, Dubb L, Benveniste EN, Ransohoff RM. Cytokine-induced expression of vascular cell adhesion molecule-1 (VCAM-1) by astrocytes and astrocytoma cell lines. The Journal of Immunology. 1995;**154**:1888-1899

[143] Shaked I, Tchoresh D, Gersner R, Meiri G, Mordechai S, Xiao X, Hart R, Schwartz M. Protective autoimmunity: Interferon-γ enables microglia to remove glutamate without evoking inflammatory mediators. Journal of Neurochemistry. 2005;**92**:997-1009

[144] Kawanokuchi J, Mizuno T, Takeuchi H, Kato H, Wang J, Mitsuma N, Suzumura A. Production of interferon-y by microglia. Multiple Sclerosis Journal. 2006;**12**:558-564

[145] Holmin S, Höjeberg B. In situ detection of intracerebral cytokine expression after human brain contusion. Neuroscience Letters. 2004;**369**:108-114

[146] Yan EB, Satgunaseelan L, Paul E, Bye N, Nguyen P, Agyapomaa D, Kossmann T, Rosenfeld JV, Morganti-Kossmann MC. Post-traumatic hypoxia is associated with prolonged cerebral cytokine production, higher serum biomarker levels, and poor outcome in patients with severe traumatic brain injury. Journal of Neurotrauma. 2014;**31**:618-629

[147] Holmin S, Schalling M, Höjeberg B, Sandberg Nordqvist A-C, Skeftruna A-K, Mathiesen T. Delayed cytokine expression in rat brain following experimental contusion. Journal of Neurosurgery. 1997;**86**:493-504

[148] Wei HH, Lu X-CM, Shear DA, Waghray A, Yao C, Tortella FC, Dave JR. NNZ-2566 treatment inhibits neuroinflammation and pro-inflammatory cytokine expression induced by experimental penetrating ballistic-like brain injury in rats. Journal of Neuroinflammation. 2009;**6**:19

[149] Williams AJ, Wei HH, Dave JR, Tortella FC. Acute and delayed neuroinflammatory response following experimental penetrating ballistic brain injury in the rat. Journal of Neuroinflammation. 2007;**4**:17

[150] Lagraoui M, Latoche JR, Cartwright NG, Sukumar G, Dalgard CL, Schaefer BC. Controlled cortical impact and craniotomy induce strikingly similar profiles of inflammatory gene expression, but with distinct kinetics. Frontiers in Neurology. Article: 155 2012;**3**:1-14

[151] Tomimoto H, Akiguchi I, Wakita H, Kinoshita A, Ikemoto A, Nakamura S, Kimura J. Glial expression of cytokines in the brains of cerebrovascular disease patients. Acta Neuropathologica. 1996;**92**:281-287

[152] Yilmaz G, Arumugam TV, Stokes KY, Granger DN. Role of T lymphocytes and interferon-γ in ischemic stroke. Circulation. 2006;**113**:2105-2112

[153] Li H-L, Kostulas N, Huang Y-M, Xiao B-G, van der Meide P, Kostulas V, Giedraitas V, Link H. IL-17 and IFN-γ mRNA expression is increased in the brain and systemically after permanent middle cerebral artery occlusion in the rat. Journal of Neuroimmunology. 2001;**116**:5-14

[154] Chung HK, Lee IK, Kang H, Suh JM, Kim H, Park KC, Kim DW, Kim YK, Ro HK, Shong M. Statin inhibits interferon-[gamma]-induced expression of intercellular adhesion molecule-1 (ICAM-1) in vascular endothelial and smooth muscle cells. Experimental & Molecular Medicine. 2002;**34**:451

[155] Pawate S, Shen Q, Fan F, Bhat NR. Redox regulation of glial inflammatory response to lipopolysaccharide and interferonγ. Journal of Neuroscience Research. 2004;**77**:540-551

[156] Stokes KY, Clanton EC, Clements KP, Granger DN. Role of interferon-γ in hypercholesterolemia-induced leukocyte- endothelial cell adhesion. Circulation. 2003;**107**:2140-2145

[157] Tellides G, Tereb DA, Kirkiles-Smith NC, Kim RW. Interferon-gamma elicits arteriosclerosis in the absence of leukocytes. Nature. 2000;**403**:207

[158] Sabat R, Grütz G, Warszawska K, Kirsch S, Witte E, Wolk K, Geginat J. Biology of interleukin-10. Cytokine & Growth Factor Reviews. 2010;**21**:331-344

[159] Moore KW, de Waal Malefyt R, Coffman RL, O'Garra A. Interleukin-10 and the interleukin-10 receptor. Annual Review of Immunology. 2001;**19**:683-765

[160] Aloisi F, Simone RD, Columba-Cabezas S, Levi G. Opposite effects of interferon-γ and prostaglandin E2 on tumor necrosis factor and interleukin-10 production in microglia: A regulatory loop controlling microglia pro- and anti-inflammatory activities. Journal of Neuroscience Research. 1999;**56**:571-580

[161] Mesples B, Plaisant F, Gressens P. Effects of interleukin-10 on neonatal excitotoxic brain lesions in mice. Developmental Brain Research. 2003;**141**:25-32

[162] Wu Z, Zhang J, Nakanishi H. Leptomeningeal cells activate microglia and astrocytes to induce IL-10 production by releasing pro-inflammatory cytokines during systemic inflammation. Journal of Neuroimmunology. 2005;**167**:90-98

[163] Koscsó B, Csóka B, Selmeczy Z, Himer L, Pacher P, Virág L, Haskó G. Adenosine augments IL-10 production by microglial cells through an A2B adenosine receptor-mediated process. The Journal of Immunology. 2012;**188**:445-453

[164] Jungi TW, Brcic M, Eperon S, Albrecht S. Transforming growth factor-beta and interleukin-10, but not interleukin-4, down-regulate procoagulant activity and tissue factor expression in human monocyte-derived macrophages. Thrombosis Research. 1994;**76**:463-474

[165] Knoblach SM, Faden AI. Interleukin-10 improves outcome and alters proinflammatory cytokine expression after experimental traumatic brain injury. Experimental Neurology. 1998;**153**:143-151

[166] Kremlev SG, Palmer C. Interleukin-10 inhibits endotoxin-induced pro-inflammatory cytokines in microglial cell cultures. Journal of Neuroimmunology. 2005;**162**:71-80

[167] de Waal Malefyt R, Abrams J, Bennett B, Figdor CG, De Vries JE. Interleukin 10 (IL-10) inhibits cytokine synthesis by human monocytes: An autoregulatory role of IL-10 produced by monocytes. Journal of Experimental Medicine. 1991;**174**:1209-1220

[168] Mizuno T, Sawada M, Marunouchi T, Suzumura A. Production of interleukin-10 by mouse glial cells in culture. Biochemical and Biophysical Research Communications. 1994;**205**:1907-1915

[169] Bell-Temin H, Culver-Cochran AE, Chaput D, Carlson CM, Kuehl M, Burkhardt BR, Bickford PC, Liu B, Stevens SM. Novel molecular insights into classical and alternative activation states of microglia as revealed by stable isotope labeling by amino acids in cell culture (SILAC)-based proteomics. Molecular & Cellular Proteomics. 2015;**14**: 3173-3184

[170] Colton CA. Heterogeneity of microglial activation in the innate immune response in the brain. Journal of Neuroimmune Pharmacology. 2009;**4**:399-418

[171] Xu H, Wang Z, Li J, Wu H, Peng Y, Fan L, Chen J, Gu C, Yan F, Wang L. The polarization states of microglia in TBI: A new paradigm for pharmacological intervention. Neural Plasticity. Article ID: 5405104 2017;**2017**:1-11

[172] Bell MJ, Kochanek PM, Doughty LA, Carcillo JA, Adelson PD, Clark RS, Wisniewski SR, Whalen MJ, Dekosky ST. Interleukin-6 and interleukin-10 in cerebrospinal fluid after severe traumatic brain injury in children. Journal of Neurotrauma. 1997;**14**: 451-457

[173] Schneider Soares FM, Menezes de Souza N, Libório Schwarzbold M, Paim Diaz A, Costa Nunes J, Hohl A, Nunes Abreu da Silva P, Vieira J, Lisboa de Souza R, Moré Bertotti M, et al. Interleukin-10 is an independent biomarker of severe traumatic brain injury prognosis. Neuroimmunomodulation. 2012;**19**:377-385

[174] Yang Y, Liu H, Zhang H, Ye Q, Wang J, Yang B, Mao L, Zhu W, Leak RK, Xiao B. ST2/IL-33-dependent microglial response limits acute ischemic brain injury. Journal of Neuroscience. 2017:3233-3216

[175] Pérez-de Puig I, Miró F, Salas-Perdomo A, Bonfill-Teixidor E, Ferrer-Ferrer M, Márquez-Kisinousky L, Planas AM. IL-10 deficiency exacerbates the brain inflammatory response to permanent ischemia without preventing resolution of the lesion. Journal of Cerebral Blood Flow & Metabolism. 2013;**33**:1955-1966

[176] Allaman I, Belanger M, Magistretti PJ. Astrocyte-neuron metabolic relationships: For better and for worse. Trends in Neurosciences. 2011;**34**:76-87

[177] Shichita T, Ago T, Kamouchi M, Kitazono T, Yoshimura A, Ooboshi H. Novel therapeutic strategies targeting innate immune responses and early inflammation after stroke. Journal of Neurochemistry. 2012;**123**:29-38

[178] Bonifati DM, Kishore U. Role of complement in neurodegeneration and neuroinflammation. Molecular Immunology. 2007;**44**:999-1010

[179] Spera PA, Ellison JA, Feuerstein GZ, Barone FC. IL-10 reduces rat brain injury following focal stroke. Neuroscience Letters. 1998;**251**:189-192

[180] Vila N, Castillo J, Dávalos A, Esteve A, Planas AM, Chamorro Á. Levels of anti-inflammatory cytokines and neurological worsening in acute ischemic stroke. Stroke. 2003;**34**:671-675

[181] Protti GG, Gagliardi RJ, Forte WC, Sprovieri SRS. Interleukin-10 may protect against progressing injury during the acute phase of ischemic stroke. Arquivos de neuro-psiquiatria. 2013;**71**:846-851

[182] Conway SE, Roy-O'Reilly M, Friedler B, Staff I, Fortunato G, McCullough LD. Sex differences and the role of IL-10 in ischemic stroke recovery. Biology of Sex Differences. 2015;**6**:17

[183] Fouda AY, Kozak A, Alhusban A, Switzer JA, Fagan SC. Anti-inflammatory IL-10 is upregulated in both hemispheres after experimental ischemic stroke: Hypertension blunts the response. Experimental & Translational Stroke Medicine. 2013;**5**:12

[184] Barone F, Price W, White R, Willette R, Feuerstein G. Genetic hypertension and increased susceptibility to cerebral ischemia. Neuroscience & Biobehavioral Reviews. 1992;**16**:219-233

[185] Gadani SP, Walsh JT, Smirnov I, Zheng J, Kipnis J. The glia-derived alarmin IL-33 orchestrates the immune response and promotes recovery following CNS injury. Neuron. 2015;**85**:703-709

[186] Korhonen P, Kanninen KM, Lehtonen Š, Lemarchant S, Puttonen KA, Oksanen M, Dhungana H, Loppi S, Pollari E, Wojciechowski S. Immunomodulation by interleukin-33 is protective in stroke through modulation of inflammation. Brain, Behavior, and Immunity. 2015;**49**:322-336

[187] Luo Y, Zhou Y, Xiao W, Liang Z, Dai J, Weng X, Wu X. Interleukin-33 ameliorates ischemic brain injury in experimental stroke through promoting Th2 response and suppressing Th17 response. Brain Research. 2015;**1597**:86-94

[188] Yasuoka S, Kawanokuchi J, Parajuli B, Jin S, Doi Y, Noda M, Sonobe Y, Takeuchi H, Mizuno T, Suzumura A. Production and functions of IL-33 in the central nervous system. Brain Research. 2011;**1385**:8-17

[189] Sinz EH, Kochanek PM, Dixon CE, Clark RS, Carcillo JA, Schiding JK, Chen M, Wisniewski SR, Carlos TM, Williams D. Inducible nitric oxide synthase is an endogenous neuroprotectant after traumatic brain injury in rats and mice. The Journal of Clinical Investigation. 1999;**104**:647-656

[190] Qian L, Yuanshao L, Wensi H, Yulei Z, Xiaoli C, Brian W, Wanli Z, Zhengyi C, Jie X, Wenhui Z. Serum IL-33 is a novel diagnostic and prognostic biomarker in acute ischemic stroke. Aging and Disease. 2016;**7**:614

[191] Liu J, Xing Y, Gao Y, Zhou C. Changes in serum interleukin-33 levels in patients with acute cerebral infarction. Journal of Clinical Neuroscience. 2014;**21**:298-300

[192] Luzina IG, Keegan AD, Heller NM, Rook GA, Shea-Donohue T, Atamas SP. Regulation of inflammation by interleukin-4: A review of "alternatives". Journal of Leukocyte Biology. 2012;**92**:753-764

[193] Derecki NC, Cardani AN, Yang CH, Quinnies KM, Crihfield A, Lynch KR, Kipnis J. Regulation of learning and memory by meningeal immunity: A key role for IL-4. Journal of Experimental Medicine. 2010;**207**:1067-1080

[194] Gadani SP, Cronk JC, Norris GT, Kipnis J. IL-4 in the brain: A cytokine to remember. The Journal of Immunology. 2012;**189**:4213-4219

[195] Ansari MA. Temporal profile of M1 and M2 responses in the hippocampus following early 24h of neurotrauma. Journal of the Neurological Sciences. 2015;**357**:41-49

[196] Butovsky O, Ziv Y, Schwartz A, Landa G, Talpalar AE, Pluchino S, Martino G, Schwartz M. Microglia activated by IL-4 or IFN-γ differentially induce neurogenesis and oligodendrogenesis from adult stem/progenitor cells. Molecular and Cellular Neuroscience. 2006;**31**:149-160

[197] Zhou X, Spittau B, Krieglstein K. TGFβ signalling plays an important role in IL4-induced alternative activation of microglia. Journal of Neuroinflammation. 2012;**9**:210

[198] Liu X, Liu J, Zhao S, Zhang H, Cai W, Cai M, Ji X, Leak RK, Gao Y, Chen J. Interleukin-4 is essential for microglia/macrophage M2 polarization and long-term recovery after cerebral ischemia. Stroke. 2016;**47**:498-504

[199] García-Berrocoso T, Giralt D, Bustamante A, Llombart V, Rubiera M, Penalba A, Boada C, Espadaler M, Molina C, Montaner J. Role of beta-defensin 2 and interleukin-4 receptor as stroke outcome biomarkers. Journal of Neurochemistry. 2014;**129**:463-472

[200] Helmy A, De Simoni M-G, Guilfoyle MR, Carpenter KL, Hutchinson PJ. Cytokines and innate inflammation in the pathogenesis of human traumatic brain injury. Progress in Neurobiology. 2011;**95**:352-372

[201] Burda JE, Sofroniew MV. Reactive gliosis and the multicellular response to CNS damage and disease. Neuron. 2014;**81**:229-248

[202] Erta M, Quintana A, Hidalgo J. Interleukin-6, a major cytokine in the central nervous system. International Journal of Biological Sciences. 2012;**8**:1254-1266

[203] Collingridge GL, Peineau S. Strippers reveal their depressing secrets: Removing AMPA receptors. Neuron. 2014;**82**:3-6

[204] Schindler R, Mancilla J, Endres S, Ghorbani R, Clark S, Dinarello CA. Correlations and interactions in the production of interleukin-6 (IL-6), IL-1, and tumor necrosis factor (TNF) in human blood mononuclear cells: IL-6 suppresses IL-1 and TNF. Blood. 1990;**75**:40-47

[205] Tilg H, Trehu E, Atkins MB, Dinarello CA, Mier JW. Interleukin-6 (IL-6) as an anti-inflammatory cytokine: Induction of circulating IL-1 receptor antagonist and soluble tumor necrosis factor receptor p55. Blood. 1994;**83**:113-118

[206] Biber K, Lubrich B, Fiebich BL, Boddeke HW, van Calker D. Interleukin-6 enhances expression of adenosine A1 receptor mRNA and signaling in cultured rat cortical astrocytes and brain slices. Neuropsychopharmacology. 2001;**24**:86-96

[207] Campbell IL, Erta M, Lim SL, Frausto R, May U, Rose-John S, Scheller J, Hidalgo J. Trans-signaling is a dominant mechanism for the pathogenic actions of interleukin-6 in the brain. Journal of Neuroscience. 2014;**34**:2503-2513

[208] Gertz K, Kronenberg G, Kälin RE, Baldinger T, Werner C, Balkaya M, Eom GD, Hellmann-Regen J, Kröber J, Miller KR, et al. Essential role of interleukin-6 in post-stroke angiogenesis. Brain. 2012;**135**:1964-1980

[209] Woodroofe M, Sarna G, Wadhwa M, Hayes G, Loughlin A, Tinker A, Cuzner M. Detection of interleukin-1 and interleukin-6 in adult rat brain, following mechanical injury, by in vivo microdialysis: Evidence of a role for microglia in cytokine production. Journal of Neuroimmunology. 1991;**33**:227-236

[210] Klein MA, Möller JC, Jones LL, Bluethmann H, Kreutzberg GW, Raivich G. Impaired neuroglial activation in interleukin-6 deficient mice. Glia. 1997;**19**:227-233

[211] Penkowa M, Moos T, Carrasco J, Hadberg H, Molinero A, Bluethmann H, Hidalgo J. Strongly compromised inflammatory response to brain injury in interleukin-6-deficient mice. Glia. 1999;**25**:343-357

[212] Galiano M, Liu ZQ, Kalla R, Bohatschek M, Koppius A, Gschwendtner A, Xu S, Werner A, Kloss CU, Jones LL. Interleukin-6 (IL6) and cellular response to facial nerve injury: Effects on lymphocyte recruitment, early microglial activation and axonal outgrowth in IL6-deficient mice. European Journal of Neuroscience. 2001;**14**:327-341

[213] Hans VH, Kossmann T, Lenzlinger PM, Probstmeier R, Imhof H-G, Trentz O, Morganti-Kossmann MC. Experimental axonal injury triggers interleukin-6 mRNA, protein synthesis and release into cerebrospinal fluid. Journal of Cerebral Blood Flow & Metabolism. 1999;**19**:184-194

[214] Penkowa M, Giralt M, Carrasco J, Hadberg H, Hidalgo J. Impaired inflammatory response and increased oxidative stress and neurodegeneration after brain injury in interleukin-6-deficient mice. Glia. 2000;**32**:271-285

[215] Swartz KR, Liu F, Sewell D, Schochet T, Campbell I, Sandor M, Fabry Z. Interleukin-6 promotes post-traumatic healing in the central nervous system. Brain Research. 2001;**896**:86-95

[216] Penkowa M, Giralt M, Lago N, Camats J, Carrasco J, Hernández J, Molinero A, Campbell IL, Hidalgo J. Astrocyte-targeted expression of IL-6 protects the CNS against a focal brain injury. Experimental Neurology. 2003;**181**:130-148

[217] Poulsen CB, Penkowa M, Borup R, Nielsen FC, Cáceres M, Quintana A, Molinero A, Carrasco J, Giralt M, Hidalgo J. Brain response to traumatic brain injury in wild-type and interleukin-6 knockout mice: A microarray analysis. Journal of Neurochemistry. 2005;**92**:417-432

[218] Quintana A, Molinero A, Borup R, Nielsen FC, Campbell IL, Penkowa M, Hidalgo J. Effect of astrocyte-targeted production of IL-6 on traumatic brain injury and its impact on the cortical transcriptome. Developmental Neurobiology. 2008;**68**:195-208

[219] Woiciechowsky C, Schöning B, Cobanov J, Lanksch WR, Volk H-D, Döcke W-D. Early IL-6 plasma concentrations correlate with severity of brain injury and pneumonia in brain-injured patients. Journal of Trauma and Acute Care Surgery. 2002;**52**:339-345

[220] McClain C, Cohen D, Phyllips R, Ott L, Young B. Increased plasma and ventricular interleukin-6 levels in head injured patients. The Journal of Laboratory and Clinical Medicine.1991;**118**:225-230

[221] Ikonomidis I, Andreotti F, Economou E, Stefanadis C, Toutouzas P, Nihoyannopoulos P. Increased proinflammatory cytokines in patients with chronic stable angina and their reduction by aspirin. Circulation. 1999;**100**:793-798

[222] Dalla Libera AL, Regner A, De Paoli J, Centenaro L, Martins TT, Simon D. IL-6 polymorphism associated with fatal outcome in patients with severe traumatic brain injury. Brain Injury. 2011;**25**:365-369

[223] Lambertsen KL, Biber K, Finsen B. Inflammatory cytokines in experimental and human stroke. Journal of Cerebral Blood Flow & Metabolism. 2012;**32**:1677-1698

[224] Loddick SA, Turnbull AV, Rothwell NJ. Cerebral interleukin-6 is neuroprotective during permanent focal cerebral ischemia in the rat. Journal of Cerebral Blood Flow & Metabolism. 1998;**18**:176-179

[225] Herrmann O, Tarabin V, Suzuki S, Attigah N, Coserea I, Schneider A, Vogel J, Prinz S, Schwab S, Monyer H. Regulation of body temperature and neuroprotection by endogenous interleukin-6 in cerebral ischemia. Journal of Cerebral Blood Flow & Metabolism. 2003;**23**:406-415

[226] Ding D. Endovascular mechanical thrombectomy for acute ischemic stroke: A new standard of care. Journal of Stroke. 2015;**17**:123

[227] Bye N, Habgood MD, Callaway JK, Malakooti N, Potter A, Kossmann T, Morganti-Kossmann MC. Transient neuroprotection by minocycline following traumatic brain injury is associated with attenuated microglial activation but no changes in cell apoptosis or neutrophil infiltration. Experimental Neurology. 2007;**204**:220-233

[228] Yang Y, Salayandia VM, Thompson JF, Yang LY, Estrada EY, Yang Y. Attenuation of acute stroke injury in rat brain by minocycline promotes blood-brain barrier remodeling and alternative microglia/macrophage activation during recovery. Journal of Neuroinflammation. 2015;**12**:26

[229] Switzer JA, Sikora A, Ergul A, Waller JL, Hess DC, Fagan SC. Minocycline prevents IL-6 increase after acute ischemic stroke. Translational Stroke Research. 2012;**3**:364-368

[230] Fagan SC, Waller JL, Nichols FT, Edwards DJ, Pettigrew LC, Clark WM, Hall CE, Switzer JA, Ergul A, Hess DC. Minocycline to Improve Neurologic Outcome in Stroke (MINOS). Stroke. 2010;**41**:2283-2287

[231] Lampl Y, Boaz M, Gilad R, Lorberboym M, Dabby R, Rapoport A, Anca-Hershkowitz M, Sadeh M. Minocycline treatment in acute stroke an open-label, evaluator-blinded study. Neurology. 2007;**69**:1404-1410

[232] Srivastava MP, Bhasin A, Bhatia R, Garg A, Gaikwad S, Prasad K, Singh MB, Tripathi M. Efficacy of minocycline in acute ischemic stroke: A single-blinded, placebo-controlled trial. Neurology India. 2012;**60**:23

[233] Amiri-Nikpour MR, Nazarbaghi S, Hamdi-Holaso M, Rezaei Y. An open-label evaluator-blinded clinical study of minocycline neuroprotection in ischemic stroke: Gender-dependent effect. Acta Neurologica Scandinavica. 2015;**131**:45-50

[234] Kohler E, Prentice DA, Bates TR, Hankey GJ, Claxton A, van Heerden J, Blacker D. Intravenous minocycline in acute stroke. Stroke. 2013;**44**:2493-2499

[235] Baki SGA, Schwab B, Haber M, Fenton AA, Bergold PJ. Minocycline synergizes with N-acetylcysteine and improves cognition and memory following traumatic brain injury in rats. PloS One. 2010;**5**:e12490

[236] Sanchez Mejia R, Ona V, Li M, Friedlander R. Minocycline reduces traumatic brain injury-mediated caspase-1 activation, tissue damage, and neurological dysfunction. Neurosurgery. 2001;**48**:1393-1399

[237] Kovesdi E, Kamnaksh A, Wingo D, Ahmed F, Grunberg NE, Long JB, Kasper CE, Agoston DV. Acute minocycline treatment mitigates the symptoms of mild blast-induced traumatic brain injury. Frontiers in Neurology. 2012;**3**:111

[238] Hanlon L, Raghupathi R, Huh J. Differential effects of minocycline on microglial activation and neurodegeneration following closed head injury in the neonate rat. Experimental Neurology. 2017;**290**:1-14

[239] Fox C, Dingman A, Derugin N, Wendland MF, Manabat C, Ji S, Ferriero DM, Vexler ZS. Minocycline confers early but transient protection in the immature brain following focal cerebral ischemia-reperfusion. Journal of Cerebral Blood Flow & Metabolism. 2005;**25**:1138-1149

[240] Arvin KL, Han BH, Du Y, Lin S-Z, Paul SM, Holtzman DM. Minocycline markedly protects the neonatal brain against hypoxic-ischemic injury. Annals of Neurology. 2002;**52**:54-61

[241] McCann SK, Cramond F, Macleod MR, Sena ES. Systematic review and meta-analysis of the efficacy of interleukin-1 receptor antagonist in animal models of stroke: An update. Translational Stroke Research. 2016;**7**:395-406

[242] Pradillo JM, Murray KN, Coutts GA, Moraga A, Oroz-Gonjar F, Boutin H, Moro MA, Lizasoain I, Rothwell NJ, Allan SM. Reparative effects of interleukin-1 receptor antagonist in young and aged/co-morbid rodents after cerebral ischemia. Brain, Behavior, and Immunity. 2017;**61**:117-126

[243] Lee JH, Kam EH, Kim JM, Kim SY, Kim EJ, Cheon SY, Koo B-N. Intranasal administration of interleukin-1 receptor antagonist in a transient focal cerebral ischemia rat model. Biomolecules & Therapeutics. 2017;**25**:149

[244] Emsley H, Smith C, Georgiou R, Vail A, Hopkins S, Rothwell N, Tyrrell P. A randomised phase II study of interleukin-1 receptor antagonist in acute stroke patients. Journal of Neurology, Neurosurgery & Psychiatry. 2005;**76**:1366-1372

[245] Tobinick E, Kim NM, Reyzin G, Rodriguez-Romanacce H, DePuy V. Selective TNF inhibition for chronic stroke and traumatic brain injury: An observational study involving 629 consecutive patients treated with perispinal etanercept. CNS Drugs. 2012;**26**(12): 1051-1070

[246] Cheong C-U, Chang C-P, Chao C-M, Cheng B-C, Yang C-Z, Chio C-C. Etanercept attenuates traumatic brain injury in rats by reducing brain TNF-α contents and by stimulating newly formed neurogenesis. Mediators of inflammation. Article ID: 620837 2013;**2013**:1-9

[247] Chio C-C, Chang C-H, Wang C-C, Cheong C-U, Chao C-M, Cheng B-C, Yang C-Z, Chang C-P. Etanercept attenuates traumatic brain injury in rats by reducing early microglial expression of tumor necrosis factor-α. BMC Neuroscience. 2013;**14**:33

[248] Chio C-C, Lin J-W, Chang M-W, Wang C-C, Kuo J-R, Yang C-Z, Chang C-P. Therapeutic evaluation of etanercept in a model of traumatic brain injury. Journal of Neurochemistry. 2010;**115**:921-929

[249] Sumbria RK, Boado RJ, Pardridge WM. Brain protection from stroke with intravenous TNFα decoy receptor-trojan horse fusion protein. Journal of Cerebral Blood Flow & Metabolism. 2012;**32**:1933-1938

[250] Clausen BH, Degn M, Martin NA, Couch Y, Karimi L, Ormhøj M, Mortensen M-LB, Gredal HB, Gardiner C, Sargent II. Systemically administered anti-TNF therapy ameliorates functional outcomes after focal cerebral ischemia. Journal of Neuroinflammation. 2014;**11**:203

[251] Baratz R, Tweedie D, Wang J-Y, Rubovitch V, Luo W, Hoffer BJ, Greig NH, Pick CG. Transiently lowering tumor necrosis factor-α synthesis ameliorates neuronal cell loss and cognitive impairments induced by minimal traumatic brain injury in mice. Journal of Neuroinflammation. 2015;**12**:45

[252] Yoon JS, Lee J-H, Tweedie D, Mughal MR, Chigurupati S, Greig NH, Mattson MP. 3, 6′-dithiothalidomide improves experimental stroke outcome by suppressing neuroinflammation. Journal of Neuroscience Research. 2013;**91**:671-680

[253] de Barros Bruno R, Marques TF, Batista TMT, Lima JCSS, de Arruda KG, Lima PFSF, da Silva Santos N, Cunha GM, Vitor HVN, de Barros Viana GS. Pentoxifylline treatment improves neurological and neurochemical deficits in rats subjected to transient brain ischemia. Brain Research. 2009;**1260**:55-64

[254] Vakili A, Mojarrad S, Akhavan MM, Rashidy-Pour A. Pentoxifylline attenuates TNF-α protein levels and brain edema following temporary focal cerebral ischemia in rats. Brain Research. 2011;**1377**:119-125

[255] Iwata N, Takayama H, Xuan M, Kamiuchi S, Matsuzaki H, Okazaki M, Hibino Y. Effects of etanercept against transient cerebral ischemia in diabetic rats. BioMed Research International. Article ID: 189292 2015;**2015**:1-10

[256] Wang J-Y, Huang Y-N, Chiu C-C, Tweedie D, Luo W, Pick CG, Chou S-Y, Luo Y, Hoffer BJ, Greig NH. Pomalidomide mitigates neuronal loss, neuroinflammation, and behavioral impairments induced by traumatic brain injury in rat. Journal of Neuroinflammation. 2016;**13**:168

[257] Doyle KP, Quach LN, Solé M, Axtell RC, Nguyen T-VV, Soler-Llavina GJ, Jurado S, Han J, Steinman L, Longo FM. B-lymphocyte-mediated delayed cognitive impairment following stroke. Journal of Neuroscience. 2015;**35**:2133-2145

[258] Sayeed I, Stein DG. Progesterone as a neuroprotective factor in traumatic and ischemic brain injury. Progress in Brain Research. 2009;**175**:219-237

[259] Liu A, Margaill I, Zhang S, Labombarda F, Coqueran B, Delespierre B, Liere P, Marchand-Leroux C, O'malley BW, Lydon JP. Progesterone receptors: A key for neuroprotection in experimental stroke. Endocrinology. 2012;**153**:3747-3757

[260] Wright DW, Kellermann AL, Hertzberg VS, Clark PL, Frankel M, Goldstein FC, Salomone JP, Dent LL, Harris OA, Ander DS. ProTECT: A randomized clinical trial of progesterone for acute traumatic brain injury. Annals of Emergency Medicine. 2007;**49**:391-402. e392

[261] Xiao G, Wei J, Yan W, Wang W, Lu Z. Improved outcomes from the administration of progesterone for patients with acute severe traumatic brain injury: A randomized controlled trial. Critical Care. 2008;**12**:R61

[262] Skolnick BE, Maas AI, Narayan RK, van der Hoop RG, MacAllister T, Ward JD, Nelson NR, Stocchetti N. A clinical trial of progesterone for severe traumatic brain injury. New England Journal of Medicine. 2014;**371**:2467-2476

[263] Wright DW, Yeatts SD, Silbergleit R, Palesch YY, Hertzberg VS, Frankel M, Goldstein FC, Caveney AF, Howlett-Smith H, Bengelink EM. Very early administration of progesterone for acute traumatic brain injury. New England Journal of Medicine. 2014;**371**:2457-2466

[264] Lin C, Chao H, Li Z, Xu X, Liu Y, Bao Z, Hou L, Liu Y, Wang X, You Y. Omega-3 fatty acids regulate NLRP3 inflammasome activation and prevent behavior deficits after traumatic brain injury. Experimental Neurology. 2017;**290**:115-122

[265] Chowdhury R, Stevens S, Gorman D, Pan A, Warnakula S, Chowdhury S, Ward H, Johnson L, Crowe F, Hu FB. Association between fish consumption, long chain omega 3 fatty acids, and risk of cerebrovascular disease: Systematic review and meta-analysis. BMJ. 2012;**345**:e6698

[266] Katayama Y, Katsumata T, Muramatsu H, Usuda K, Obo R, Terashi A. Effect of long-term administration of ethyl eicosapentate (EPA-E) on local cerebral blood flow and glucose utilization in stroke-prone spontaneously hypertensive rats (SHRSP). Brain Research. 1997;**761**:300-305

[267] Tanaka K, Ishikawa Y, Yokoyama M, Origasa H, Matsuzaki M, Saito Y, Matsuzawa Y, Sasaki J, Oikawa S, Hishida H. Reduction in the recurrence of stroke by eicosapentaenoic acid for hypercholesterolemic patients. Stroke. 2008;**39**:2052-2058

[268] Chen G, Shi J, Hu Z, Hang C. Inhibitory effect on cerebral inflammatory response following traumatic brain injury in rats: A potential neuroprotective mechanism of N-acetylcysteine. Mediators of Inflammation. Article ID: 716458 2008;**2008**:1-8

[269] Hicdonmez T, Kanter M, Tiryaki M, Parsak T, Cobanoglu S. Neuroprotective effects of N-acetylcysteine on experimental closed head trauma in rats. Neurochemical Research. 2006;**31**:473-481

[270] Choi S-H, Aid S, Kim H-W, Jackson SH, Bosetti F. Inhibition of NADPH oxidase promotes alternative and anti-inflammatory microglial activation during neuroinflammation. Journal of Neurochemistry. 2012;**120**:292-301

[271] Shen W-H, Zhang C-Y, Zhang G-Y. Antioxidants attenuate reperfusion injury after global brain ischemia through inhibiting nuclear factor-kappa B activity in rats. Acta Pharmacologica Sinica. 2003;**24**:1125-1130

[272] Şenol N, Nazıroğlu M, Yürüker V. N-acetylcysteine and selenium modulate oxidative stress, antioxidant vitamin and cytokine values in traumatic brain injury-induced rats. Neurochemical Research. 2014;**39**:685-692

[273] Eakin K, Baratz-Goldstein R, Pick CG, Zindel O, Balaban CD, Hoffer ME, Lockwood M, Miller J, Hoffer BJ. Efficacy of N-acetyl cysteine in traumatic brain injury. PloS One. 2014;**9**:e90617

[274] Haber M, Baki SGA, Grin'kina NM, Irizarry R, Ershova A, Orsi S, Grill RJ, Dash P, Bergold PJ. Minocycline plus N-acetylcysteine synergize to modulate inflammation and prevent cognitive and memory deficits in a rat model of mild traumatic brain injury. Experimental Neurology. 2013;**249**:169-177

[275] Hoffer ME, Balaban C, Slade MD, Tsao JW, Hoffer B. Amelioration of acute sequelae of blast induced mild traumatic brain injury by N-acetyl cysteine: A double-blind, placebo controlled study. PloS One. 2013;**8**:e54163

[276] Khan M, Sekhon B, Jatana M, Giri S, Gilg AG, Sekhon C, Singh I, Singh AK. Administration of N-acetylcysteine after focal cerebral ischemia protects brain and reduces inflammation in a rat model of experimental stroke. Journal of Neuroscience Research. 2004;**76**:519-527

[277] Knuckey NW, Palm D, Primiano M, Epstein MH, Johanson CE. N-acetylcysteine enhances hippocampal neuronal survival after transient forebrain ischemia in rats. Stroke. 1995;**26**:305-311

[278] Shohami E, Gallily R, Mechoulam R, Bass R, Ben-Hur T. Cytokine production in the brain following closed head injury: Dexanabinol (HU-211) is a novel TNF-α inhibitor and an effective neuroprotectant. Journal of Neuroimmunology. 1997;**72**:169-177

[279] Lavie G, Teicher A, Shohami E. Dexanabinol (HU-211) improves long-term outcome in rats subjected to transient focal brain ischemia. Abstracts - Society for Neuroscience. 2000;**30**:771

[280] Knoller N, Levi L, Shoshan I, Reichenthal E, Razon N, Rappaport ZH, Biegon A. Dexanabinol (HU-211) in the treatment of severe closed head injury: A randomized, placebo-controlled, phase II clinical trial. Critical Care Medicine. 2002;**30**:548-554

[281] Maas AI, Murray G, Henney H, Kassem N, Legrand V, Mangelus M, Muizelaar J-P, Stocchetti N, Knoller N. Efficacy and safety of dexanabinol in severe traumatic brain injury: Results of a phase III randomised, placebo-controlled, clinical trial. The Lancet Neurology. 2006;**5**:38-45

[282] Panikashvili D, Na'ama AS, Mechoulam R, Trembovler V, Kohen R, Alexandrovich A, Shohami E. The endocannabinoid 2-AG protects the blood-brain barrier after closed head injury and inhibits mRNA expression of proinflammatory cytokines. Neurobiology of Disease. 2006;**22**:257-264

[283] Panikashvili D, Simeonidou C, Ben-Shabat S, Hanuš L, Breuer A, Mechoulam R, Shohami E. An endogenous cannabinoid (2-AG) is neuroprotective after brain injury. Nature. 2001;**413**:527-531

[284] Lloyd E, Somera-Molina K, Van Eldik LJ, Watterson DM, Wainwright MS. Suppression of acute proinflammatory cytokine and chemokine upregulation by post-injury administration of a novel small molecule improves long-term neurologic outcome in a mouse model of traumatic brain injury. Journal of Neuroinflammation. 2008;**5**:28

Chapter 10

Role of Kynurenine Pathway in Glioblastoma

Gustavo Ignacio Vázquez Cervantes,
Nora Karen Olascoaga Arellano,
Daniela Ramírez Ortega, Alelí Salazar Ramiro,
Dinora F. González Esquivel, Camilo Ríos,
Benjamín Pineda Olvera and
Verónica Pérez de la Cruz

Additional information is available at the end of the chapter

http://dx.doi.org/10.5772/intechopen.68939

Abstract

In brain, the tryptophan degradation products through the kynurenine pathway exhibit neuromodulatory and inflammatory effects and have been related to the progression of neurodegenerative disorders, furthermore, their protagonism on the modulation of immune response and in cancer development has been reported. The immunosuppressive role of kynurenines has been described on glioblastoma models. In patients, the elevated activity of indoleamine-2,3-dioxygenase (IDO) such as the increase of kynurenine/tryptophan ratio have been also reported, suggesting that activation of kynurenine pathway is present during glioblastoma formation and can be related with tumor progression. The importance of the kynurenine pathway during cancer development has encouraged recent studies to the use of IDO inhibitors as a therapeutic strategy for treatment of breast, lung and ovarian cancer, until to get its use in clinical trials. IDO inhibitors also have been used in in vitro and in vivo models of glioblastoma showing promising results. The effect of kynurenines on glioblastoma offer a new perspective about the tryptophan metabolism during cancer. Due to the relevance of the kynurenine pathway in brain homeostasis, immunomodulation and cancer, we discuss the relevance of the kynurenine pathway on the development of glioblastoma multiforme as well as a possible molecular target for glioblastoma treatment.

Keywords: glioblastoma, tryptophan catabolism, immune response, immunoedition

1. Introduction

Tryptophan (Trp) is considered as an essential amino acid, which is required for life and growth but is not synthesized by the organism. Although approximately 1% of tryptophan dietary intake is used for protein synthesis, the rest 99% is metabolized through the 5-hydroxyindole pathway for the production of melatonin and serotonin, decarboxylated to tryptamine, transaminated to indol-3-pyruvic acid, or oxidized by the so-named kynurenine pathway (KP), for the new synthesis of NAD+ and NADP+ (**Figure 1**) [1–3].

The KP degrades over 95% of whole tryptophan intake; its rate-limiting enzymes, tryptophan 2,3-dioxygenase (TDO), and indoleamine 2,3-dioxygenase (IDO), catalyze the cleavage of the tryptophan pyrrole ring to produce N-formylkynurenine [1, 4]. Among mammals, TDO is mainly expressed in liver and only uses L-tryptophan as a specific substrate; instead of that, IDO is expressed in extrahepatic tissues, such as brain, lung, kidney, and immune cells [1, 4]. Furthermore, IDO's substrate span is wider than TDO's, being D- or L-tryptophan, D- or L-hydroxytryptophan, tryptamine, serotonin, and melatonine available for the catalytic activity of IDO [5]. An IDO isoenzyme has been reported, IDO2 is expressed in the murine kidney, liver, and reproductive system, and the gene encoding IDO2 is adjacent to the IDO gene and has similar affinity for substrates than IDO [6, 7]. N-formylkynurenine is transformed

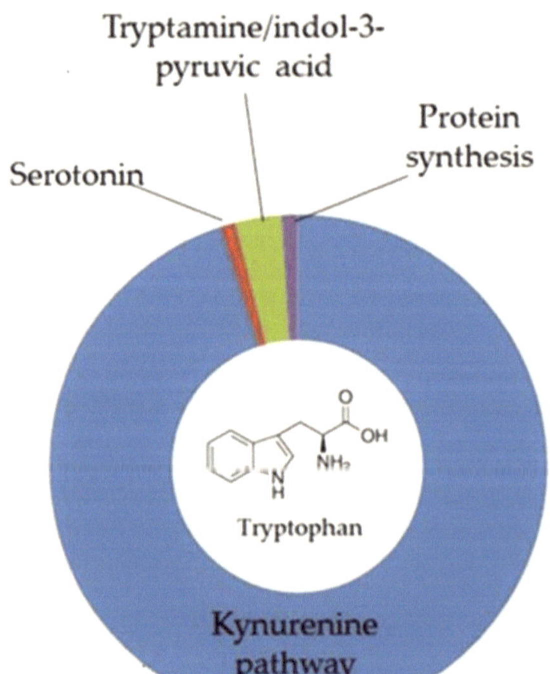

Figure 1. Tryptophan catabolism occurs by different pathways. Ninety-five percent of the dietary uptake of tryptophan is catabolized mainly by the kynurenine pathway. About 3% is decarboxylated to tryptamine or transaminated to indol-3-pyruvic acid, 1% is intended for serotonin and melatonin synthesis, and resting 1% is for protein synthesis.

http://dx.doi.org/10.5772/intechopen.68939

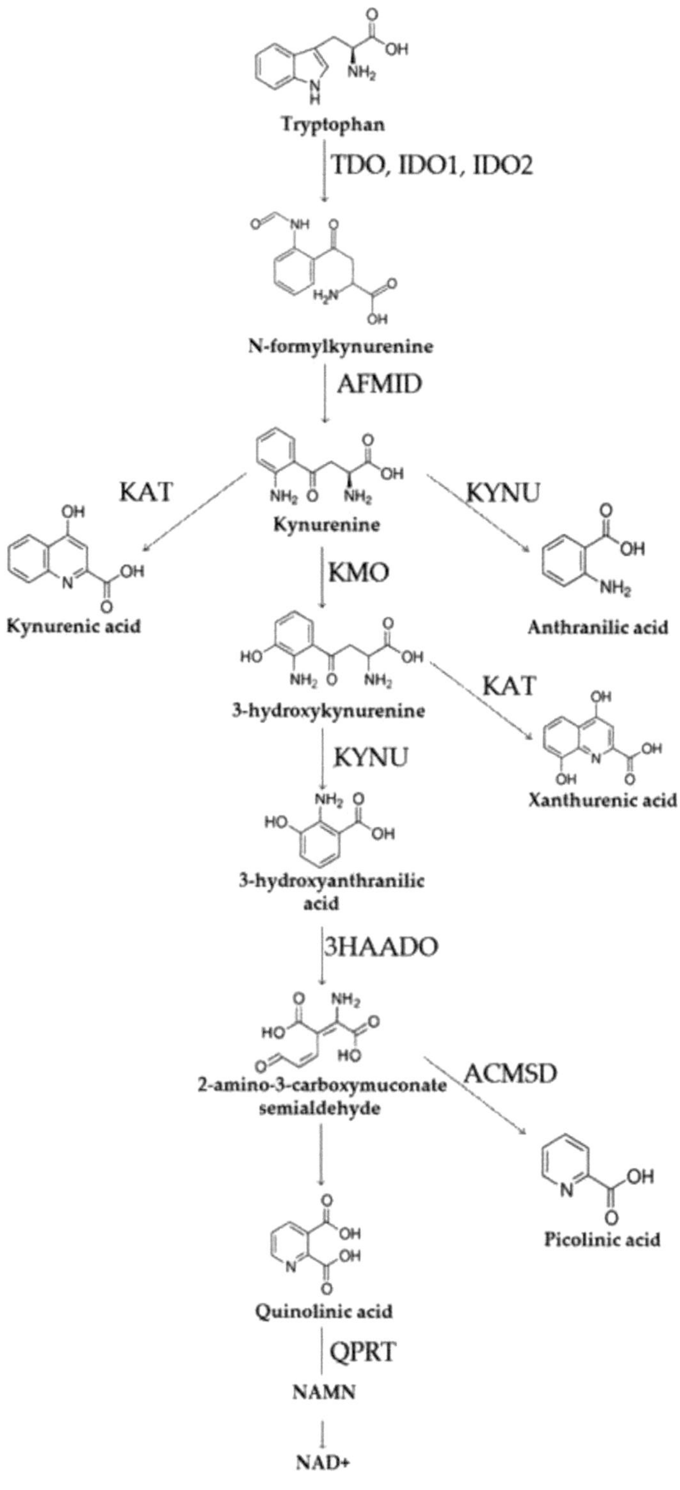

Figure 2. The kynurenine pathway.

to L-kynurenine (L-kyn) by the arylformidase (AFMID); kynurenine aminotransferases (KAT I, KAT II), and kynureninase (KYNU), with pyridoxal-5′-phosphate as a cofactor, as well as kynurenine monooxygenase (KMO), which uses FAD as a cofactor, transform L-kyn into kynurenic acid (Kyna), anthranilic acid (AA), or 3-hydroxykynurenine (3-HK), respectively [8–10]. KMO is located in mitochondrial outer membrane and it has been shown to have high affinity by the substrate suggesting that KMO metabolizes more L-kyn than other enzymes [11]. KATs and KYNU can also use 3-HK as a substrate to produce xanthurenic acid (Xanth) or 3-hydroxyanthranilic acid (3HAA) [8, 12]. Oxidation of 3HAA by the 3HAA dioxygenase (3HAADO) produces 2-amino-3-carboxymuconate semialdehyde (Acms) which is transformed by non-enzymatic dehydration into quinolinic acid (Quin), or into picolinic acid (Pic) by the Acms decarboxylase (ACMSD). Finally, Quin phosphoribosyltransferase (QPRT) uses Quin as a substrate for the formation of nicotinamine-adenine-mononucleotide (NaMN), the nicotinamine-adenine-dinucleotide (NAD+) precursor (**Figure 2**) [13, 14]. Enzyme kinetics of the whole KP have been determined, giving a wide perspective of the kynurenine pathway and its functionality [13], enzyme kinetics data of the KP are summarized in **Table 1**.

Enzyme	Substrate	K_M (mM)	K_{cat} (s^{-1})	Reference
IDO	5-Hydroxytriptamine	0.02	0.043	[5, 13, 15]
	Serotonin	0.1	0.002	
	Tryptophan	0.045	1.65	
	Oxygen	0.042		
TDO	Tryptophan	0.222	1.4	[16]
	Oxygen	0.037		
AFMID	N-formylkynurenine	0.05	100	[17, 18]
KAT I	L-kynurenine	4.7	3.35	[19]
KAT II	L-kynurenine	4.7	9.76	[20]
	3-hydroxykynurenine	3.8	1.7	
KAT III	L-kynurenine	1.5	2.3	[21]
KMO	L-kynurenine	0.89	1.88	[22]
	Oxygen	0.071		
	NADPH	0.82		
KYNU	L-kynurenine	0.495	0.23	[23]
	3-hydroxykynurenine	0.028	3.5	
3HAADO	3-hydroxyanthranilic acid	0.016	64	[24]
	Oxygen	0.615		
ACMSD	2-amino-3-carboxy muconate semialdehyde	0.0065	1	[25]
QPRT	Quinolinic acid	0.022	0.05	[26]

Table 1. Enzyme kinetics parameters for the kynurenine pathway enzymes.

2. Role of kynurenine pathway in brain

Although NAD+ is a final product of the KP, many of the intermediary metabolites, the so-called kynurenines, have demonstrated to exert many effects on cellular homeostasis and bioenergetics resulting on changes in organism behavior or immune response. In brain, Trp is transported through the blood-brain barrier by the large neutral amino acids transporter [27]. The imbalance on the levels of its metabolites (kynurenines) has been related with the progression of neurodegenerative disorders, such as Huntington, Alzheimer, and Parkinson due to their redox nature and their capacity to exert neuromodulatory mechanisms [28].

On a redox perspective, both 3-HK and 3-HAA represent a double-edged sword. Reports show that 3-HK is able to promote cell death due to the increase in reactive oxygen species (ROS) production; also, 3-HK interaction with metallic ions promotes protein aggregation as well as cataract formation and toxicity in neuronal cultures without region selectivity [29–32] pointing this kynurenine as a pro-oxidant and cytotoxic compound. In the same way, 3-HAA is able to cause protein damage due to interaction with metals producing $OH^{\bullet}$; furthermore, this metabolite causes oxidative phosphorylation uncoupling and decreased oxygen consumption [31, 33]. On the other hand, there are reports pointing to the antioxidant and protective side of these molecules, demonstrating a 3-HK-induced decrease of oxidative stress parameters; also, it has been observed that 3-HK acts as a free radical scavenger of radicals like $O_2^{\bullet-}$ [34, 35]; the antioxidant activity of 3-HAA also has been reported showing free radical scavenging and ROS production decrease [36]. Finally, the protective effect of 3-HK and 3-HAA on the inhibited mitochondrial electron transport chain, as electron carriers, also has been reported [37].

On the other hand, Kyna is the only endogenous antagonist to N-methyl-D-aspartate (NMDA) receptors known so far, it inhibits the α7-nicotinic receptors, showing anticonvulsant effects on murine models as well as in human patients [38]. Recently, it was found that Kyna is a free radical scavenger of radicals, such as superoxide anion ($O_2^{\bullet-}$), hydroxyl radical ($OH^{\bullet}$), and peroxynitrite (ONOO–), besides it is able to reduce oxidative damage caused by pro-oxidants, so it is considered an endogenous antioxidant [39]. Furthermore, it has been shown that Kyna binds selectively to GPR35 receptor [40]; Kyna-mediated activation of GPR35 leads to intracellular Ca^{2+} influx, inositol phosphate production and, attenuates LPS-induced TNF-α release and reduces acetic acid-induced pain, suggesting that GPR35 could be mediating Kyna excitatory, anti-inflammatory, and antinociceptive functions [40–42]. Contributing with the anti-inflammatory response, Kyna also has been described as an agonist of the intracellular aryl hydrocarbon receptor (AHR); AHR translocation into the nucleus modulates the production of proinflammatory mediators and, as discussed below, inhibits T immune responses [43]. Because of Kyna is unable to cross the blood-brain barrier, systemic L-kyn administration has been used to show the protective effect of Kyna in 6-hydroxidopamine-induced Parkinson disease models, hippocampal β-amyloid, and glutamate toxicity [44–46].

Contrasting with Kyna, Quin has been described as an agonist of NMDA receptors; in fact, it has been demonstrated that Quin is a pro-convulsive agent which generates mitochondrial progressive dysfunction by reducing activity of respiratory complexes II and III [47], increases ROS production and lipid peroxidation in presence of Fe^{2+} [48], induces Ca^{2+} cellular influx increase, release of glutamate, and apoptosis [49–51]. Recently, the decrease in autophagy inhibition by Beclin-1 reported in human astrocytes and neurons has been attributed to Quin toxicity [52]. Because of the selective damage that exerts in striatal spiny neurons with γ-amino butyric acid and substance P, Quin has also been a good model to mimic early symptoms of Huntington's disease [53–55]. In addition, increases in Quin concentrations were observed in the cerebral cortex of macaques infected with retroviruses, particularly those with local inflammatory lesions [56]. Moreover, Quin levels are increased in cerebrospinal fluid in the acquired immunodeficiency syndrome and in HIV patients; also in humans, Quin levels are elevated after traumatic brain injury [57].

2.1. Inflammatory process and kynurenine pathway components

Moreover, kynurenine pathway has been related to inflammatory processes. It has been shown that IDO, KMO, and KYNU expression is strongly induced by proinflammatory cytokines, mainly interferon-ɣ (IFN-ɣ), interleukin 1 (IL1), interleukin 17 (IL17), or the tumor necrosis factor α (TNF-α) during bacterial and viral infections in immune privileged tissues, such as brain [58, 59]. Thus, activation of the KP by proinflammatory molecules inhibits bacterial proliferation through tryptophan depletion, avoids autoimmune responses by limiting T cell activation and recruiting of immune regulatory cells [60–62]. The immunoregulatory role of the KP could act as a double-edged sword, meanwhile it is inhibiting pathogen growth and regulating immune responses to avoid an autoimmune damage, the same activation during cancer supports tumor immune evasion and promotes tumor growth and invasiveness.

Beyond their role on neurodegenerative disorders, kynurenines have also been related with cancer progression in more than one way. It has been described that IDO expression is high in all thyroid carcinomas [63]. Moreover, L-kyn and Quin promote neoplastic cell proliferation *in vitro* and the formation of larger tumors *in vivo*, in a colorectal cancer model, through the Wnt/β-catenin signaling, despite of the ablation of IDO [64]. L-kyn modulates the repairing enzyme DNA polymerase kappa, protecting tumor cells from DNA damage and propitiating genomic instability [65]. Also, Quin produced by microglial cells in glioma models confers tumor tolerance to oxidative stress due to the production of NAD+, promotes cell proliferation by the modulation of the fibroblast growth factor-1 (FGF-1) release, and it is elevated in children with central nervous system tumors [66–68]. Kyna also promotes glioma cell proliferation through FGF-1 release [67]. The high expression and activity of the KP in the tumor microenvironment will be reflected on the maintenance of the NAD+/NADH supply, NAD+ and its reduced form NADH participate in several metabolic, redox, and stress response signals, providing favorable growing conditions for cancer cells. Finally, IDO expression and activity as well as the kynurenines promote cancer development by affecting the host's immune responsiveness. The effects of the KP on cancer immunosuppressive mechanisms will be detailed below.

2.2. Cancer immunoedition

All the cancer cells must possess a series of characters that allow them to develop tumors, these "hallmarks" let cancer cells to rapidly grow, evade cell death, migrate through the organism and colonize new tissues, modify their metabolic program, and to avoid immune destruction [69].

Before the establishment and development of a tumor, cancer cells must overcome elements of the immune system of the organism that can recognize, induce cellular signals, and finally, destroy exogenous agents or defective cells within the organism. In the early twentieth century, Paul Ehrlich formulated the idea that the immune system of an organism is able to recognize, destroy, and then protect against tumor cells. Later in the mid-twentieth century, the "immunosurveillance" hypothesis was then postulated by Sir Macfarlane Burnet and Lewis Thomas, based on this original idea and in experimental evidence of that, mouse lacking of interferon-γ responsiveness or with adaptive immunity defects, were susceptible to develop cancer [69, 70]. More recent evidence has demonstrated that the immune system not only protects against cancer progression, immune cells, and signaling but also promotes tumor cell establishment, and furthermore, cancer cells modulate immune mechanisms favoring tumor progression, transforming the idea of "immunosurveillance" into the "cancer immunoediting" hypothesis [69–70].

The cancer immunoediting hypothesis postulates that cancer cells and immune system create a set of dynamical interactions during the formation of a tumor; these interactions are arranged in three stages of the "cancer immunoediting," or "The three E's hypothesis" process named: elimination, equilibrium, and escape [70]. During the elimination phase, cancer cells are recognized by the immune system and cytotoxic reactions induce cancer cell death; in the equilibrium phase, the cytotoxic mechanisms of the immune system act as selective pressure on tumor cells; cancer cells that survive, remain proliferating and establishing the tumor. Finally, at the escape phase, cancer cells are able to evade and suppress the immune mechanisms leading to the formation of tumors [70–72].

Cancer immunoediting mechanisms could be given by genetic alterations, proper of the cancer cells, which induce overexpression and secretion of suppressive molecules, such as the transforming growth factor-β, the vascular endothelial growth factor, prostaglandin E2, and the soluble MHCI-related gene A; cancer cells also recruit immune regulatory cells like T regulatory cells (Tregs), myeloid-derived suppressor cells (MDSC), and tolerogenic dendritic cells (TDC); and finally, by induction of immune checkpoint, inhibitory molecules, such as PD-L1 [73]. A second type of immunoediting is carried out by cytotoxic T cells of the own adaptive immune system, while exerting their protective role against cancer, T cells release cytokines like IFN-γ which can also induce the production of immune suppressive molecules by tumor cells, during the equilibrium phase of the "cancer immunoediting" [73]. Remarkably, IFN-γ is a strong inducer of IDO expression and activity which leads tryptophan metabolism through the KP in tumor microenvironment, and then to the triggering of the kynurenines' immunosuppressive effects [73, 74]. In cultured human glioma, stimulation with IFN-γ significantly increased the expression of IDO-1, IDO-2, kynureninase, and kynurenine hydroxylase, which potentiate the KP; whereas significantly decreased 2-amino-3-carboxymuconate semialdehyde decarboxylase (ACMSD) and kynurenine aminotransferase-I (KAT-I), which reduce the neuroprotective metabolites [75].

2.2.1. The kynurenines in cancer immunoediting

As mentioned above, the own immune response against tumors could propitiate the formation of an immunosuppressive microenvironment, one of these mechanisms is carried out by IFN-γ and other proinflammatory cytokines secreted by cytotoxic lymphocytes which strongly induce IDO expression. Beyond the increase of IDO levels in tumor cells, the formation and accumulation of different kynurenines have demonstrated immunosuppressive and immunoinhibitory effects [76].

Recent works have demonstrated that tryptophan starvation is able to inhibit T cell and macrophage cell viability and proliferation [77–80]. Furthermore, KP metabolites have also shown direct effects as immunosuppressive molecules. L-kyn is able to activate the aryl hydrocarbon receptor (AHR) and thus to promote the generation of Tregs from naive T cells [81]. Moreover, there are reports showing that 3-HAA, 3-HK, and Quin promote Treg generation and that 3-HAA and 3-HK block T cell activation and induce cell death of CD4+ T and CD8+ T cells as well as of natural killer cells (NK) and B lymphocytes [82–86]. All these reports settle down the idea that immunosuppressive mechanisms carried out through the KP activation may be due to tryptophan deprivation of the tumor microenvironment or secondly, by the direct effect of the kynurenines on Treg recruitment and the impact on viability of effector T cells. Finally, both tryptophan depletion and the presence of the KP intermediates could enhance an immunosuppressive environment. It has been showed that L-kyn, Pic, 3-HK, 3-HAA, and Quin reduced cell viability and induced apoptosis on CD4+ in absence of tryptophan [82, 83]; besides at lower concentrations were able to increase Treg-mediated immunotolerance [84].

It is relevant to note that in some cases, the kynurenines are not produced by cancer cells but by other components of the tumor microenvironment, such as dendritic cells (DCs) or mesenchymal stem cells and also by microglial cells in the case of brain tumors [83, 87, 88]. Regarding dendritic cells expressing IDO, they can suppress effective immune responses through diverse strategies: by inhibiting the proliferation and effector functions of cytotoxic cells, such as NK and CD8+ T lymphocytes, as well as plasma cells; by inducing of CD4+ CD25+ FOXP3+ regulatory T cells from naive CD4+ cells; and by triggering immunosuppressive activity in adjacent IDO-expressing DCs [89]. Possible implication of IDO2 in cancer immunosuppression has been suggested due to reports showing its ability to mobilize the nuclear factor interleukin 6 inhibitor, LIP [6].

Thus, locating the IDO expression and the kynurenines in the "Three E's" context, it would be in this way: IFNɣ, TNFα, and proinflammatory cytokines secreted by cytotoxic lymphocytes, while killing recognized tumor cells during Elimination and Equilibrium phases, induce IDO expression of tumor cells, those that survived to immune response, and of other infiltrating cells, such as DCs and macrophages. Tumor cells expressing IDO, deplete tryptophan from the tumor microenvironment and begin to produce kynurenines and NAD+; tryptophan depletion from, and release of kynurenines to the tumor microenvironment, inhibit T cells and NK proliferation; induce apoptosis, while promote differentiation and proliferation of Tregs, and recruiting of DCs and macrophages. NAD+ production allows cancer cells to overcome DNA damage and oxidative stresses, promoving their proliferation during the Escape phase.

Because of the importance of the KP in brain and the relationship of tryptophan catabolism with immune modulation during cancer, researchers have begun to clarify the role of the activation of this pathway on glioblastoma progression for further development of new strategies to treat this illness.

2.3. The glioblastoma multiforme

Astrocytes are non-excitable nervous cells of great importance for the physiological maintenance that exert on neurons, by regulating ions and excitatory amino-acids concentrations on synaptic regions, forming the brain-blood-barrier (BBB)-mediating neuron-blood stream signaling and regulating the transport of nutrients into and out of the brain [90, 91]. Beyond this, astrocytes can be differentiated on a wide span of morphological, physiological, and genomic subtypes [90–91].

Deregulation of cell proliferation and uncontrolled proliferation caused by mutations of certain genes lead astrocytes to transform into astrocytomas. Astrocytomas have been classified into four subtypes depending on the rate of proliferation and the grade of malignancy: grade I pilocytic astrocytomas are non-invasive tumors, they represent the less malignant of astrocytomas; diffuse astrocytomas are grade II tumors that tend to invade peripheral tissues but their growth rate is slow; anaplastic astrocytomas grow faster than diffuse astrocytomas and tend to form tentacle-like projections into surrounding tissues, instead of grade III anaplastic astrocytomas, their frequency is low; finally, glioblastomas (GBM), also known as glioblastoma multiforme, are grade IV tumors, these are the most malignant of astrocytomas [92]. GBM can be originated *de novo* from mature astrocytes, primary GBM, or from a less malignant astrocytoma, secondary GBM; they represent 15.1% of all brain primary tumors and 55.1% of all gliomas [93].

Incidence rate of GBM is 3.19 per 100,000 people with a median age at diagnosis of 64 years old for primary GBM, and 45 years old for secondary GBM, the median survival overall for diagnosed and treated GBM ranges between 12 and 14 months [94, 95]. Furthermore, GBM represent 2.8% of brain tumors during childhood [96]; however, its frequency is lower in adults, high-grade astrocytic tumor incidence rate is 0.85 per 100,000 people being more frequent in children between 5 and 9 years old, also, the median survival overall is over 43 months [97–99]. The most common treatment for GBM is surgical resection of the tumor, followed by temozolomide-based chemotherapy, and 5000–6000 Gy radiotherapy which prolongs the lifespan 202 weeks [100–102]. Despite the treatment, the survival of afflicted patients is no longer than 14 months and only 5% of the patients have a survival rate of 5 years. It is believed that the lack of response of GBM to the multimodal treatment is due to multiple factors that combined, make GBM resistance and aggressiveness.

A major character among GBM is a loss-of-function mutation of Retinoblastoma (Rb) gene, a cell cycle regulator protein at the phase G to phase S checkpoint, that also regulates apoptosis and differentiation, which occurs on 77% of GBM [103, 104]. Instead of that, another genetic mutations and genomic expression patterns differ among GBM, integrated genomic analysis originated four types of GBM named: proneural, associated with PDGFRA, IDH1, and TP53 mutations; neural, expressing neuronal markers, such as NEFL, GABRA1, SYT1, and SLC12A5; classical, showing amplifications on EGFR expression and deletions of Ink4a/ARF locus; and mesenchymal, characterized by overexpression of CHI3L1 and MET so as deletion of NF1 [103]. Several other mutations in key oncogenic signaling pathways, such as the receptor tyrosine kinase (RTK)/RAS/PI3K, p53 pathways, lead to uncontrolled tumor cell proliferation, genomic instability, and resistance to therapeutic strategies.

GBM may have a wide cellular diversity, more than tumor cells which are polygonal or spindled small sized with big nuclei, GBM-initiating cells (also called glioma stem cells) are responsible for cell proliferation and renewal of GBM cells, also confer chemo- and radioresistance; infiltrating multinucleated cells, such as lymphocytes, macrophages, and neutrophils, and cells with lipid vacuoles are present in these tumors [105]. Because GBM are highly angiogenic tumors, blood vessels surrounded by pericytes are also present in tumors. GBM also show necrotic regions among the central body tumor and some other necrotic foci in outer regions of the tumor [105, 106]. In addition to all these mechanisms, the GBM has the ability to create an immunosuppressive environment that prevents the response lead by the immune system against GBM.

2.3.1. *Immunosuppressive environment in GBM*

Historically, the brain has been considered an immune privileged organ due to the inability of reject exo-grafts and the lack of response in case of infection [107], as well as, absence of a normal response of the lymphatic system and the extremely distinctiveness of antigen-presenting cells (APCs) in brain tissue [108, 109]. However, diverse studies have recently found that there is not an absolute isolation of the rest of the organism; moreover, within the dural sinuses is located a lymphatic system that connect with the deep cervical lymph nodes, able of taking immune cells and macromolecules into the CNS [108].

Even with this lymphatic system, the access to CNS is highly regulated, mostly by the BBB [110]. The BBB is a highly selective layer composed of basement membranes, brain pericytes, astrocytes, and neurons, which have the ability to reject more than the 90% of small molecules, allowing the entrance just to certain lipophilic molecules [111]. However, it has been observed that when a GBM appears, this tumor easily disrupts the BBB due to this abnormal structure, which has as consequence the free-crossing of a more varied group of substances into the CNS [111] and also cells of the immune system.

GBM is infiltrated by several cell types, such as monocyte-derived cells, microglia, and activated T cells. These immune cells are recruited by chemotaxis to the tumor and together with molecules secreted by GBM itself, such as IL-10, prostaglandins, and TGF-β1 (**Table 2**), playing a major role in the immunosuppression of the tumor [112–113]. Specifically, several studies have found that the infiltration of T cells subtypes is higher in GBM than any other CNS tumor [114], comprising between 10 and 30% of cells within the tumor mass [115–116]. Due to the production of immunosuppressive cytokines, inhibition of T cell proliferation, activation of Tregs and hypoxia, an immunosuppressive environment, is made in GBM, which can be enhanced by the activation of the KP.

Because of the high immunosuppressive conditions in the GBM, new therapies have begun to being developed, focusing on antitumoral immune response for improvement of GBM patients. Thus, epidermal growth factor receptor (EGFR) variant III-specific peptide vaccination and autologous tumor lysate-DC vaccination have been tested with successful results on phase I and phase II clinical trials [117–120]. However, a better understanding of the immunosuppressive mechanisms occurring during GBM development, including those carried out by IDO activity and the kynurenines, could impulse the furtherance of new tools and strategies for GBM treatment.

http://dx.doi.org/10.5772/intechopen.68939

Molecule	Effect	Mechanism
Interleukin-10 (IL-10)	Induce apoptosis in T cells, possibly through the expression of Fas-ligand	[121–123]
Tumor-promoting cytokines	Dampen the antitumor immune response	[124, 125]
Interleukin-6 (IL-6)	Shifting adaptive immunity to humoral response (TH2)	[124, 126]
Prostaglandin E2 (PGE2)	Dampen the antitumor immune response suppressing lymphocyte proliferation	[124, 125, 127–129]
TGF-β1	Ability to polarize TAMs toward M2 phenotype	
CD70 and ganglioside	Promotion of T cells apoptosis	[130, 131]
Colony stimulating factor-1 (CSF-1)	Stimulating of monocytic cells	[124, 126]
	Ability to polarize TAMs toward M2 phenotype	
Basic fibroblast growth factor (BFGF),	Dampen the antitumor immune response	[124, 125]
Vascular endothelial growth factor (VEGF)	Proangiogenic factor.	[132]
	Support of vascularity and tumor growth	
Factor-1α (HIF-1α)	Activation of Tregs and production of vascular endothelial growth factor (VEGF)	[133]
Transcription 3 (STAT3)	Synthesis of hypoxia-inducible factor -1α (HIF-1α) that subsequently induces activation of Tregs and production of vascular endothelial growth factor (VEGF).	[133]
	Promotion of angiogenesis	

Table 2. Molecules implicated in the immunosuppression of GBM.

2.3.2. Implications of kynurenine pathway in GBM development

Kynurenine pathway enzymes are overexpressed in GBM. Upregulated expression of these enzymes has been related to severity of gliomas and patient survival. The IDO expression in 343 glioma specimens and correlated to patient survival has been analyzed [134], this expression was associated with poor prognosis and was more frequently observed in high-grade glioma. Moreover, in an orthotopic GL261 cell tumor model was shown that IDO-competent brain tumors increased the recruitment of immunosuppressive Tregs, and decreased the frequency of CD8+ T cells compared with IDO-deficient brain tumors [134]. Another study, including 75 gliomas, showed higher expression of IDO in malignant gliomas compared with low-grade gliomas. Moreover, stronger IDO expression was associated with shortened survival time in GBM patients [135]. Additionally, it has been reported that glioma cells have increased mRNA expression of IDO1 and IDO2 compared with human fetal astrocytes and human adult astrocytes cultures as well as decreased Kats mRNA expression, and these expression enhanced when cells were stimulated with IFNɣ [75]; the same work also reported increased Kyn/Trp ratios and decreased Kyna/Kyn ratios in the plasma of glioblastoma patients compared with healthy people [75]. The levels of Trp and Kyn were evaluated in GBM patients before and after tumor resection. Interestingly, both Trp and Kyn significantly decreased after 48 h and 10 weeks after surgery. In addition, patients with a high-ratio Kyn/Trp had worse mean overall survival compared with patients with lower ratio [136].

The significantly increased expression of IDO in cancer cells and in the tumor microenvironment has arisen as a promising target for GBM treatment, based on the inhibition of IDO as a potential therapy for cancer patients. Among the first strategies, is the systemic administration of 1-methyl tryptophan (1-MT), a competitive inhibitor of the IDO, which delayed tumor development in a murine model of Lewis lung carcinoma [137]. Subsequently, it was described that the expression of IDO in immunogenic cells (P815B) avoided their rejection by preimmunized mice, an effect that was associated with the inhibition of specific T cell response [138]. This effect was partially reversed when preimmunized mice were administered with 1-MT [138]. Due to the results observed in animal models, 1-MT has been tested and approved on phase I clinical trials in patients with solid and solid metastatic neoplasms, lung, ovarian, Fallopian tube, and breast cancer showing disease stabilization in most cases [89, 139–141].

Concerning to GBM, at least three clinical trials involving IDO inhibitors are in recruiting status (Feb. 2017), but the use of 1-MT on *in vivo* GBM models has shown that when is used in combination with classical chemotherapeutic agents, such as temozolomide or cyclophosphamide, and additional radiotherapy, increases the overall survival as well as reduces the tumor volume [142, 143]. Additionally to this effect, inhibition of IDO has also shown increased complement component C3 deposition on the tumor region, which is necessary for tumor volume reduction [142], as well as increased CD4+ and CD8+ T cell population from animal spleens, treated with 1-MT [143], indicating that IDO inhibition rescues the host's immune activation.

Despite reports pointing that 1-MT has a greater affinity for IDO2 than for IDO [6, 7], it is of mention that the majority of reports about the targeting of the KP for cancer treatment are focused on IDO inhibition. But IDO is just one of the enzymes that fuel this catabolic route, so the better understanding of the roles of both IDO2 and TDO in cancer development and immunosuppression would result in better ways for combating cancer [144].

As mentioned above, in most cases, IDO expression as well as kynurenines production and immunosuppressive mechanisms are carried out by infiltrating tumor cells. For GBM, microglial cells are an important source of kynurenines so, the microglial depletion could be another important strategy for tumor mitigation. Studies focusing in microglial depletion through the use of CSF-1 receptor inhibitors have shown prolonged mice survival and enhanced antitumoral immune response when animals were treated in combination with DC vaccination [145, 146]. The effect of microglial elimination on IDO expression and on the levels of KP metabolites, still remains to be elucidated, but the immune response reported with the use of the CSF-1 receptor inhibitors settle down some clues about what could happen in the KP context.

Thus, the use of IDO inhibitors and microglial elimination in combination with classical chemotherapy and radiotherapy in GBM murine models, as well as the clinical trials that have tested 1-MT in different kinds of solid and metastatic tumors has shown promising results for targeting IDO and the KP against GBM.

2.4. Concluding remarks

GBM is an astrocyte-derived tumor, the most common of brain tumors, characterized by its high proliferation rates, genomic instability, and invasiveness, as well as to being a high immunosuppressive tumor. The nature of GBM results in a rapid expansion into the surrounding tissues, associated with poor prognosis and patient low survival despite classical treatment of these tumors, tumor extirpation, temozolomide therapy, and radiotherapy, which only prolongs median survival over 2 months.

In this chapter, we have discussed the importance of the tryptophan catabolism through the KP during GBM development. Activation of this catabolic route provides cancer cells a constant

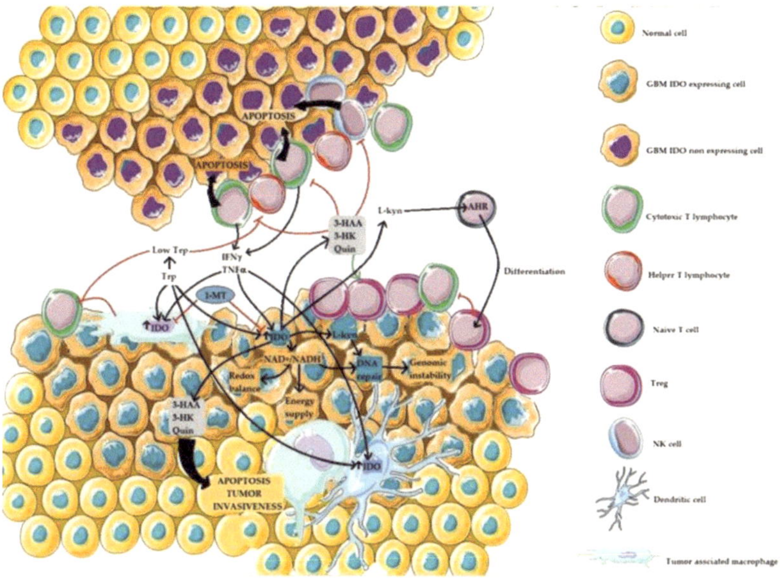

Figure 3. Global scheme of the role of IDO expression and the kynurenine pathway on glioblastoma development. During glioblastoma formation, a population of tumor cells is recognized and eliminated by the host immune system (cytotoxic T lymphocytes, helper T lymphocytes, and natural killer cells). While eliminating the recognized tumor cells, cytotoxic T lymphocytes secrete IF Nγ, TNFα, and other proinflammatory cytokines which strongly induce IDO expression and the kynurenine pathway activation in survivor glioblastoma cells and tumor infiltrating cells (dendritic cells and tumor-associated macrophages). Glioblastoma IDO expressing cells maintain a rich NAD+/NADH pool which provides redox balance, energy supply, and active DNA repairing mechanisms, facilitating genomic instability and tumor growth; also in glioblastoma cells, L-kyn also contributes to genomic instability by modulating DNA polymerase κ. In the tumor microenvironment, released L-kyn promotes Treg differentiation from naïve T cells. While 3-HAA, 3-HK, and Quin promote Treg recruitment and inhibit both cytotoxic and helper T lymphocytes activation and proliferation; and also promote T lymphocytes, natural killer cells, and nontumor cells apoptosis, promoting more invasiveness. Microenvironmental tryptophan depletion caused by high tryptophan uptake by IDO expressing cells enhances the kynurenines effect against T cell activation proliferation. Finally, the use of IDO inhibitor 1-methyl-tryptophan rises as a promising strategy for glioblastoma treatment.

supply of NAD+ and promotes the expression of damaged DNA repairing enzymes, which allow cancer cells to have an active metabolism, and to bypass redox stress and DNA damage pressure (**Figure 3**).

Furthermore, IDO expression and elevated Kyn/Trp ratios are related with poor prognosis and low survival of GBM patients. The expression of key enzymes of the KP is induced by stimulation of cytokines secreted during antitumoral immune responses, after this, tryptophan depletion and kynurenines production inhibit effector CD4+ and CD8+ T cell and NK cell proliferation, meanwhile promote Treg differentiation and MDSC infiltration into the tumor, attenuating antitumor responses. It is of note that IDO expression and immunosuppressive mechanisms are not carried out by cancer cells alone, but tumor infiltrating cells are also able to synthesize IDO and to promote an immunosuppressive environment (**Figure 3**).

The results of the use of IDO inhibitors, like 1-MT, in *in vivo* GBM models and in phase I and phase II clinical trials against lung, breast, and ovarian cancer, arise them as a promising strategy for combating GBM. However, detailed information about the role of key enzymes of the KP, KYNU, KAT, KMO, and QPRT, could provide more information for the development of more truthful treatments against GBM.

Conflict of interests

The authors report no conflicts of interest. The authors alone are responsible for the content and writing of the chapter.

Acknowledgements

This work was supported by CONACYT Grant 262010.

Author details

Gustavo Ignacio Vázquez Cervantes[1,2], Nora Karen Olascoaga Arellano[3], Daniela Ramírez Ortega[1], Alelí Salazar Ramiro[3], Dinora F. González Esquivel[1], Camilo Ríos[1], Benjamín Pineda Olvera[3] and Verónica Pérez de la Cruz[1]*

*Address all correspondence to: veped1981@gmail.com

1 Departamento de Neuroquímica, Instituto Nacional de Neurología y Neurocirugía "Manuel Velasco Suárez", Mexico

2 Doctoral Program in Biological Sciences, Universidad Nacional Autónoma de México (UNAM), Mexico

3 Laboratorio de Neuroinmunología, Instituto Nacional de Neurología y Neurocirugía "Manuel Velasco Suarez", Mexico

References

[1] Bender DA. Biochemistry of tryptophan in health and disease. Molecular Aspects of Medicine. 1982;**6**:101-197

[2] Green AR, Aronson JK, Curzon G, Woods HF. Metabolism of an oral tryptophan load. I: Effects of dose and pretreatment with tryptophan. British Journal of Clinical Pharmacology. 1980;**10**(6):603-610

[3] Heuther G, Hajak G, Reimer A, Poeggeler B, Blömer B, Rodenbeck A, Rüther E. The metabolic fate of infused l-tryptophan in men: Possible clinical implications of the accumulation of circulating tryptophan and tryptophan metabolites. Psychopharmacology. 1992;**109**(4):422-432

[4] Chen Y, Guillemin GJ. Kynurenine pathway metabolites in humans: Disease and healthy states. International Journal of Tryptophan Research. 2009;**2**:1-19

[5] Hayaishi O. Properties and function of indoleamine 2,3-dioxygenase. Journal of Biochemistry. 1976;**79**(4):13P-21P

[6] Metz R, Duhadaway JB, Kamasani U, Laury-Kleintop L, Muller AJ, Prendergast GC. Novel tryptophan catabolic enzyme IDO2 is the preferred biochemical target of the antitumor indoleamine 2,3-dioxygenase inhibitory compound D-1-methyl-tryptophan. Cancer Research. 2007;**67**(15):7082-7087. DOI: 10.1158/0008-5472.CAN-07-

[7] Ball HJ, Yuasa HJ, Austin CJ, Weiser S, Hunt NH. Indoleamine 2,3-dioxygenase-2; a new enzyme in the kynurenine pathway. The International Journal of Biochemistry and Cell Biology. 2009;**41**(3):467-471. DOI: 10.1016/j.biocel.2008.01.005

[8] Phillips RS. Structure and mechanism of kynureninase. Archives of Biochemistry and Biophysics. 2014;**544**:69-74. DOI: 10.1016/j.abb.2013.10.020

[9] Majewski M, Kozlowska A, Thoene M, Lepiarczyk E, Grzegorzewski WJ. Overview of the role of vitamins and minerals on the kynurenine pathway in health and disease. Journal of Physiology and Pharmacology. 2016;**67**(1):3-19

[10] Nematollahi A, Sun G, Harrop SJ, Hanrahan JR, Church WB. Structure of the PLP-Form of the human kynurenine aminotransferase II in a novel spacegroup at 1.83 Å resolution. International Journal of Molecular Sciences. 2016;**17**(4):446. DOI: 10.3390/ijms17040446

[11] Wang Q, Liu D, Song P, Zou MH. Deregulated tryptophan-kynurenine pathway is linked to inflammation, oxidative stress, and immune activation pathway in cardiovascular diseases. Frontiers in Bioscience. 2015;**20**:1116-1143

[12] Han Q, Fang J, Li J. Kynurenine aminotransferase and glutamine transaminase K of Escherichia coli: Identity with aspartate aminotransferase. The Biochemical Journal. 2001;**360**(Pt 3):617-623. DOI: 10.1042/BSR20100117

[13] Stavrum AK, Heiland I, Schuster S, Puntervoll P, Ziegler M. Model of tryptophan metabolism, readily scalable using tissue-specific gene expression data. The Journal of Biological Chemistry. 2013;**288**(48):34555-34566. DOI: 10.1074/jbc.M113.474908

[14] Badawy AA. Tryptophan availability for kynurenine pathway metabolism across the life span: Control mechanisms and focus on aging, exercise, diet and nutritional supplements. Neuropharmacology. 2017;**112**(Pt B):248-263. DOI: 10.1016/j.neuropharm.2015.11.015

[15] Kudo Y, Boyd CA. Human placental indoleamine 2,3-dioxygenase: Cellular localization and characterization of an enzyme preventing fetal rejection. Biochimica et Biophysica Acta. 2000;**1500**(1):119-124

[16] Basran J, Rafice SA, Chauhan N, Efimov I, Cheesman MR, Ghamsari L, Raven EL. A kinetic, spectroscopic, and redox study of human tryptophan 2,3-dioxygenase. Biochemistry. 2008;**47**(16):4752-4760. DOI: 10.1021/bi702393b

[17] Shinohara R, Ishiguro I. The purification and properties of formamidase from rat liver. Biochimica et Biophysica Acta. 1970;**198**(2):324-331

[18] Krisch K, Arndt R, Junge W, Menge U, Michelssen K. Purification and some properties of formamidase from rat and pig liver. Acta Vitaminologica et Enzymologica. 1975;**29**(1-6):302-306

[19] Han Q, Li J, Li J. pH dependence, substrate specificity and inhibition of human kynurenine aminotransferase I. European Journal of Biochemistry. 2004;**271**(23-24):4804-4814. DOI: 10.1186/1471-2091-11-19

[20] Han Q, Cai T, Tagle DA, Robinson H, Li J. Substrate specificity and structure of human aminoadipate aminotransferase/kynurenine aminotransferase II. Bioscience Reports. 2008;**28**(4):205-215. DOI: 10.1042/BSR20080085

[21] Han Q, Robinson H, Cai T, Tagle DA, Li J. Biochemical and structural properties of mouse kynurenine aminotransferase III. Molecular and Cellular Biology. 2009;**29**(3):784-793. DOI: 10.1128/MCB.01272-08

[22] Han Q, Calvo E, Marinotti O, Fang J, Rizzi M, James AA, Li J. Analysis of the wild-type and mutant genes encoding the enzyme kynurenine monooxygenase of the yellow fever mosquito, Aedes aegypti. Insect Molecular Biology. 2003;**12**(5):483-490

[23] Lima S, Kristoforov R, Momany C, Phillips RS. Crystal structure of Homo sapiens kynureninase. Biochemistry. 2008;**46**(10):2735-2744. DOI: 10.1021/bi0616697

[24] Malherbe P, Köhler C, Da Prada M, Lang G, Kiefer V, Schwarcz R, Lahm HW, Cesura AM. Molecular cloning and functional expression of human 3-hydroxyanthranilic-acid dioxygenase. The Journal of Biological Chemistry. 1994;**29**(19):13792-13797

[25] Pucci L, Perozzi S, Cimadamore F, Orsomando G, Raffaelli N. Tissue expression and biochemical characterization of human 2-amino 3-carboxymuconate 6-semialdehyde decarboxylase, a key enzyme in tryptophan catabolism. The FEBS Journal. 2007;**274**(3):827-840. DOI: 10.1111/j.1742-4658.2007.05635.x

[26] Liu H, Woznica K, Catton G, Crawford A, Botting N, Naismith JH. Structural and kinetic characterization of quinolinate phosphoribosyltransferase (hQPRTase) from Homo sapiens. Journal of Molecular Biology. 2007;**373**(3):755-763. DOI: 10.1016/j.jmb.2007.08.043

[27] Boado RJ, Li JY, Nagaya M, Zhang C, Pardridge WM. Selective expression of the large neutral amino acid transporter at the blood-brain barrier. Procedures of the National Academy of Sciences of the United States of America. 1999;**96**(21):12079-12084

[28] Schwarcz R, Stone TW. The kynurenine pathway and the brain: Challenges, controversies and promises. Neuropharmacology. 2017;**112**(Pt B):237-247. DOI: 10.1016/j.neuropharm.2016.08.003

[29] Okuda S, Nishiyama S, Saito H, Katsuki H. 3-Hydroxykynurenine, an endogenous oxidative stress generator, causes neuronal cell death with apoptotic features and region selectivity. Journal of Neurochemistry. 1998;**70**(1):299-307

[30] Nakagami Y, Saito H, Katsuki H. 3-Hydroxykynurenine toxicity on the rat striatum *in vivo*. Japanese Journal of Pharmacology. 1996;**71**(2):183-186

[31] Goldstein LE, Leopold MC, Huang X, Atwood CS, Saunders AJ, Hartshorn M, Lim JT, Faget KY, Muffat JA, Scarpa RC, Chylack Jr LT, Bowden EF, Tanzi RE, Bush AI. 3-Hydroxykynurenine and 3-hydroxyanthranilic acid generate hydrogen peroxide and promote alpha-crystallin cross-linking by metal ion reduction. Biochemistry. 2000;**39**(24):7266-7275

[32] Vazquez S, Aquilina JA, Jamie JF, Sheil MM, Truscott RJ. Novel protein modification by kynurenine in human lenses. The Journal of Biological Chemistry. 2002;**277**(7):4867-4873. DOI: 10.1074/jbc.M107529200

[33] Quagliariello E, Papa S, Saccone C, Alifano A. Effect of 3-hydroxyanthranilic acid on the mitochondrial respiratory system. The Biochemical Journal. 1964;**91**(1):137-146

[34] Goshima N, Wadano A, Miura K. 3-Hydroxykynurenine as O2- scavenger in the blowfly, Aldrichina grahami. Biochemichal and Biophysical Research Communications. 1986;**139**(2):666-672. DOI: 10.1016/S0006-291X(86)80042-0

[35] Wadano A, Takenaka Y, Matumoto M. 3-Hydroxykynurenine as a radical scavenger in the blowfly, Aldrichina grahami. Insect Biochemistry and Molecular Biology. 1993;**23**(8):919-925. DOI: 10.1016/0965-1748(93)90109-6

[36] Leipnitz G, Schumacher C, Dalcin KB, Scussiato K, Solano A, Funchal C, Dutra-Filho CS, Wyse AT, Wannmacher CM, Latini A, Wajner M. *In vitro* evidence for an antioxidant role of 3-hydroxykynurenine and 3-hydroxyanthranilic acid in the brain. Neurochemistry International. 2007;**50**(1):83-94. DOI: 10.1016/j.neuint.2006.04.017

[37] Quagliariello E, Palmieri F, Alifano A, Papa S. 3-hydroxyanthranilic acid-mediated respiration in the inhibited respiratory chain. Biochimica et Biophysica Acta. 1966;**113**(3): 482-489

[38] Foster AC, Vezzani A, French ED, Schwarcz R. Kynurenic acid blocks neurotoxicity and seizures induced in rats by the related brain metabolite quinolinic acid. Neuroscience Letters. 1984;**48**(3):273-278

[39] Lugo-Huitrón R, Blanco-Ayala T, Ugalde-Muñiz P, Carrillo-Mora P, Pedraza-Chaverrí J, Silva-Adaya D, Maldonado PD, Torres I, Pinzón E, Ortiz-Islas E, López T, García E,

Pineda B, Torres-Ramos M, Santamaría A, La Cruz VP. On the antioxidant properties of kynurenic acid: Free radical scavenging activity and inhibition of oxidative stress. Neurotoxicology and Teratology. 2011;**33**(5):538-347. DOI: 10.1016/j.ntt.2011.07.002

[40] Wang J, Simonavicius N, Wu X, Swaminath G, Reagan J, Tian H, Ling L. Kynurenic acid as a ligand for orphan G protein-coupled receptor GPR35. The Journal of Biological Chemistry. 2006;**281**(31):22021-22028. DOI: 10.1074/jbc.M603503200

[41] Cosi C, Mannaioni G, Cozzi A, Carlà V, Sili M, Cavone L, Maratea D, Moroni F. G-protein coupled receptor 35 (GPR35) activation and inflammatory pain: Studies on the antinociceptive effects of kynurenic acid and zaprinast. Neuropharmacology. 2011;**60**(7-8):1227-1231. DOI: 10.1016/j.neuropharm.2010.11.014

[42] Berlinguer-Palmini R, Masi A, Narducci R, Cavone L, Maratea D, Cozzi A, Sili M, Moroni F, Mannaioni G. GPR35 activation reduces Ca2+ transients and contributes to the kynurenic acid-dependent reduction of synaptic activity at CA3-CA1 synapses. PloS One. 2013;**8**(11):e82180. DOI: 10.1371/journal.pone.0082180

[43] Moroni F1, Cozzi A, Sili M, Mannaioni G. Kynurenic acid: a metabolite with multiple actions and multiple targets in brain and periphery. Journal of Neural Transmission. 2012;**119**(2):133-139. DOI: 10.1007/s00702-011-0763-x

[44] Kumar A, Babu GN. *In vivo* neuroprotective effects of peripheral kynurenine on acute neurotoxicity induced by glutamate in rat cerebral cortex. Neurochemical Research. 2010;**35**(4):636-644. DOI: 10.1007/s11064-009-0114-6

[45] Carrillo-Mora P, Méndez-Cuesta LA, Pérez-De La Cruz V, Fortoul-van Der Goes TI, Santamaría A. Protective effect of systemic L-kynurenine and probenecid administration on behavioural and morphological alterations induced by toxic soluble amyloid beta (25-35) in rat hippocampus. Behavioural Brain Research. 2010;**210**(2):240-250. DOI: 10.1016/j.bbr.2010.02.041

[46] Silva-Adaya D, Pérez-De La Cruz V, Villeda-Hernández J, Carrillo-Mora P, González-Herrera IG, García E, Colín-Barenque L, Pedraza-Chaverrí J, Santamaría A. Protective effect of L-kynurenine and probenecid on 6-hydroxydopamine-induced striatal toxicity in rats: Implications of modulating kynurenate as a protective strategy. Neurotoxicology and Teratology. 2011;**33**(2):303-312. DOI: 10.1016/j.ntt.2010.10.002

[47] Ribeiro CA, Grando V, Dutra Filho CS, Wannmacher CM, Wajner M. Evidence that quinolinic acid severely impairs energy metabolism through activation of NMDA receptors in striatum from developing rats. Journal of Neurochemistry. 2006;**99**(6):1531-1542

[48] Goda K, Kishimoto R, Shimizu S, Hamane Y, Ueda M. Quinolinic acid and active oxygens. Possible contribution of active Oxygens during cell death in the brain. Advances in Experimental Medicine and Biology. 1996;**398**:247-254

[49] Moroni F, Lombardi G, Moneti G, Aldinio C. The excitotoxin quinolinic acid is present in the brain of several mammals and its cortical content increases during the aging process. Neuroscience Letters. 1984;**47**(1):51-55

[50] Bordelon YM, Chesselet MF, Nelson D, Welsh F, Erecińska M. Energetic dysfunction in quinolinic acid-lesioned rat striatum. Journal of Neurochemistry. 1997;**69**(4):1629-1639

[51] Tavares RG, Tasca CI, Santos CE, Alves LB, Porciúncula LO, Emanuelli T, Souza DO. Quinolinic acid stimulates synaptosomal glutamate release and inhibits glutamate uptake into astrocytes. Neurochemistry International. 2002;**40**(7):621-627

[52] Braidy N, Brew BJ, Inestrosa NC, Chung R, Sachdev P, Guillemin GJ. Changes in Cathepsin D and Beclin-1 mRNA and protein expression by the excitotoxin quinolinic acid in human astrocytes and neurons. Metabolic Brain Disease. 2014;**29**(3):873-883. DOI: 10.1007/s11011-014-9557-9

[53] Beal MF, Kowall NW, Ellison DW, Mazurek MF, Swartz KJ, Martin JB. Replication of the neurochemical characteristics of Huntington's disease by quinolinic acid. Nature. 1986;**321**(6066):168-171. DOI: 10.1038/321168a0

[54] Stone TW. Neuropharmacology of quinolinic and kynurenic acids. Pharmacological Reviews. 1993;**45**(3):309-379

[55] Lugo-Huitrón R, Ugalde Muñiz P, Pineda B, Pedraza-Chaverrí J, Ríos C, Pérez-de la Cruz V. Quinolinic acid: an endogenous neurotoxin with multiple targets. Oxidative Medicine and Celular Longevity. 2013;**2013**:104024. DOI: 10.1155/2013/104024

[56] Heyes MP, Saito K, Jacobowitz D, Markey SP, Takikawa O, Vickers JH. Poliovirus induces indoleamine-2,3-dioxygenase and quinolinic acid synthesis in macaque brain. FASEB Journal. 1992;**6**(11):2977-2989

[57] Yan EB, Frugier T, Lim CK, Heng B, Sundaram G, Tan M, Rosenfeld JV, Walker DW, Guillemin GJ, Morganti-Kossmann MC. Activation of the kynurenine pathway and increased production of the excitotoxin quinolinic acid following traumatic brain injury in humans. Journal of Neuroinflammation. 2015;**12**:110. DOI: 10.1186/s12974-015-0328-2

[58] Brooks AK, Lawson MA, Smith RA, Janda TM, Kelley KW, McCusker RH. Interactions between inflammatory mediators and corticosteroids regulate transcription of genes within the Kynurenine Pathway in the mouse hippocampus. Journal of Neuroinflammation. 2016;**13**(1):98. DOI: 10.1186/s12974-016-0563-1

[59] Ueland PM, McCann A, Midttun Ø, Ulvik A. Inflammation, vitamin B6 and related pathways. Molecular Aspects of Medicine. 2017;**53**:10-17. DOI: 10.1016/j.mam.2016.08.001

[60] Müller A, Heseler K, Schmidt SK, Spekker K, Mackenzie CR, Däubener W. The missing link between indoleamine 2,3-dioxygenase mediated antibacterial and immunoregulatory effects. Journal of Cellular and Molecular Medicine. 2009;**13**(6):1125-1135. DOI: 10.1111/j.1582-4934.2008.00542.x

[61] Wang Q, Liu D, Song P, Zou MH. Tryptophan-kynurenine pathway is dysregulated in inflammation, and immune activation. Frontiers in Bioscience. 2015b;**20**:1116-1143

[62] Routy JP, Routy B, Graziani GM, Mehraj V. The kynurenine pathway is a Double-Edged sword in Immune-Privileged sites and in cancer: Implications for immunotherapy. International Journal of Tryptophan Research. 2016;**9**:67-77. DOI: 10.4137/IJTR.S38355

[63] Moretti S, Menicali E, Voce P, Morelli S, Cantarelli S, Sponziello M, Colella R, Fallarino F, Orabona C, Alunno A, de Biase D, Bini V, Mameli MG, Filetti S, Gerli R, Macchiarulo A, Melillo RM, Tallini G, Santoro M, Puccetti P, Avenia N, Puxeddu E. Indoleamine 2,3-dioxygenase 1 (IDO1) is up-regulated in thyroid carcinoma and drives the development of an immunosuppressant tumor microenvironment. The Journal of Clinical Endocrinology and Metabolism. 2014;**99**(5):E832-E840. DOI: 10.1210/jc.2013-3351

[64] Thaker AI, Rao MS, Bishnupuri KS, Kerr TA, Foster L, Marinshaw JM, Newberry RD, Stenson WF, Ciorba MA. IDO1 metabolites activate β-catenin signaling to promote cancer cell proliferation and colon tumorigenesis in mice. Gastroenterology. 2013;**145**(2):416-425. DOI: 10.1053/j.gastro.2013.05.002

[65] Bostian AC, Eoff RL. Aberrant kynurenine signaling modulates DNA replication stress factors and promotes genomic instability in gliomas. Chemical Research in Toxicology. 2016;**29**(9):1369-1380. DOI: 10.1021/acs.chemrestox.6b00255

[66] Heyes MP, Saito K, Milstien S, Schiff SJ. Quinolinic acid in tumors, hemorrhage and bacterial infections of the central nervous system in children. Journal of the Neurological Sciences. 1995;**133**(1-2):112-118

[67] Di Serio C, Cozzi A, Angeli I, Doria L, Micucci I, Pellerito S, Mirone P, Masotti G, Moroni F, Tarantini F. Kynurenic acid inhibits the release of the neurotrophic fibroblast growth factor (FGF)-1 and enhances proliferation of glia cells, *in vitro*. Cellular and Molecular Neurobiology. 2005;**25**(6): 981-993. DOI: 10.1007/s10571-005-8469-y

[68] Sahm F, Oezen I, Opitz CA, Radlwimmer B, von Deimling A, Ahrendt T, Adams S, Bode HB, Guillemin GJ, Wick W, Platten M. The endogenous tryptophan metabolite and NAD+ precursor quinolinic acid confers resistance of gliomas to oxidative stress. Cancer Research. 2013;**73**(11):3225-3234. DOI: 10.1158/0008-5472.CAN-12-3831

[69] Pecorino L. 2012. Molecular Biology of Cancer. Mechanisms, Targets and Therapeutics. 3rd ed. Italy: Oxford University Press

[70] Rabinovich GA, Gabrilovich D, Sotomayor EM. Immunosuppressive strategies that are mediated by tumor cells. Annual Review of Immunology. 2007;**25**:267-296. DOI: 10.1146/annurev.immunol.25.022106.141609

[71] Dunn GP, Bruce AT, Ikeda H, Old LJ, Schreiber RD. Cancer immunoediting: From immunosurveillance to tumor escape. Nature Immunology. 2002;**3**(11):991-998. DOI: 10.1038/ni1102-991

[72] Dunn GP, Old LJ, Schreiber RD. The three Es of cancer immunoediting. Annual Review of Immunology. 2004;**22**:329-360. DOI: 10.1146/annurev.immunol.22.012703.104803

[73] Yaguchi T, Kawakami Y. Cancer-induced heterogeneous immunosuppressive tumor microenvironments and their personalized modulation. International Immunology. 2016;**28**(8):393-399. DOI: 10.1093/intimm/dxw030

[74] van Baren N, Van den Eynde BJ. Tumoral immune resistance mediated by enzymes that degrade tryptophan. Cancer Immunology Research. 2015;**3**(9):978-985. DOI: 10.1158/2326-6066.CIR-15-0095

[75] Adams S, Teo C, McDonald KL, Zinger A, Bustamante S, Lim CK, Sundaram G, Braidy N, Brew BJ, Guillemin GJ. Involvement of the kynurenine pathway in human glioma pathophysiology. PloS One. 2014;**9**(11):e112945. DOI: 10.1371/journal.pone.0112945

[76] Munn DH, Mellor AL. IDO in the tumor microenvironment: Inflammation, Counter-Regulation, and tolerance. Trends in Immunology. 2016;**37**(3):193-207. DOI: 10.1016/j.it.2016.01.002

[77] Mellor AL, Munn DH. Tryptophan catabolism and T-cell tolerance: Immunosuppression by starvation? Immunology Today. 1999;**20**(10):469-473

[78] Munn DH, Shafizadeh E, Attwood JT, Bondarev I, Pashine A, Mellor AL. Inhibition of T cell proliferation by macrophage tryptophan catabolism. The Journal of Experimental Medicine. 1999;**189**(9):1363-1372

[79] Poormasjedi-Meibod MS, Jalili RB, Hosseini-Tabatabaei A, Hartwell R, Ghahary A. Immuno-regulatory function of indoleamine 2,3 dioxygenase through modulation of innate immune responses. PloS One. 2013;**8**(8):e71044. DOI: 10.1371/journal.pone.0071044

[80] Jochems C, Fantini M, Fernando RI, Kwilas AR, Donahue RN, Lepone LM, Grenga I, Kim YS, Brechbiel MW, Gulley JL, Madan RA, Heery CR, Hodge JW, Newton R, Schlom J, Tsang KY. The IDO1 selective inhibitor epacadostat enhances dendritic cell immunogenicity and lytic ability of tumor antigen-specific T cells. Oncotarget. 2016;**7**(25):37762-37772. DOI: 10.18632/oncotarget.9326

[81] Mezrich JD, Fechner JH, Zhang X, Johnson BP, Burlingham WJ, Bradfield CA. An interaction between kynurenine and the aryl hydrocarbon receptor can generate regulatory T cells. Journal of Immunology. 2010;**185**(6):3190-3198. DOI: 10.4049/jimmunol.0903670

[82] Frumento G, Rotondo R, Tonetti M, Damonte G, Benatti U, Ferrara GB. Tryptophan-derived catabolites are responsible for inhibition of T and natural killer cell proliferation induced by indoleamine 2,3-dioxygenase. The Journal of Experimental Medicine. 2002;**196**(4):459-468

[83] Terness P, Bauer TM, Röse L, Dufter C, Watzlik A, Simon H, Opelz G. Inhibition of allogeneic T cell proliferation by indoleamine 2,3-dioxygenase-expressing dendritic cells: Mediation of suppression by tryptophan metabolites. The Journal of Experimental Medicine. 2002;**196**(4):447-457

[84] Belladonna ML, Puccetti P, Orabona C, Fallarino F, Vacca C, Volpi C, Gizzi S, Pallotta MT, Fioretti MC, Grohmann U. Immunosuppression via tryptophan catabolism: The role of kynurenine pathway enzymes. Transplantation. 2007;**84**(1 Suppl):S17-S20. DOI: 10.1097/01.tp.0000269199.16209.22

[85] Zaher SS, Germain C, Fu H, Larkin DF, George AJ. 3-hydroxykynurenine suppresses CD4+ T-cell proliferation, induces T-regulatory-cell development, and prolongs corneal

allograft survival. Investigative Ophthalmology and Visual Science. 2011;**52**(5):2640-2648. DOI: 10.1167/iovs.10-5793

[86] Ninomiya S, Narala N, Huye L, Yagyu S, Savoldo B, Dotti G, Heslop HE, Brenner MK, Rooney CM, Ramos CA. Tumor indoleamine 2,3-dioxygenase (IDO) inhibits CD19-CAR T cells and is downregulated by lymphodepleting drugs. Blood. 2015;**125**(25):3905-3916. DOI: 10.1182/blood-2015-01-621474

[87] Ochs K, Sahm F, Opitz CA, Lanz TV, Oezen I, Couraud PO, von Deimling A, Wick W, Platten M. Immature mesenchymal stem cell-like pericytes as mediators of immunosuppression in human malignant glioma. Journal of Neuroimmunology. 2013;**265**(1-2):106-116. DOI: 10.1016/j.jneuroim.2013.09.011

[88] Ling W, Zhang J, Yuan Z, Ren G, Zhang L, Chen X, Rabson AB, Roberts AI, Wang Y, Shi Y. Mesenchymal stem cells use IDO to regulate immunity in tumor microenvironment. Cancer Research. 2014;**74**(5):1576-1587. DOI: 10.1158/0008-5472.CAN-13-1656

[89] Vacchelli E, Aranda F, Eggermont A, Sautès-Fridman C, Tartour E, Kennedy EP, Platten M, Zitvogel L, Kroemer G, Galluzzi L. Trial watch: IDO inhibitors in cancer therapy. Oncoimmunology. 2014;**3**(10):e957994. DOI: 10.4161/21624011.2014.957994

[90] Kimelberg HK. The problem of astrocyte identity. Neurochemistry International. 2004;**45**(2-3):191-202. DOI: 10.1016/j.neuint.2003.08.015

[91] Matyash V, Kettenmann H. Heterogeneity in astrocyte morphology and physiology. Brain Research Reviews. 2010;**63**(1-2):2-10. DOI: 10.1016/j.brainresrev.2009.12.001

[92] American Brain Tumor Association. Astrocytoma [Internet]. 2017. Available from: http://www.abta.org/brain-tumor-information/types-of-tumors/astrocytoma.html [Accessed: 16-February-2017]

[93] American Brain Tumor Association. Glioblastoma [Internet]. 2017. Available from: http://www.abta.org/brain-tumor-information/types-of-tumors/glioblastoma.html [Accessed: 16-February-2017]

[94] Ostrom QT, Gittleman H, Farah P, Ondracek A, Chen Y, Wolinsky Y, Stroup NE, Kruchko C, Barnholtz-Sloan JS. CBTRUS statistical report: Primary brain and central nervous system tumors diagnosed in the United States in 2006-2010. Neuro-oncology. 2013;**15**(Suppl 2):ii1-ii56. DOI: 10.1093/neuonc/not151

[95] Thakkar JP, Dolecek TA, Horbinski C, Ostrom QT, Lightner DD, Barnholtz-Sloan JS, Villano JL. Epidemiologic and molecular prognostic review of glioblastoma. Cancer Epidemiology, Biomarkers & Prevention: A publication of the American Association of Cancer Research, cosponsored by the American Society of Preventive Oncology. 2014;**23**(10):1985-1996. DOI: 10.1158/1055-9965.EPI-14-0275

[96] MacDonald TJ, Aguilera D, Kramm CM. Treatment of high-grade glioma in children and adolescents. Neuro-oncology. 2011;**13**(10):1049-1058. DOI: 10.1093/neuonc/nor092

[97] Fangusaro J. Pediatric high grade glioma: A review and update on tumor clinical characteristics and biology. Frontiers in Oncology. 2012;**2**:105. DOI: 10.3389/fonc.2012.00105

[98] Song KS, Phi JH, Cho BK, Wang KC, Lee JY, Kim DG, Kim IH, Ahn HS, Park SH, Kim SK. Long-term outcomes in children with glioblastoma. Journal of Neurosurgery. Pediatrics. 2010;**6**(2):145-149. DOI: 10.3171/2010.5.PEDS09558

[99] Dana Farber Cancer Institute [Internet]. 2017. Available from: http://www.dana-farber.org/Adult-Care/Treatment-and-Support/Glioblastoma.aspx [Accessed: February 20, 2017]

[100] Simpson JR, Horton J, Scott C, Curran WJ, Rubin P, Fischbach J, Isaacson S, Rotman M, Asbell SO, Nelson JS, Weinstein AS, Nelson DF. Influence of location and extent of surgical resection on survival of patients with glioblastoma multiforme: Results of three consecutive Radiation Therapy Oncology Group (RTOG) clinical trials. International Journal of Radiation Oncology, Biology, Physics. 1993;**26**(2):239-244

[101] Stupp R, Mason WP, van den Bent MJ, Weller M, Fisher B, Taphoorn MJ, Belanger K, Brandes AA, Marosi C, Bogdahn U, Curschmann J, Janzer RC, Ludwin SK, Gorlia T, Allgeier A, Lacombe D, Cairncross JG, Eisenhauer E, Mirimanoff RO. European Organisation for Research and Treatment of Cancer Brain Tumor and Radiotherapy Groups; National Cancer Institute of Canada Clinical Trials Group. Radiotherapy plus concomitant and adjuvant temozolomide for glioblastoma. The New England Journal of Medicine. 2005;**352**(10):987-996. DOI: 10.1056/NEJMoa043330

[102] Mahvash M, Hugo HH, Maslehaty H, Mehdorn HM, Stark AM. Glioblastoma multiforme in children: Report of 13 cases and review of the literature. Pediatric Neurology. 2011;**45**(3):178-180. DOI: 10.1016/j.pediatrneurol.2011.05.004

[103] Verhaak RG, Hoadley KA, Purdom E, Wang V, Qi Y, Wilkerson MD, Miller CR, Ding L, Golub T, Mesirov JP, Alexe G, Lawrence M, O'Kelly M, Tamayo P, Weir BA, Gabriel S, Winckler W, Gupta S, Jakkula L, Feiler HS, Hodgson JG, James CD, Sarkaria JN, Brennan C, Kahn A, Spellman PT, Wilson RK, Speed TP, Gray JW, Meyerson M, Getz G, Perou CM, Hayes DN. Cancer Genome Atlas Research Network. Integrated genomic analysis identifies clinically relevant subtypes of glioblastoma characterized by abnormalities in PDGFRA, IDH1, EGFR, and NF1. Cancer Cell. 2010;**17**(1):98-110. DOI: 10.1016/j.ccr.2009.12.020

[104] Herwig S, Strauss M. The retinoblastoma protein: A master regulator of cell cycle, differentiation and apoptosis. European Journal of Biochemistry. 1997;**246**(3):581-601

[105] Urbańska K, Sokołowska J, Szmidt M, Sysa P. Glioblastoma multiforme—An overview. Contemporary Oncology. 2014;**18**(5):307-312. DOI: 10.5114/wo.2014.40559

[106] Linkous AG, Yazlovitskaya EM. Angiogenesis in glioblastoma multiforme: Navigating the maze. Anti-cancer Agents in Medicinal Chemistry. 2011;**11**(8):712-718

[107] Forrester JV, Xu H, Lambe T, Cornall R. Immune privilege or privileged immunity? Mucosal Immunology. 2008;**1**(5):372-381. DOI: 10.1038/mi.2008.27

[108] Loveau A, Harris TH, Kipnis J. Revisiting the concept of CNS immune privilege. Trends in Immunology. 2015;**36**(10):569-577. DOI: 10.1016/j.it.2015.08.006

[109] Razavi SM, Lee KE, Jin BE, Aujla PS, Gholamin S, Li G. Immune evasion strategies of hlioblastoma. Frontiers in Surgery. 2016;**3**:11. DOI: 10.3389/fsurg.2016.00011

[110] Galea I, Bernardes-Silva M, Forse PA, van Rooijen N, Liblau RS, Perry VH. An antigen-specific pathway for CD8 T cells across the blood-brain barrier. The Journal of Experimental Medicine. 2007;**204**(9):2023-2030. DOI: 10.1084/jem.20070064

[111] Woodworth GF, Dunn GP, Nance EA, Hanes J, Brem H. Emerging insights into barriers to effective brain tumor therapeutics. Frontiers in Oncology. 2014;**4**:126. DOI: 10.3389/fonc.2014.00126

[112] Gorbachev, AV, Kobayashi H, Kudo D, Tannenbaum CS, Finke JH, Shu S, Farber JM, Fairchild RL. CXC chemokine ligand 9/monokine induced by IFN-gamma production by tumor cells is critical for T cell-mediated suppression of cutaneous tumors. Journal of Immunology. 2007;**178**(4):2278-2286

[113] Sakai K, Shimodaira S, Maejima S, Udagawa N, Sano K, Higuchi Y, Koya T, Ochiai T, Koide M, Uehara S, Nakamura M, Sugiyama H, Yonemitsu Y, Okamoto M, Hongo K. Dendritic cell-based immunotherapy targeting Wilms' tumor 1 in patients with recurrent malignant glioma. Journal of Neurosurgery. 2015;**123**(4):989-997. DOI: 10.3171/2015.1.JNS141554

[114] Yang I, Han SJ, Sughrue ME, Tihan T, Parsa AT. Immune cell infiltrate differences in pilocytic astrocytoma and glioblastoma: Evidence of distinct immunological microenvironments that reflect tumor biology. Journal of Neurosurgery. 2011;**115**(3):505-511. DOI: 10.3171/2011.4.JNS101172

[115] Prins RM, Soto H, Konkankit V, Odesa SK, Eskin A, Yong WH, Nelson SF, Liau LM. Gene expression profile correlates with T-cell infiltration and relative survival in glioblastoma patients vaccinated with dendritic cell immunotherapy. Clinical Cancer Research. 2011;**17**(6):1603-1615. DOI: 10.1158/1078-0432.CCR-10-2563

[116] Prins RM, Wang X, Soto H, Young E, Lisiero DN, Fong B, Everson R, Yong WH, Lai A, Li G, Cloughesy TF, Liau LM. Comparison of glioma-associated antigen peptide-loaded versus autologous tumor lysate-loaded dendritic cell vaccination in malignant glioma patients. Journal of Immunotherapy. 2013;**36**(2):152-157. DOI: 10.1097/CJI.0b013e3182811ae4

[117] Schmittling RJ, Archer GE, Mitchell DA, Heimberger A, Pegram C, Herndon JE 2nd, Friedman HS, Bigner DD, Sampson JH. Detection of humoral response in patients with glioblastoma receiving EGFRvIII-KLH vaccines. Journal of Immunological Methods. 2008;**339**(1):74-81. DOI: 10.1016/j.jim.2008.08.004

[118] Fadul CE, Fisher JL, Hampton TH, Lallana EC, Li Z, Gui J, Szczepiorkowski ZM, Tosteson TD, Rhodes CH, Wishart HA, Lewis LD, Ernstoff MS. Immune response in patients with newly diagnosed glioblastoma multiforme treated with intranodal autologous tumor lysate-dendritic cell vaccination after radiation chemotherapy. Journal of Immunotherapy. 2011;**34**(4):382-389. DOI: 10.1097/CJI.0b013e318215e300. DOI: 10.1097/CJI.0b013e318215e300

[119] Sampson JH, Heimberger AB, Archer GE, Aldape KD, Friedman AH, Friedman HS, Gilbert MR, Herndon 2nd JE, McLendon RE, Mitchell DA, Reardon DA, Sawaya R, Schmittling RJ, Shi W, Vredenburgh JJ, Bigner DD. Immunologic escape after prolonged progression-free survival with epidermal growth factor receptor variant III peptide vaccination in patients with newly diagnosed glioblastoma. Journal of Clinical Oncology. 2010;**28**(31):4722-2729. DOI: 10.1200/JCO.2010.28.6963. DOI: 10.1200/JCO.2010.28.6963

[120] Sampson JH, Aldape KD, Archer GE, Coan A, Desjardins A, Friedman AH, Friedman HS, Gilbert MR, Herndon JE, McLendon RE, Mitchell DA, Reardon DA, Sawaya R, Schmittling R, Shi W, Vredenburgh JJ, Bigner DD, Heimberger AB. Greater chemotherapy-induced lymphopenia enhances tumor-specific immune responses that eliminate EGFRvIII-expressing tumor cells in patients with glioblastoma. Neuro-oncology. 2011;**13**(3):324-333. DOI: 10.1093/neuonc/noq157

[121] Huettner C, Palaus W, Roggendorf W. Messenger RNA expression of the immunosuppressive cytokine IL-10 in human gliomas. American Journal of Patjology. 1995;**146**(2): 317-322

[122] Yang I, Han SJ, Kaur G, Crane C, Parsa AT. The role of microglia in central nervous system immunity and glioma immunology. Journal of Clinical Neuroscience. 2010;**17**(1):6-10. DOI: 10.1016/j.jocn.2009.05.006

[123] Badie B, Schartner J, Prabakaran S, Paul J, Vorpahl J. Expression of Fas ligand by microglia: Possible role in glioma immune evasion. Journal of Neuroimmunology. 2001;**120**(1-2):19-24

[124] Hao C, Parney IF, Roa WH, Turner J, Petruk KC, Ramsay DA. Cytokine and cytokine receptor mRNA expression in human glioblastomas: Evidence of Th1, Th2 and Th3 cytokine dysregulation. Acta Neuropathologica. 2002;**103**(2):171-178. DOI: 10.1007/s004010100448

[125] Jackson C, Ruzevick J, Phallen J, Belcaid Z, Lim M. Challenges in immunotherapy presented by the glioblastoma multiforme microenvironment. Clinical and Developmental Immunology. 2011;**2011**:732413. DOI: 10.1155/2011/732413

[126] Parney IF, Farr-Jones MA, Chang LJ, Petruk KC. Human glioma immunobiology *in vitro*: Implications for Immunogene Therapy. Neurosurgery. 2000;**46**(5):1169-1177

[127] Fontana A, Kristensen F, Dubs R, Gemsa D, Weber E. Production of prostaglandin E and an interleukin-1 like factor by cultured astrocytes and C6 glioma cells. Journal of Immunology. 1982;**129**(6):2413-2419

[128] Siepl C, Bodmer S, Frei K, MacDonald HR, De Martin R, Hofer E, Fontana A. The glioblastoma-derived T cell suppressor factor/transforming growth factor-beta 2 inhibits T cell growth without affecting the interaction of interleukin 2 with its receptor. Eurpean Journal of Immunology. 1988;**18**(4):593-600. DOI: 10.1002/eji.1830180416

[129] Kuppner MC, Hamou MF, Sawamura Y, Bodmer S, de Tribolet N. Inhibition of lymphocyte function by glioblastoma-derived transforming growth factor beta 2. Journal of Neurosurgery. 1989;**71**(2):211-217. DOI: 10.3171/jns.1989.71.2.0211

[130] Wischhusen J, Jung G, Radovanovic I, Beier C, Steinbach JP, Rimner A, Huang H, Schulz JB, Ohgaki H, Aguzzi A, Rammensee HA, Weller M. Identification of CD70-mediated apoptosis of immune effector cells as a novel immune escape pathway of human glioblastoma. Cancer Research. 2002;**62**(9):2592-2599

[131] Chahlavi A, Rayman P, Richmond AL, Biswas K, Zhang R, Vogelbaum M, Tannenbaum C, Barnett G, Finke JH. Glioblastomas induce T-lymphocyte death by two distinct pathways involving gangliosides and CD70. Cancer Research. 2005;**65**(12):5428-5438. DOI: 10.1158/0008-5472.CAN-04-4395

[132] Weathers SP, de Groot J. VEGF manipulation in glioblastoma. Oncology (Williston Park). 2015;**29**(10):720-727

[133] Lin EY, Li JF, Gnatovskiy L, Deng Y, Zhu L, Grzesik DA, Qian H, Xue XN, Pollard JW. Macrophages regulate the angiogenic switch in a mouse model of breast cancer. Cancer Research. 2006;**66**(23):11238-11246. DOI: 10.1158/0008-5472.CAN-06-1278

[134] Wainwright DA, Balyasnikova IV, Chang AL, Ahmed AU, Moon KS, Auffinger B, Tobias AL, Han Y, Lesniak MS. IDO expression in brain tumors increases the recruitment of regulatory T cells and negatively impacts survival. Clinical Cancer Research. 2012;**18**(22):6110-6121. DOI: 10.1158/1078-0432.CCR-12-2130

[135] Mitsuka K, Kawataki T, Satoh E, Asahara T, Horikoshi T, Kinouchi H. Expression of indoleamine 2,3-dioxygenase and correlation with pathological malignancy in gliomas. Neurosurgery. 2013;**72**(6):1031-1038. DOI: 10.1227/NEU.0b013e31828cf945

[136] Zhai L, Dey M, Lauing KL, Gritsina G, Kaur R, Lukas RV, Nicholas MK, Rademaker AW, Dostal CR, McCusker RH, Raizer JJ, Parsa AT, Bloch O, Wainwright DA. The kynurenine to tryptophan ratio as a prognostic tool for glioblastoma patients enrolling in immunotherapy. Journal of Clinical Neuroscience. 2015a;**22**(12):1964-1968. DOI: 10.1227/NEU.0b013e31828cf945

[137] Friberg M, Jennings R, Alsarraj M, Dessureault S, Cantor A, Extermann M, Mellor AL, Munn DH, Antonia SJ. Indoleamine 2,3-dioxygenase contributes to tumor cell evasion of T cell-mediated rejection. International Journal of Cancer. 2002;**101**(2):151-155. DOI: 10.1002/ijc.10645

[138] Uyttenhove C, Pilotte L, Théate I, Stroobant V, Colau D, Parmentier N, Boon T, Van den Eynde BJ. Evidence for a tumoral immune resistance mechanism based on tryptophan

degradation by indoleamine 2,3-dioxygenase. Nature Medicine. 2003;**9**(10):1269-1274. DOI: 10.1038/nm934

[139] Iversen TZ, Engell-Noerregaard L, Ellebaek E, Andersen R, Larsen SK, Bjoern J, Zeyher C, Gouttefangeas C, Thomsen BM, Holm B, Thor Straten P, Mellemgaard A, Andersen MH, Svane IM. Long-lasting disease stabilization in the absence of toxicity in metastatic lung cancer patients vaccinated with an epitope derived from indoleamine 2,3 dioxygenase. Clinical Cancer Research. 2014;**20**(1):221-232. DOI: 10.1158/1078-0432.CCR-13-1560

[140] A Phase 2 Study of the IDO Inhibitor INCB024360 Versus Tamoxifen for Subjects With Biochemical-recurrent-only EOC, PPC or FTC Following Complete Remission With First-line Chemotherapy [Internet]. 2017. Available from: https://clinicaltrials.gov/ct2/show/NCT01685255?term=NCT01685255&rank=1 [Accessed: February 25, 2017]

[141] Vaccination with Peptides in Combination with Either Ipilimumab or Vemurafenib for the Treatment of Unresectable Stage III or IV Malignant Melanoma [Internet]. 2017. Available from: https://clinicaltrials.gov/ct2/show/NCT02077114?term=NCT02077114&rank=1 [Accessed: February 25, 2017]

[142] Li M, Bolduc AR, Hoda MN, Gamble DN, Dolisca SB, Bolduc AK, Hoang K, Ashley C, McCall D, Rojiani AM, Maria BL, Rixe O, MacDonald TJ, Heeger PS, Mellor AL, Munn DH, Johnson TS. The indoleamine 2,3-dioxygenase pathway controls complement-dependent enhancement of chemo-radiation therapy against murine glioblastoma. Journal of Immunotherapy for Cancer. 2014;**2**:21. DOI: 10.1186/2051-1426-2-21

[143] Hanihara M, Kawataki T, Oh-Oka K, Mitsuka K, Nakao A, Kinouchi H. Synergistic antitumor effect with indoleamine 2,3-dioxygenase inhibition and temozolomide in a murine glioma model. Journal of Neurosurgery. 2016;**124**(6):1594-1601. DOI: 10.3171/2015.5.JNS141901

[144] Zhai L, Spranger S, Binder DC, Gritsina G, Lauing KL, Giles FJ, Wainwright DA. Molecular pathways: Targeting IDO1 and other tryptophan dioxygenases for cancer immunotherapy. Clinical Cancer Research. 2015b;**21**(24):5427-5433. DOI: 10.1158/1078-0432.CCR-15-0420

[145] Antonios JP, Soto H, Everson RG, Moughon D, Orpilla JR, Shin NP, Sedighim S, Treger J, Odesa S, Tucker A, Yong WH, Li G, Cloughesy TF, Liau LM, Prins RM. Immunosuppressive tumor-infiltrating myeloid cells mediate adaptive immune resistance via a PD-1/PD-L1 mechanism in glioblastoma.Neuro-oncology. 2017;**19**(6): 796-807.

[146] Zhai L, Ladomersky E, Dostal CR, Lauing KL, Swoap K, Billingham LK, Gritsina G, Wu M, McCusker RH, Binder DC, Wainwright DA. Non-tumor cell IDO1 predominantly contributes to enzyme activity and response to CTLA-4/PD-L1 inhibition in mouse glioblastoma. Brain, Behavior, and Immunity. 2017. **62**:S0889-1591(17)30020-X. DOI: 10.1016/j.bbi.2017.01.022

Chapter 11

Neuroinflammatory Signals during Acute and Chronic Liver Diseases

Matthew McMillin and Sharon DeMorrow

Additional information is available at the end of the chapter

http://dx.doi.org/10.5772/intechopen.68938

Abstract

A spectrum of neurological complications can result from acute and chronic liver diseases and is termed hepatic encephalopathy. The precise pathogenic mechanisms by which hepatic encephalopathy occurs is unclear. However, it is commonly accepted that the development of hepatic encephalopathy shares a long-standing relationship with neuroinflammation. This chapter will outline the evidence for a role of neuroinflammation and proinflammatory cytokines in the pathogenesis of hepatic encephalopathy. Furthermore, we will identify the possible circulating factors, released from the liver after damage, that may contribute to the neurological complications of hepatic encephalopathy, including neuroinflammation. Lastly, we discuss the current and experimental treatment options aimed at reducing neuroinflammation for the management of hepatic encephalopathy.

Keywords: hepatic encephalopathy, microglia, acute liver disease, liver cirrhosis, cytokines

1. Introduction

Hepatic encephalopathy (HE) describes a spectrum of neurological complications that arise during acute liver failure or chronic liver diseases and can be classified depending upon the underlying liver pathology. Specifically, Type A HE is associated with acute liver failure. Acute liver failure, or fulminant hepatic failure, is a rapid deterioration of liver function without any pre-existing liver disease. It can arise due to drug-induced liver injury (e.g., acetaminophen overdose), viral hepatitis or ischemic hepatitis. Type B HE arises from a portal-systemic bypass without underlying liver disease. This occurs when blood bypasses the liver, thereby bypassing the detoxification function of the liver, resulting in an increased buildup of toxic substances in the blood stream and subsequent neurological impairment. Lastly, type C HE is a result of liver cirrhosis. In late stage chronic liver diseases, when severe fibrosis is evident, the liver decompensates leading to the development of HE. Recently, it was suggested that a 4th type of HE exists that results from acute-on-chronic liver failure. This occurs when an acute liver insult (e.g., an infection) occurs in a patient with an existing chronic liver condition. The HE that may arise has features in common with both Type A and Type C HE and therefore perhaps should be characterized as its own entity.

Regardless of the type of HE, clinical symptoms of HE range from altered cognitive function, mood changes, disorientation, and neuromuscular problems such as asterixis and ataxia, which ultimately culminate in hepatic coma. Associated with these symptoms are cerebral edema, leading to increased intracranial pressure (evident only in HE due to acute liver failure), astrocyte swelling, neuronal dysfunction and neuroinflammation.

The neurological changes during HE are thought to arise due to the buildup of toxic or inflammatory substance in the blood stream as a result of impaired liver function. With the increased permeability of the blood-brain barrier observed in patients and in animal models of HE, these substances are able to cross the blood-brain barrier and alter cognitive function. While the full scope of liver-derived substances may not yet be fully appreciated, some of these include ammonia buildup, increased bile acids and circulating proinflammatory cytokines. The consequences of these agents on the brain, and neuroinflammation in particular, will be discussed in detail below.

2. Microglia activation during HE

Neuroinflammation is a key feature in common with all types of HE and is predominantly modulated by microglia, the resident macrophage-like cell in the brain. Microglia are normally found in their quiescent or ramified form, characterized morphologically by small cell body and long, branching processes. The cell body typically remains stationary, whereas the processes are constantly moving and surveying their microenvironment for proinflammatory signals released by surrounding damaged neurons, infectious agents etc. Upon activation, microglia undergo morphological changes, including a thickening and retraction of the branches and increased cell body volume, and produce increased amounts of proinflammatory cytokines and recruitment molecules (e.g., chemokines). A schematic diagram of these morphological changes can be seen in **Figure 1**. Furthermore, reactive microglia undergo rapid proliferation to increase their number. The increased microglia number at a site of trauma is thought to be a combination of proliferation of resident microglia and recruitment of microglia from neighboring areas.

Microglial activation has been demonstrated to be a key feature in the pathogenesis of HE regardless of the type. Indirect clinical evidence for microglial activation has been demonstrated by an upregulation of the microglial marker Ionized calcium binding adaptor molecule 1 (Iba-1) in postmortem cortical brain tissue from patients with liver cirrhosis and HE, when compared to cirrhotic patients without HE [1]. In addition, data from a comprehensive gene expression profile analysis demonstrated an upregulation of markers for both the

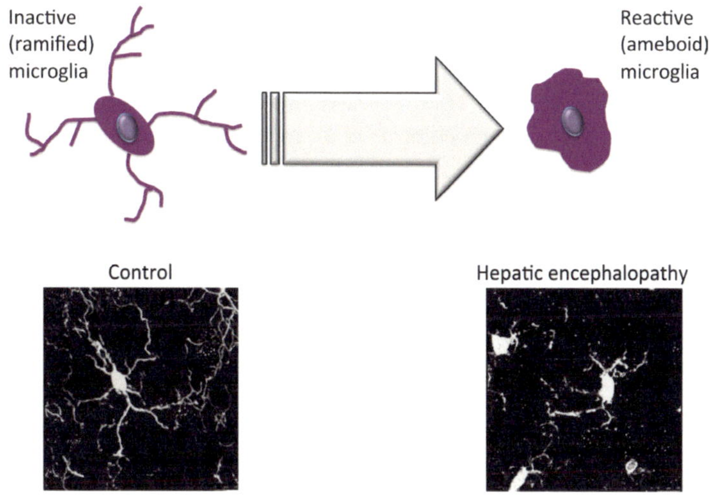

Figure 1. Schematic diagram depicting changes in microglia morphology during neuroinflammation. Lower panels show immunofluorescent staining of microglia using an Iba1-specific antibody in a mouse model of HE.

proinflammatory M1 and anti-inflammatory M2 microglial phenotypes, suggesting that both subpopulations of microglia may be present in patients with HE due to cirrhosis [2]. Taken together, these clinical data indirectly support a role of microglia activation in HE.

In contrast, evidence for a direct role for microglia activation in the neurological consequences of both acute liver failure and liver cirrhosis is more striking in animal models of these diseases. Furthermore, in many of the models used, treatment modalities shown to inhibit microglia activation also alleviated or prevented the cognitive impairment and neurological decline observed during HE. Specific details are described below.

2.1. Toxic liver injury

A range of hepatotoxic agents have been used to uncover basic mechanisms responsible for the CNS complications of liver failure. This topic was reviewed by a panel of experts nominated by The International Society for Hepatic Encephalopathy and Nitrogen Metabolism (ISHEN) who, after careful deliberation, recommended two toxic models based upon the extent of their characterization. The two models of acute liver failure were the azoxymethane (AOM) mouse model and the thioacetamide (TAA) rat model [3]***. Very elegant and detailed analyses of the morphological changes in microglia and real-time analysis of microglial dysmotility after AOM have been demonstrated [4]. Both microglia activation (as demonstrated by an ameboidal phenotype) and motility (as demonstrated by analysis of the turnover rate) were shown to be altered in the cerebral cortex at late stages of HE when severe neurological symptoms were evident, coinciding with the appearance of brain edema [4]. Furthermore, increased number of microglia [5–7] and increased reactive phenotype [6] has been demonstrated in the cerebral cortex of AOM-injected mice. This HE-associated microgliosis could be attenuated with anti-inflammatory treatment modalities [5–7], which also attenuated or delayed various neurocognitive deficits observed in this model of Type A HE, indicating that microglia activation may be contributing to the behavioral abnormalities observed in HE rather than as a consequence.

While microglia activation has not been assessed specifically in the ISHEN-recommended TAA rat model of acute liver failure, Faleiros et al. recently assessed this phenomenon using the relatively uncharacterized TAA mouse model of acute liver failure [8]. While mice injected with TAA displayed a significant reduction in locomotor activity, which was accompanied by increased expression of certain proinflammatory cytokines and chemokines, no microglia activation was observed [8]. However, it is conceivable that this observation may be an anomaly of this model rather than evidence of a lack of microglia involvement.

2.2. Ischemic liver failure

Experimental acute liver failure can be induced by the performing an end-to-side portacaval anastomosis followed by hepatic artery ligation and is thought to mimic ischemic liver failure. Rats undergoing this surgery exhibit key clinical features of HE, including cerebral edema and hyperammonemia, which ultimately result in grade 4 HE (hepatic coma). An increase in the number of OX-42/CD11b positive microglia has been demonstrated in the frontal cortex, thalamus, hippocampus and cerebellum starting 6 h after surgery (early stage HE) and worsening at the time of coma/edema [9, 10]. These pathological effects, to include brain edema and HE progression, could be alleviated by either mild hypothermia [9] or treatment with minocycline [10].

2.3. Portal-systemic (bypass) encephalopathy

In a related, more subtle model of HE induced by end-to-side portacaval shunt surgery without subsequent hepatic artery ligation, rats develop mild cognitive impairment over the following 3–4 weeks. Associated with this mild form of HE (or minimal HE) is a change in the microglia morphology to a more ameboid, activated phenotype [11, 12]. Curiously, these changes were restricted to cerebellum. Chronic infusion of a p38 mitogen-activated protein kinase inhibitor [11] or the phosphodiesterase inhibitor Sildenafil [12] reversed the morphological changes observed in microglia and prevented the cognitive impairment.

2.4. Biliary cirrhosis

Obstruction of the common bile duct induces a reproducible model of biliary cirrhosis in rats. Bile duct-ligated (BDL) animals have liver failure, developing jaundice, portal hypertension, portal-systemic shunting, bacterial translocation and immune system dysfunction. BDL rats are hyperammonemic but show only low-grade or minimal encephalopathy (decreased locomotor activities) [3]. Using this model, microglia are activated predominantly in the cerebellum with only traces of activation in the striatum and thalamus [13]. Treatment with ibuprofen reduced microglia activation and reversed the concomitant cognitive impairments observed [13]. Similarly, microglia activation has been shown after BDL in mice, as demonstrated by morphological changes in Iba-1 positive microglia [14]. However, in contrast to

http://dx.doi.org/10.5772/intechopen.68938

the rat model, the activation of microglia was localized to the cerebral cortex rather than the cerebellum. The cause of these region-and species-selective changes remains unknown. The activation of microglia in BDL mice is thought to subsequently recruit monocytes to the brain that contribute to the cognitive impairment observed [15].

3. Mechanism of microglia activation during HE

As mentioned above, the development of HE appears to be due to the buildup of toxic or inflammatory substances in the blood stream as a result of impaired liver function. While the identity of all of these substances is likely unknown, a summary of the identified factors and their involvement in HE is shown in **Figure 2** and is described in greater detail as follows:

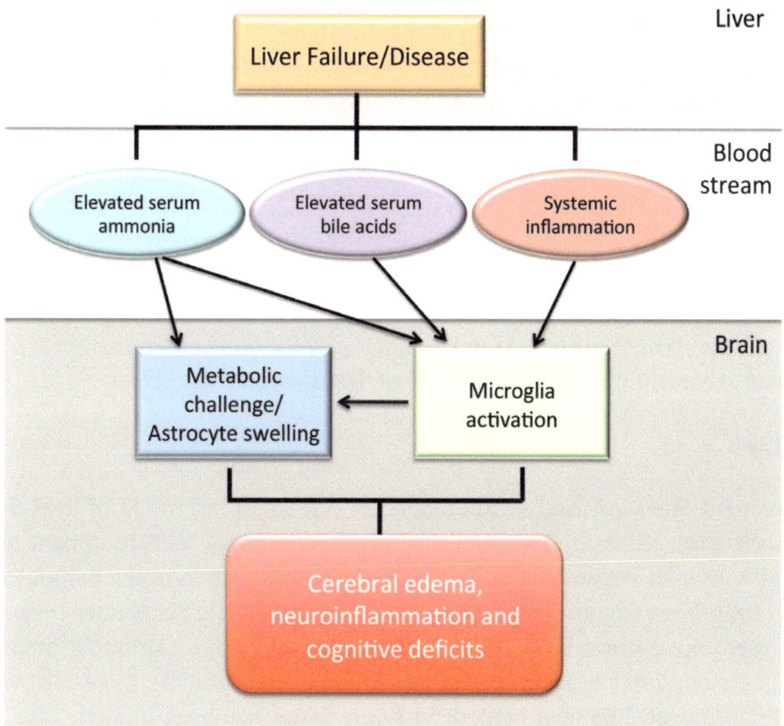

Figure 2. Schematic diagram depicting the current knowledge of the pathogenic mechanisms of HE. Following liver failure or chronic liver disease, there are elevations of serum ammonia, circulating bile acids and systemic inflammation. All of these are able to promote microglia activation as has been shown by numerous studies. In addition, elevated cerebral ammonia leads to an elevation of glutamine in astrocytes causing a metabolic challenge and swelling of astrocytes. There are potential mechanisms at play in which activated microglia promote astrocyte swelling. Both astrocyte swelling and microglia activation promote the development of HE.

3.1. Ammonia

Ammonia is a nitrogenous compound that is the best-characterized neurotoxin that contributes to the development of HE. Ammonia is generated through both gut bacteria and enterocytes and is subsequently metabolized by the liver into urea after its passage through the portal tract [16, 17]. Urea, unlike ammonia, can be excreted from the body via the kidney. However, when the liver is damaged or diseased, this detoxification of ammonia into urea by the liver is impaired leading to significant elevations of ammonia in the bloodstream. Ammonia has the capability to cross the blood-brain barrier during HE and once in the brain, ammonia is taken up by astrocytes [18]. Astrocytes metabolize ammonia into glutamate and subsequently into glutamine via glutamine synthetase. The increased levels of glutamine inside of astrocytes cause an osmotic gradient which results in the swelling of astrocytes and cytotoxic edema [19]. This results in a morphological change in astrocytes, which have been characterized as Alzheimer type II astrocytes, which are a neuropathological marker of this disease state [20].

Ammonia can contribute to other aspects of pathology other than the swelling of astrocytes as this metabolite has been shown to induce oxidative stress and neuroinflammation, which contribute to the pathology of HE. This is evident in cell culture studies where treating rat primary microglia with 5 mM of ammonia was found to induce the expression of reactive nitrogen and oxygen species [21]. In addition, treating rat primary astrocytes with conditioned media from these ammonia-treated microglia induced cell swelling [22]. The idea that ammonia was the primary factor necessary to induce encephalopathy is not be the case in every circumstance. Injection of LPS into sham-operated, ammonia-fed and BDL rats determined that significant neurological deficits and cytotoxic brain edema were observed only in the BDL rats administered LPS [22]. This gives support that inflammation induced by organ injury works in tandem with LPS-induced inflammation to contribute to HE. Therefore, while ammonia does play a significant role in HE, microglia-induced inflammation is a synergistic partner that also contributes to the pathology of this disorder.

3.2. Bile acids

It is well accepted that increased serum bile acids can be an indication of liver damage [23] and have been observed in the cerebrospinal fluid of patients with fulminant hepatic failure [24], and with liver cirrhosis [25], however, their contribution to the pathogenesis of HE has only recently been suggested [26, 27]. Increased serum bile acids have been implicated in the increased blood-brain barrier permeability observed in a rat model of chronic liver disease [28] hereby allowing access of bile acids and other signaling molecules to the brain. Furthermore, increased bile acid content in brain tissue has been demonstrated in rodent models of both acute and chronic liver diseases [26, 27]. In the AOM mouse model of Type A HE, increased total bile acid content was observed in the frontal cortex, and strategies to reduced circulating bile acids (e.g., cholestyramine feeding or the use of a genetically modified mouse with impaired bile acid synthesis) proved neuroprotective [26].

Activation of microglia is a delicate balance between the proinflammatory chemokine ligand 2 (CCL2) and the anti-inflammatory chemokine fractalkine, which in physiological conditions favors the dampening of microglia activation [6]. However, during type A HE, this balance is dysregulated leading to an increased production of CCL2 [5] and a downregulation of fractalkine [6] and subsequent microglia activation [5, 6]. This imbalance may, at least in part, be attributable to aberrant bile acid signaling in the frontal cortex during acute liver failure [29].

3.3. Proinflammatory cytokines

It is commonly accepted that systemic inflammation contributes to the progression of HE. Indeed, in patients and in animal models of HE, systemic inflammation causes worsening of the encephalopathy, and it has been proposed that proinflammatory signals act synergistically with ammonia toxicity to bring about the neurological complications of acute and chronic liver failure [30–32].

Because the proinflammatory cytokines released from the liver during liver damage are often identical to those released from activated microglia, it is difficult to determine the precise origin and role of each source of cytokine during HE. However, a number of liver-derived proinflammatory cytokines have been definitively demonstrated.

Tumor necrosis factor-alpha (TNFα) is a potent proinflammatory cytokine. Circulating levels of TNFα are increased as a function of the severity of HE in both patients [33] and experimental animals [10] with liver failure. Moreover, the presence of TNFα gene polymorphisms is known to influence the clinical outcome in patients with acute liver failure [34]. In experimental models of acute liver failure, mice lacking the TNF receptor 1 gene had a delayed onset of encephalopathy and an attenuation of brain edema [35]. TNFα has been shown to activate microglia in a number of experimental models of neuroinflammation [36, 37]. With respect to HE, systemic levels of TNFα are increased in the AOM model of acute liver failure [7]. Inhibition of TNFα signaling by systemic treatment with etanercept reduced systemic inflammation, attenuated the neurological decline, and prevented microglial activation in the cerebral cortex [7]. These data support the hypothesis that peripherally derived TNFα, at least in part, contributes to the microglial activation and subsequent neurological decline in liver failure. In support of this concept, neurological complications occurring in the BDL model of biliary cirrhosis were shown to be the consequence of monocyte recruitment in response to TNFα signaling and occurred via microglial activation. Specifically, peripheral TNFα signaling stimulates microglia to produce CCL2, which subsequently mediates monocyte recruitment into the brain [14]. These findings were suggested to constitute a novel immune-to-brain communication pathway with the potential to result in altered neuronal excitability and neurological complications during cholestatic liver disease.

The role of transforming growth factor β (TGFβ) in the inflammatory response is largely context dependent. Specifically, TGFβ has both anti-inflammatory and proinflammatory effects on various immune cells in the body, including microglial activation. Increased levels of TGFβ have been demonstrated in the liver and serum in the AOM model of acute liver failure [38]. The authors demonstrated that peripheral TGFβ has implications on microglial activation [39]. Specifically, systemic treatment of mice with a neutralizing anti-TGFβ antibody, that did not significantly alter the underlying liver damage, but inhibited the actions of circulating TGFβ delayed the neurological decline observed in AOM-induced acute liver failure [38], and attenuated the morphological changes in Iba-1 positive microglia [39]. However, whether liver-derived TGFβ is acting directly on microglia to regulate the neuroinflammatory response in these models of HE, or whether the changes in microglial activation are an indirect effect of the protective effect of anti-TGFβ neutralizing antibodies remains to be established.

3.4. Neuron and astrocyte crosstalk with microglia

Microglia activation does not occur in an isolated system, and various studies have demonstrated that both neurons and astrocytes have the capability to crosstalk with microglia and promote their activation during neuroinflammatory states. This does occur in conditions other than HE. For example, in a mouse model of Alzheimer's disease, astrocytes have upregulated CCAAT/enhancer-binding protein and proinflammatory cytokines, which are associated with microglia activation and migration [40]. During hyperammonemia in rats, it was found that ammonia induces both astrocyte and microglia activation along with increased production of interleukin-1 beta (IL-1β) and interleukin-6 (IL-6) [41]. In a recent report, LPS-stimulated microglia have increased production of proinflammatory cytokines including IL-1β, IL-6 and TNFα which were reduced when microglia were co-cultured with astrocytes indicating that astrocytes may play an immunomodulatory role [42].

In contrast, neurons have been demonstrated to induce the activation of microglia during HE. In the cortex of mice with acute liver failure, there is an elevation of CCL2 in neurons, which signals through chemokine receptor 2 (CCR2) and chemokine receptor 4 (CCR4) [5]. Antagonism of CCR2 or CCR4 was found to improve HE outcomes and reduce microglia activation compared to controls [5]. In physiological states, neurons are able to inhibit microglia expression by producing fractalkine, which signals through CX3CR1 on microglia [6]. Fractalkine in neurons was found to be suppressed in the cortex during HE in mice with acute liver failure and infusion of soluble fractalkine into the brain led to reduced microglia activation [6].

4. Treatment strategies to reduce neuroinflammation during liver disease

At this time, most therapies used for the treatment and management of HE are not targeted directly at neuroinflammation, per se. As ammonia was the first identified neurotoxin to play a role in HE, current treatment strategies are aimed at reducing circulating ammonia levels during this disease state. Some of these treatments appear to have efficacy in certain conditions, while others do not. Current treatments and future potential therapeutic strategies will be discussed below.

4.1. Current treatments for HE

A majority of current therapies are aimed at reducing the levels of circulating ammonia by targeting the bacteria of the gut. It should be noted that these treatments may indirectly reduce inflammation due to the synergism of ammonia and neuroinflammation during HE described above. The non-absorbable disaccharides lactulose and lactitol are commonly used for HE treatment. These are metabolized by the gut microbiota, which acidifies the colon, reduces the number of ammonia producing bacteria, and converts ammonia to ammonium, which cannot be absorbed [43]. While studies have reported improved outcomes of HE patients during lactulose treatment [44], a meta-analysis assessing 30 studies determined that lactulose treatment did not significantly reduce mortality in HE patients though it did reduce the risk of no improvement [45]. Lactitol has been shown to be just as efficacious as lactulose and has less severe side effects but is not available in the United States [46].

Non-digestible antibiotics are another therapy targeted at reducing ammonia production of intestinal bacteria and can be used in conjunction with lactulose. Rifaximin has the least number of side effects and is the most well-characterized [47]. Rifaximin is effective against both Gram-positive and Gram-negative bacteria of the gastrointestinal tract. Rifaximin works by disrupting transcription by binding RNA polymerase and has been demonstrated to reduce ammonia concentrations and improve mental status to a greater degree than lactulose or other antibiotics in HE patients [48].

L-Ornithine-L-aspartate (LOLA) is aimed at reducing ammonia concentrations by increasing the generation of urea through the urea cycle. Oral administration of LOLA is not recommended for the management of HE as the studies assessing its efficacy have been conflicting with some stating no benefit compared to placebo [49]. Newer studies have identified that intravenous administration of LOLA is more efficacious at lowering ammonia levels and is recommended for patients that do not respond to lactulose treatment [50].

Probiotics are dietary supplements containing viable bacteria that are designed to deprive pathogenic bacteria of nutrients, while supplying beneficial bacteria with growth-promoting substrates. While there have not been definitive studies during acute liver failure, probiotics have shown efficacy during type C HE. A meta-analysis of probiotics usage in patients with minimal HE described that they are associated with significantly improved outcomes [51]. In another study, it was found that the probiotic VSL#3 improved outcomes in patients with minimal HE and had comparable efficacy to lactulose [52].

Other treatments employed are designed to minimize the complications of HE. Two of these are mannitol and hypertonic saline which aim to reduce cerebral edema and intracranial pressures that are a result of cytotoxic edema and inflammation [50].

4.2. Pre-clinical therapies targeting inflammation

While the current therapies being employed are largely focused on ammonia, there are prospective therapeutic approaches that are targeted at reducing neuroinflammation with many of the studies reporting improved HE outcomes.

Therapeutic hypothermia has been employed in rodent models and in patients. In rats with end-to-side portacaval anastomosis, moderate hypothermia (33°C) was found to reduce cerebral edema and TNFα, IL-1β and IL-6 concentrations in the cortex [9]. A similar finding was observed in HE patients where reducing their core temperature to 32–33°C was able to decrease levels of circulating TNFα, IL-1β and IL-6 as well as reduce cerebral edema and intracranial pressure [53]. However, a recent report investigating moderate hypothermia (33–34°C) in HE patients from acute liver failure determined that this treatment strategy did little to reduce increased intracranial pressures or mortality [54]. Therefore, more studies are necessary to determine the clinical potential of therapeutic hypothermia in patients with HE.

Chemokines and cytokines may also be a potential target for the management of HE. Systemic antagonism of CCR2 or CCR4 was found to reduce neuroinflammation and neurological decline in AOM-treated mice [5]. In addition, supplementation of CX3CR1-mediated signaling via soluble fractalkine infusion in the brain reduced microglia activation and neuroinflammation in AOM-treated mice [6]. TNFα-mediated signaling seems to play a significant role in neuroinflammation and outcomes during HE as infliximab, etanercept and p38 inhibitors all reduced serum and brain levels of proinflammatory cytokines and improved cognitive and motor functions in rodent models of HE [7, 11, 55].

N-acetylcysteine is a therapeutic agent that is known to be efficacious in the treatment of hepatotoxic acetaminophen overdose by increasing bioavailability of the antioxidant glutathione. In regard to HE, it has been shown that in acute liver failure not due to acetaminophen overdose that N-acetylcysteine is able to reduce IL-17 and improve outcomes but this occurs only in patients with grade 0-II HE [56, 57]. These beneficial effects of N-acetylcysteine were not observed in children with minimal HE due to non-acetaminophen-induced acute liver failure as there was no change in 1-year survival [58]. In fact, it was observed that children younger than 2 years old actually had a significantly reduced 1-year transplant free survival compared to controls [58].

Non-steroidal anti-inflammatory drugs (NSAIDs) also show promise at mitigating neuroinflammation and improving outcomes during HE. Ibuprofen has been shown to reduce microglia activation, cerebellar IL-1β concentrations and improved learning and motor functions in BDL rats [13]. In portacaval shunt rats with HE, ibuprofen treatment reduced inducible nitric oxide synthase expression and improved motor and cognitive function compared to controls [59]. Indomethacin has shown conflicting results with this treatment reducing intracranial pressures in patients with acute liver failure while increasing TNFα and mortality in TAA-induced liver failure in rats [60]. More studies are necessary with NSAIDs in patient populations before these agents should be used for the treatment of HE [61].

The elevation of bile acids in the brain and CSF of HE patients due to acute liver failure has been previously described [24]. Recently, we published a report that bile acids are elevated in the cortex of AOM treated mice, and the use of cholestyramine (to promote fecal excretion of bile acids) or Cyp7A1-null mice (that have reduced bile acid synthesis) were protected from neurological decline [26]. This is not unique to this model as BDL rats 3 weeks after surgery have significant elevations of lithocholic acid in the brain [62]. Bile acids in other systems have been demonstrated to have the ability to modulate inflammation, giving support that they could contribute to neuroinflammation during HE.

4.3. Clinical trials

At this time, there are 83 open clinical trials assessing aspects of HE. That being said, the numbers directly assessing HE are only 15 and of these 15, 6 involve lactulose or rifaximin that are already being readily used in the clinic. Of these remaining studies, only 6 involve novel treatments not currently in use.

Due to the lack of efficacy for probiotics during HE due to acute liver failure, fecal microbiota transplants are being proposed to better control the makeup of the gut microbiome. Fecal microbiota transplants are taken from a health donor and are then administered in a diseased individual with the goal of altering their gut bacteria to a healthier population. The first trial is aimed at cirrhotic patients with recurrent HE that do not respond to lactulose or rifaximin (NCT02255617). The second trial is also in cirrhotic patients and is aimed at determining the feasibility and safety of fecal microbiota transplants in HE patients (NCT02862249).

GABA receptor antagonists could also be a potential therapy for HE as this neurotransmitter is modulated by both positive and negative regulators [63]. As GABA activation suppresses neural circuits, this neurotransmission pathway could suppress the CNS and promote hepatic coma. Flumazenil is a GABA receptor antagonist that is being proposed for use in non-alcoholic cirrhotic patients that have HE (NCT02048969). This trial will employ proton magnetic resonance spectroscopy to determine the metabolic and biochemical changes in these patients that are on flumazenil or placebo.

Metformin is one of the primary medications used for the treatment of type 2 diabetes. During HE, it has been shown that metformin inhibits glutaminase activity and was protective against HE in cirrhotic patients with diabetes [64]. In order to determine whether metformin is beneficial in cirrhotic patients with diabetes and minimal HE, a clinical trial is being performed that will assess neurobehavioral outcomes using psychometric tests in these patients (NCT02470546).

Albumin infusion is a method employed to scavenge substances, and proteins in the blood to improve patient outcomes. In cirrhotic patients with HE, albumin infusion has been previously used and was found to not reduce the occurrence of HE during hospitalization, but did improve survival after hospitalization [65]. The new trial is comparing infusion of human albumin into cirrhotic patients with HE and is assessing survival at 90 days and 180 days following initial dose (NCT02401490).

The last clinical trial is the joint administration of nitazoxanide and lactulose in cirrhotic patients with HE (NCT02464124). Nitazoxanide is an oral medication that is used to treat *Giardia lamblia* and *Cryptosporidium parvum* during infectious diarrhea. The outcomes of this trial are to determine the number of patients with total reversal of HE.

5. Conclusions

In conclusion, the evidence for a role of neuroinflammation in HE is unequivocal. However, the precise molecular mechanism by which neuroinflammation, and more specifically microglia, is activated is not completely understood. Targetting the neuroinflammatory aspect of HE may prove to be a useful strategy for the development of experimental therapeutics to manage the neurological complications of HE.

Funding

This work was funded by an NIH R01 award (DK082435) and a VA Merit award (BX002638) from the United States Department of Veterans Affairs Biomedical Laboratory Research and Development Service to Dr. DeMorrow and a VA Career Development award (BX003486) from the United States Department of Veterans Affairs Biomedical Laboratory Research and Development Service to Dr. McMillin.

Acknowledgements

This work was completed with support from the Veterans Health Administration and with resources and the use of facilities at the Central Texas Veterans Health Care System, Temple, Texas. The contents do not represent the views of the U.S. Department of Veterans Affairs or the United States Government.

Author details

Matthew McMillin[1,2] and Sharon DeMorrow[1,2]*

*Address all correspondence to: demorrow@medicine.tamhsc.edu

1 Central Texas Veterans Health Care System, TX, United States

2 Department of Internal Medicine, Texas A&M University Health Science Center, College of Medicine, TX, United States

References

[1] Zemtsova I, Gorg B, Keitel V, Bidmon HJ, Schror K, Haussinger D. Microglia activation in hepatic encephalopathy in rats and humans. Hepatology. 2011;**54**:204-215

[2] Gorg B, Bidmon HJ, Haussinger D. Gene expression profiling in the cerebral cortex of patients with cirrhosis with and without hepatic encephalopathy. Hepatology. 2013;**57**:2436-2347

[3] Butterworth RF, Norenberg MD, Felipo V, Ferenci P, Albrecht J, Blei AT, Members of the ICoEMoHE. Experimental models of hepatic encephalopathy: ISHEN guidelines. Liver International. 2009;**29**:783-788

[4] Rangroo Thrane V, Thrane AS, Chang J, Alleluia V, Nagelhus EA, Nedergaard M. Real-time analysis of microglial activation and motility in hepatic and hyperammonemic encephalopathy. Neuroscience. 2012;**220**:247-255

[5] McMillin M, Frampton G, Thompson M, Galindo C, Standeford H, Whittington E, Alpini G, DeMorrow S. Neuronal CCL2 is upregulated during hepatic encephalopathy and contributes to microglia activation and neurological decline. Journal of Neuroinflammation. 2014;**11**:121

[6] McMillin M, Grant S, Frampton G, Andry S, Brown A, DeMorrow S. Fractalkine suppression during hepatic encephalopathy promotes neuroinflammation in mice. Journal of Neuroinflammation. 2016;**13**:198

[7] Chastre A, Belanger M, Beauchesne E, Nguyen BN, Desjardins P, Butterworth RF. Inflammatory cascades driven by tumor necrosis factor-alpha play a major role in the progression of acute liver failure and its neurological complications. PLoS One. 2012;**7**:e49670

[8] Faleiros BE, Miranda AS, Campos AC, Gomides LF, Kangussu LM, Guatimosim C, Camargos ER, Menezes GB, Rachid MA, Teixeira AL. Up-regulation of brain cytokines and chemokines mediates neurotoxicity in early acute liver failure by a mechanism independent of microglial activation. Brain Research. 2014;**1578**:49-59

[9] Jiang W, Desjardins P, Butterworth RF. Direct evidence for central proinflammatory mechanisms in rats with experimental acute liver failure: Protective effect of hypothermia. Journal of Cerebral Blood Flow & Metabolism. 2009;**29**:944-952

[10] Jiang W, Desjardins P, Butterworth RF. Cerebral inflammation contributes to encephalopathy and brain edema in acute liver failure: Protective effect of minocycline. Journal of Neurochemistry. 2009;**109**:485-493

[11] Agusti A, Cauli O, Rodrigo R, Llansola M, Hernandez-Rabaza V, Felipo V. p38 MAP kinase is a therapeutic target for hepatic encephalopathy in rats with portacaval shunts. Gut. 2011;**60**:1572-1579

[12] Hernandez-Rabaza V, Agusti A, Cabrera-Pastor A, Fustero S, Delgado O, Taoro-Gonzalez L, Montoliu C, Llansola M, Felipo V. Sildenafil reduces neuroinflammation and restores spatial learning in rats with hepatic encephalopathy: Underlying mechanisms. Journal of Neuroinflammation. 2015;**12**:195

[13] Rodrigo R, Cauli O, Gomez-Pinedo U, Agusti A, Hernandez-Rabaza V, Garcia-Verdugo JM, Felipo V. Hyperammonemia induces neuroinflammation that contributes to cognitive impairment in rats with hepatic encephalopathy. Gastroenterology. 2010;**139**:675-684

[14] D'Mello C, Le T, Swain MG. Cerebral microglia recruit monocytes into the brain in response to tumor necrosis factoralpha signaling during peripheral organ inflammation. Journal of Neuroinflammation. 2009;**29**:2089-2102

[15] Kerfoot SM, D'Mello C, Nguyen H, Ajuebor MN, Kubes P, Le T, Swain MG. TNF-alpha-secreting monocytes are recruited into the brain of cholestatic mice. Hepatology. 2006;**43**:154-162

[16] Richardson AJ, McKain N, Wallace RJ. Ammonia production by human faecal bacteria, and the enumeration, isolation and characterization of bacteria capable of growth on peptides and amino acids. BMC Microbiology. 2013;**13**:6

[17] Holecek M. Evidence of a vicious cycle in glutamine synthesis and breakdown in pathogenesis of hepatic encephalopathy-therapeutic perspectives. Metabolic Brain Disease. 2014;**29**:9-17

[18] Keiding S, Sorensen M, Bender D, Munk OL, Ott P, Vilstrup H. Brain metabolism of 13N-ammonia during acute hepatic encephalopathy in cirrhosis measured by positron emission tomography. Hepatology. 2006;**43**:42-50

[19] Tofteng F, Hauerberg J, Hansen BA, Pedersen CB, Jorgensen L, Larsen FS. Persistent arterial hyperammonemia increases the concentration of glutamine and alanine in the brain and correlates with intracranial pressure in patients with fulminant hepatic failure. Journal of Cerebral Blood Flow & Metabolism. 2006;**26**:21-27

[20] Norenberg MD. The role of astrocytes in hepatic encephalopathy. Neurochemical Pathology. 1987;**6**:13-33

[21] Rao KV, Brahmbhatt M, Norenberg MD. Microglia contribute to ammonia-induced astrocyte swelling in culture. Metabolic Brain Disease. 2013;**28**:139-143

[22] Wright G, Davies NA, Shawcross DL, Hodges SJ, Zwingmann C, Brooks HF, Mani AR, Harry D, Stadlbauer V, Zou Z, Williams R, Davies C, Moore KP, Jalan R. Endotoxemia produces coma and brain swelling in bile duct ligated rats. Hepatology. 2007;**45**: 1517-1526

[23] Thompson MB. Bile acids in the assessment of hepatocellular function. Toxicologic Pathology. 1996;24:62-71

[24] Bron B, Waldram R, Silk DB, Williams R. Serum, cerebrospinal fluid, and brain levels of bile acids in patients with fulminant hepatic failure. Gut. 1977;**18**:692-696

[25] Weiss N, Barbier Saint Hilaire P, Colsch B, Isnard F, Attala S, Schaefer A, Amador MD, Rudler M, Lamari F, Sedel F, Thabut D, Junot C. Cerebrospinal fluid metabolomics highlights dysregulation of energy metabolism in overt hepatic encephalopathy. Journal of Hepatology. 2016;**65**:1120-1130

[26] McMillin M, Frampton G, Quinn M, Ashfaq S, de los Santos M, 3rd, Grant S, DeMorrow S. Bile acid signaling Is involved in the neurological decline in a murine model of acute liver failure. American Journal of Pathology. 2016;**186**:312-323

[27] McMillin M, Frampton G, Quinn M, Divan A, Grant S, Patel N, Newell-Rogers K, DeMorrow S. Suppression of the HPA axis during cholestasis can be attributed to hypothalamic bile acid signaling. Molecular Endocrinology. 2015;**29**:1720-1730

[28] Quinn M, McMillin M, Galindo C, Frampton G, Pae HY, DeMorrow S. Bile acids permeabilize the blood brain barrier after bile duct ligation in rats via Rac1-dependent mechanisms. Digestive and Liver Disease. 2014;**46**:527-534

[29] McMillin M, Frampton G, Galindo C, Standeford H, Alpini G, DeMorrow S. Microglia activation during hepatic encephalopathy is driven by an imbalance of monocyte chemoattractant protein 1/fractalkine due to bile acid signaling. Hepatology. 2014;**60**:202A

[30] Shawcross DL, Davies NA, Williams R, Jalan R. Systemic inflammatory response exacerbates the neuropsychological effects of induced hyperammonemia in cirrhosis. Journal of Hepatology. 2004;**40**:247-254

[31] Butterworth RF. Hepatic encephalopathy: A central neuroinflammatory disorder? Hepatology. 2011;**53**:1372-1376

[32] Butterworth RF. The liver-brain axis in liver failure: Neuroinflammation and encephalopathy. Nature Reviews Gastroenterology & Hepatology. 2013;**10**:522-528

[33] Odeh M. Pathogenesis of hepatic encephalopathy: The tumour necrosis factor-alpha theory. European Journal of Clinical Investigation. 2007;**37**:291-304

[34] Bernal W, Donaldson P, Underhill J, Wendon J, Williams R. Tumor necrosis factor genomic polymorphism and outcome of acetaminophen (paracetamol)-induced acute liver failure. Journal of Hepatology. 1998;**29**:53-59

[35] Bemeur C, Qu H, Desjardins P, Butterworth RF. IL-1 or TNF receptor gene deletion delays onset of encephalopathy and attenuates brain edema in experimental acute liver failure. Neurochemistry International. 2010;**56**:213-215

[36] Lambertsen KL, Biber K, Finsen B. Inflammatory cytokines in experimental and human stroke. Journal of Cerebral Blood Flow & Metabolism. 2012;**32**:1677-1698

[37] Rubio-Perez JM, Morillas-Ruiz JM. A review: Inflammatory process in Alzheimer's disease, role of cytokines. Scientific World Journal. 2012;**2012**:756357

[38] McMillin M, Galindo C, Pae HY, Frampton G, Di Patre PL, Quinn M, Whittington E, DeMorrow S. Gli1 activation and protection against hepatic encephalopathy is suppressed by circulating transforming growth factor beta1 in mice. Journal of Hepatology. 2014;**61**:1260-1266

[39] McMillin M. The role of transforming growth factor beta in hepatic encephalopathy pathogenesis (Doctoral dissertation). Texas A&M University. 2013

[40] Ko CY, Wang WL, Wang SM, Chu YY, Chang WC, Wang JM. Glycogen synthase kinase-3beta-mediated CCAAT/enhancer-binding protein delta phosphorylation in astrocytes promotes migration and activation of microglia/macrophages. Neurobiology of Aging. 2014;**35**:24-34

[41] Hernandez-Rabaza V, Cabrera-Pastor A, Taoro-Gonzalez L, Malaguarnera M, Agusti A, Llansola M, Felipo V. Hyperammonemia induces glial activation, neuroinflammation and alters neurotransmitter receptors in hippocampus, impairing spatial learning: Reversal by sulforaphane. Journal of Neuroinflammation. 2016;**13**:41

[42] Karababa A, Groos-Sahr K, Albrecht U, Keitel V, Shafigullina A, Gorg B, Haussinger D. Ammonia attenuates LPS-induced upregulation of pro-inflammatory cytokine mRNA in co-cultured astrocytes and microglia. Neurochemical Research. 2017;**42**:737-749

[43] Leise MD, Poterucha JJ, Kamath PS, Kim WR. Management of hepatic encephalopathy in the hospital. Mayo Clinic Proceedings. 2014;**89**:241-253

[44] Gluud LL, Vilstrup H, Morgan MY. Non-absorbable disaccharides versus placebo/no intervention and lactulose versus lactitol for the prevention and treatment of hepatic encephalopathy in people with cirrhosis. Cochrane Database of Systematic Reviews. 2016;**4**:CD003044

[45] Als-Nielsen B, Gluud LL, Gluud C. Nonabsorbable disaccharides for hepatic encephalopathy. Cochrane Database of Systematic Reviews. 2004;2:CD003044

[46] Al Sibae MR, McGuire BM. Current trends in the treatment of hepatic encephalopathy. Therapeutics and Clinical Risk Management. 2009;**5**:617-626

[47] Patidar KR, Bajaj JS. Covert and overt hepatic encephalopathy: Diagnosis and management. Clinical Gastroenterology and Hepatology. 2015;**13**:2048-6120

[48] Bajaj JS, Riggio O. Drug therapy: Rifaximin. Hepatology. 2010;**52**:1484-1488

[49] Jiang Q, Jiang XH, Zheng MH, Chen YP. L-Ornithine-L-aspartate in the management of hepatic encephalopathy: A meta-analysis. Journal of Gastroenterology and Hepatology. 2009;**24**:9-14

[50] Wijdicks EF. Hepatic encephalopathy. The New England Journal of Medicine. 2016;**375**: 1660-1670

[51] Shukla S, Shukla A, Mehboob S, Guha S. Meta-analysis: The effects of gut flora modulation using prebiotics, probiotics and synbiotics on minimal hepatic encephalopathy. Alimentary Pharmacology & Therapeutics. 2011;**33**:662-671

[52] Pratap Mouli V, Benjamin J, Bhushan Singh M, Mani K, Garg SK, Saraya A, Joshi YK. Effect of probiotic VSL#3 in the treatment of minimal hepatic encephalopathy: A non-inferiority randomized controlled trial. Hepatology Research. 2015;**45**:880-889

[53] Jalan R, Olde Damink SW, Deutz NE, Hayes PC, Lee A. Moderate hypothermia in patients with acute liver failure and uncontrolled intracranial hypertension. Gastroenterology. 2004;**127**:1338-1346

[54] Bernal W, Murphy N, Brown S, Whitehouse T, Bjerring PN, Hauerberg J, Frederiksen HJ, Auzinger G, Wendon J, Larsen FS. A multicentre randomized controlled trial of moderate hypothermia to prevent intracranial hypertension in acute liver failure. Journal of Hepatology. 2016;**65**:273-279

[55] Dadsetan S, Balzano T, Forteza J, Cabrera-Pastor A, Taoro-Gonzalez L, Hernandez-Rabaza V, Gil-Perotin S, Cubas-Nunez L, Garcia-Verdugo JM, Agusti A, Llansola M, Felipo V. Reducing peripheral inflammation with infliximab reduces neuroinflammation and improves cognition in rats with hepatic encephalopathy. Frontiers in Molecular Neuro science. 2016;**9**:106

[56] Stravitz RT, Sanyal AJ, Reisch J, Bajaj JS, Mirshahi F, Cheng J, Lee WM. Acute liver failure study G: Effects of N-acetylcysteine on cytokines in non-acetaminophen acute

liver failure: Potential mechanism of improvement in transplant-free survival. Liver International. 2013;**33**:1324-1331

[57] Lee WM, Hynan LS, Rossaro L, Fontana RJ, Stravitz RT, Larson AM, Davern TJ, 2nd, Murray NG, McCashland T, Reisch JS, Robuck PR. Acute liver failure study G: Intravenous N-acetylcysteine improves transplant-free survival in early stage non-acetaminophen acute liver failure. Gastroenterology. 2009;**137**:856-864: 64 e1

[58] Squires RH, Dhawan A, Alonso E, Narkewicz MR, Shneider BL, Rodriguez-Baez N, Olio DD, Karpen S, Bucuvalas J, Lobritto S, Rand E, Rosenthal P, Horslen S, Ng V, Subbarao G, Kerkar N, Rudnick D, Lopez MJ, Schwarz K, Romero R, Elisofon S, Doo E, Robuck PR, Lawlor S, Belle SH. Pediatric acute liver failure study G: Intravenous N-acetylcysteine in pediatric patients with nonacetaminophen acute liver failure: A placebo-controlled clinical trial. Hepatology. 2013;**57**:1542-1549

[59] Cauli O, Rodrigo R, Piedrafita B, Boix J, Felipo V. Inflammation and hepatic encephalopathy: Ibuprofen restores learning ability in rats with portacaval shunts. Hepatology. 2007;**46**:514-519

[60] Tofteng F, Larsen FS. The effect of indomethacin on intracranial pressure, cerebral perfusion and extracellular lactate and glutamate concentrations in patients with fulminant hepatic failure. Journal of Cerebral Blood Flow & Metabolism. 2004;**24**:798-804

[61] Chu CJ, Hsiao CC, Wang TF, Chan CY, Lee FY, Chang FY, Chen YC, Huang HC, Wang SS, Lee SD. Prostacyclin inhibition by indomethacin aggravates hepatic damage and encephalopathy in rats with thioacetamide-induced fulminant hepatic failure. World Journal of Gastroenterology. 2005;**11**:232-236

[62] Tripodi V, Contin M, Fernandez MA, Lemberg A. Bile acids content in brain of common duct ligated rats. Annals of Hepatology. 2012;**11**:930-934

[63] Sergeeva OA. GABAergic transmission in hepatic encephalopathy. Archives of Biochemistry and Biophysics. 2013;**536**:122-130

[64] Ampuero J, Ranchal I, Nunez D, Diaz-Herrero Mdel M, Maraver M, del Campo JA, Rojas A, Camacho I, Figueruela B, Bautista JD, Romero-Gomez M. Metformin inhibits glutaminase activity and protects against hepatic encephalopathy. PLoS One. 2012;**7**: e49279

[65] Simon-Talero M, Garcia-Martinez R, Torrens M, Augustin S, Gomez S, Pereira G, Guevara M, Gines P, Soriano G, Roman E, Sanchez-Delgado J, Ferrer R, Nieto JC, Sunye P, Fuentes I, Esteban R, Cordoba J. Effects of intravenous albumin in patients with cirrhosis and episodic hepatic encephalopathy: A randomized double-blind study. Journal of Hepatology. 2013;**59**:1184-1192